Renal Disease

Guest Editor

EDGAR V. LERMA, MD

CLINICS IN GERIATRIC MEDICINE

www.geriatric.theclinics.com

August 2009 • Volume 25 • Number 3

SAUNDERS an imprint of ELSEVIER, Inc.

W.B. SAUNDERS COMPANY

A Division of Elsevier Inc.

1600 John F. Kennedy Blvd., Suite 1800. Philadelphia, Pennsylvania 19103-2899

http://www.theclinics.com

CLINICS IN GERIATRIC MEDICINE Volume 25, Number 3
August 2009 ISSN 0749–0690, ISBN-13: 978-1-4377-1385-5, ISBN-10: 1-4377-1385-8

Editor: Yonah Korngold

Clinics in Geriatric Medicine (ISSN 0749-0690) is published quarterly by Elsevier Inc., 360 Park Avenue South, New York, NY 10010-1710. Months of issue are February, May, August, and November. Business and Editorial Offices: 1600 John F. Kennedy Blvd., Suite 1800, Philadelphia, PA 191023-2899. Periodicals postage paid at New York, NY, and additional mailing offices. Subscription prices is $208.00 per year (US individuals), $353.00 per year (US institutions), $271.00 per year (Canadian individuals), $440.00 per year (Canadian institutions), $288.00 per year (foreign individuals) and $440.00 per year (foreign institutions). Foreign air speed delivery is included in all *Clinics* subscription prices. All prices are subject to change without notice. POSTMASTER: Send address changes to *Clinics in Geriatric Medicine,* Elsevier Health Sciences Division, Subscription Customer Service, 3251 Riverport Lane, Maryland Heights, MO 63043. Telephone: 1-800-654-2452 (U.S. and Canada); 314-447-8871 (outside U.S. and Canada). Fax: 314-447-8029. E-mail: journalscustomerservice-usa@elsevier.com (for print support); journalsonlinesupport-usa@elsevier.com (for online support).

Reprints. For copies of 100 or more, of articles in this publication, please contact the Commercial Reprints Department, Elsevier Inc., 360 Park Avenue South, New York, New York 10010-1710. Tel.: (212) 633-3812; Fax: (212) 462-1935, E-mail: reprints@elsevier.com.

Clinics in Geriatric Medicine is covered in *MEDLINE/PubMed (Index Medicus), EMBASE/Excerpta Medica, Current Contents/Clinical Medicine (CC/CM),* and the *Cumulative Index to Nursing & Allied Health Literature.*

Printed in the United States of America.

Contributors

GUEST EDITOR

EDGAR V. LERMA, MD, FACP, FASN, FAHA
Clinical Associate Professor of Medicine, Department of Medicine, Division of Nephrology, University of Illinois at Chicago College of Medicine, Associates in Nephrology, SC, Chicago, Illinois

AUTHORS

KHALED ABDEL-KADER, MD
Postdoctoral Fellow, Renal-Electrolyte Division, Department of Medicine, University of Pittsburgh School of Medicine, Pittsburgh, Pennsylvania

MARIA CZARINA ACELAJADO, MD
Post-doctoral Fellow, Vascular Biology and Hypertension Program of the Division of Cardiovascular Disease, University of Alabama at Birmingham, Birmingham, Alabama

JAMES LYNCH BAILEY, MD
Professor of Medicine, Director of the Renal Fellowship Program, Renal, Division, Emory University School of Medicine, Emory University, WMB, Atlanta, Georgia

WILLIAM M. BENNETT, MD
Director of Renal and Pancreas Transplantation, Northwest Renal Clinic, Legacy Good Samaritan Hospital Transplant Services, Oregon

LUCIA DEL VECCHIO, MD
Department of Nephrology and Dialysis, and Renal Transplant Ospedale A. Manzoni, Lecco, Italy

ELI A. FRIEDMAN, MD, MACP
Distinguished Teaching Professor of Medicine, Renal Division, Department of Medicine, Downstate Medical Center, Brooklyn, New York

RICHARD J. GLASSOCK, MD, MACP
Emeritus Professor, The David Geffen School of Medicine at, UCLA, Laguna Niguel, Los Angeles, California

TOMAS L. GRIEBLING, MD, MPH
John P. Wolf 33° Masonic Distinguished Professor of Urology, Vice-Chair, Department of Urology, Faculty Associate, The Landon Center on Aging; and Assistant Dean for Student Affairs, The University of Kansas, Kansas City, Kansas

SARBJIT VANITA JASSAL, MB, MD(UK), FRCPC
Associate Professor of Medicine, University of Toronto; Staff Nephrologist and Clinical Director of Dialysis Rehabilitation Program, University Health Network, Toronto, Ontario, Canada

ANTHONY J. JOSEPH, MD
Assistant Professor of Medicine, Medical Director of Acute Dialysis, Renal Division, Department of Medicine, Downstate Medical Center, Brooklyn, New York

EDGAR V. LERMA, MD, FACP, FASN, FAHA
Clinical Associate Professor of Medicine, Department of Medicine, Division of Nephrology, University of Illinois at Chicago College of Medicine, Associates in Nephrology, SC, Chicago, Illinois

FRANCESCO LOCATELLI, MD
Professor, Department of Nephrology and Dialysis, and Renal Transplant Ospedale A. Manzoni, Lecco, Italy

L.E. NICOLLE, MD, FRCPC
Professor, Department of Internal Medicine, Health Sciences Centre, University of Manitoba; and Department of Medical Microbiology, Health Sciences Centre, University of Manitoba, Winnipeg, Manitoba, Canada

ALLEN R. NISSENSON, MD
Division of Nephrology, Department of Medicine, David Geffen School of Medicine at UCLA, Los Angeles; and DaVita Inc., El Segundo, California

ALI J. OLYAEI, PharmD
Associate Professor of Medicine, Division of Nephrology & Hypertension, Oregon Health and Science University, Portland, Oregon

SUZANNE OPARIL, MD
Professor, Departments of Medicine and Physiology & Biophysics; Director, Vascular Biology and Hypertension Program of the Division of Cardiovascular Disease, University of Alabama at Birmingham, Birmingham, Alabama

PAUL M. PALEVSKY, MD
Chief, Renal Section, VA Pittsburgh Healthcare System, University Drive; and Professor of Medicine, Renal-Electrolyte Division, Department of Medicine, University of Pittsburgh School of Medicine, Pittsburgh, Pennsylvania

ANJAY RASTOGI, MD
Division of Nephrology, David Geffen School of Medicine at UCLA, Los Angeles, California

JEFF M. SANDS, MD, PhD
Juha P. Kokko Professor of Medicine and Physiology, Director, Renal Division, Associate Dean for Clinical and Translational Research, Renal Division, Emory University School of Medicine, Emory University, WMB, Atlanta, Georgia

LYNN E. SCHLANGER, MD
Assistant Professor of Medicine/Chief of Nephrology, Medical Division, VAMC at Atlanta, Decatur, Georgia; Renal Division, Emory University School of Medicine, Emory University, WMB, Atlanta, Georgia

MARSHALL L. STOLLER, MD
Professor and Vice Chairman, Department of Urology, University of California San Francisco, San Francisco, California

TIMOTHY Y. TSENG, MD
Endourology and Laparoscopy Fellow, Department of Urology, University of California San Francisco, San Francisco, CA

XIAOYI YE, MD
Division of Nephrology, David Geffen School of Medicine at UCLA, Los Angeles, California

Contents

In the 1980s geriatric nephrology was introduced as a subspecialty in anticipation of the increased number of elderly and very elderly people during the 21st century. There has been more clinical research dedicated to geriatric nephrology, education on the subspecialty has been implemented at national and university level, and funds for career development have been instituted over the past two decades. Our treatment of the elderly and very elderly patients seems to be more focused on their biologic age rather than chronologic age; they undergo diagnostic tests such as kidney biopsies and are candidates for kidney transplant. Although great strides have been made in the assimilation of geriatrics into nephrology more has to be done. This article examines the areas of research that encompass geriatric nephrology and clinic observations applicable to the care of the geriatric population.

Aging is a degenerative biologic process that affects the kidneys. It is known to be associated with a decline in kidney function coincident with a progressive decrease in the number of functioning nephrons and with glomerular and tubulointerstitial scarring. These changes affect glomerular and tubular function, systemic hemodynamics, and, as a whole, body homeostasis.

The aging kidney undergoes several important anatomic and physiologic changes that increase the risk of acute kidney injury (formerly acute renal failure) in the elderly. This article reviews these changes and discusses the diagnoses frequently encountered in the elderly patient with acute kidney injury. The incidence, staging, evaluation, management, and prognosis of acute kidney injury are also examined with special focus given to older adults.

Chronic kidney disease is increasingly being recognized in elderly individuals across the world. An understanding of the methods used to estimate or to measure kidney function, the likelihood and factors associated with

progressive decline in renal function, and the clinical syndromes associated with poor renal function are key topics for individuals working across
many medical disciplines. This review addresses some of the important
aspects of chronic kidney disease, and summarizes some of the clinical
and laboratory features associated with progressive disease.

Although diabetes is clearly linked to macro- and microvasculopathy in
multiple organs resulting in cardiovascular and cerebrovascular cata-
strophic diseases, blindness, and limb amputations, it is the relentless progression of diabetic nephropathy toward becoming the major cause of
end-stage renal disease (ESRD) that now challenges budgets and treatment facilities providing hemodialysis, peritoneal dialysis, and kidney
transplantation. Nephrology, as a specialty, is now dominated by the necessity to address geriatrics and endocrinology to cope with the tidal
wave of elderly ESRD patients suffering from uremia caused by diabetes.
On the brighter side, emergence of effective renoprotective regimens now
slow the incidence rate of ESRD in those with diagnosed diabetes. There is
bona fide reason to hope that within a decade, kidney failure attributable to
diabetes will be transformed into a preventable complication of a disease
that has dominated and directed our heritage.

Hypertension is an important risk factor for cardiovascular morbidity and
mortality, particularly in the elderly. Blood pressure elevation in the elderly
is due to structural and functional changes that occur with aging. Treatment of hypertension reduces the risk of stroke, heart failure, myocardial
infarction, all-cause mortality, cognitive impairment, and dementia in elderly patients with hypertension. A healthy lifestyle helps hypertension
management, with benefits extending beyond lowering of blood pressure.
Several classes of antihypertensive drugs are effective in preventing cardiovascular events. Treatment decisions should be guided by the presence of compelling indications such as diabetes or heart failure and by
the tolerability of individual drugs or drug combinations in individual patients. The concomitant intake of certain medications that counter the effects of antihypertensive drugs and the frequent occurrence of orthostatic
hypotension complicate treatment in older patients and drive down blood
pressure control rates.

Chronic glomerular disease is a common cause of disability and mortality
in the elderly. The underlying cause of the glomerular disease in this population is diverse but can generally be divided into those that affect the kidneys primarily (primary glomerular disease) and those in which the kidney
damage is a part of a systemwide process (secondary glomerular disease).

population. Most types of kidney diseases are chronic conditions and frequently manifest at the late stages of life. Epidemiologic studies suggest that older patients are at a greater risk for renal failure if the kidney experiences insults from ischemia or exposure to pharmacologic and diagnostic nephrotoxins. Pharmacologic management of most common diseases in elderly individuals is a difficult task, particularly in older individuals with chronic kidney disease. Thus, primary care providers must proceed with caution when prescribing drugs for elderly patients with kidney disease.

Rates of chronic kidney disease and end-stage renal disease are increasing as the United States population ages. The elderly with chronic kidney disease or end-stage renal disease face specific challenges with regard to medical care. Being of elderly age should not be a contraindication for initiation of renal replacement therapy. As the United States population ages, physicians will have to face many challenges associated with aging, whether medical, psychosocial, or ethical. This article discusses issues specific to the geriatric dialysis population.

Despite the many technical advances in medical care and dialysis delivery, mortality and morbidity remain high in patients with end-stage renal disease. This is particularly true in older patients, who often have a great number of coexisting diseases. In this population, life expectancy and quality of life may be rather poor, raising a number of ethical issues about the decision of starting start or withdrawing renal replacement therapy. Unfortunately, clear behavior guidelines on these critical issues are still insufficient. Reasons for not starting dialysis include old age, neurologic impairment, end-stage organ failure other than the kidneys, metastatic cancer, multiple comorbidities, and patient or family refusal. Similar reasons often underlie dialysis withdrawal of dialysis. Often these difficult decisions are left to care givers and family members or surrogates, since only a minority of patients with severe medical conditions discuss end-of-life care before becoming mentally impaired. The final shared decision should be the result of weighing beneficence (to maximise maximize good) with non-maleficence (to not cause harm); in the presence of severe medical conditions and/or mental impairment, dialysis may represent a prolongation of death rather than life.

THE CLINICS ARE NOW AVAILABLE ONLINE!

Access your subscription at:
www.theclinics.com

Preface

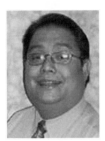

Edgar V. Lerma, MD
Guest Editor

In the United States, the average life expectancy in 2004 was 75.2 years for men and 80.4 years for women; by 2015, it is expected to be 76.2 and 82.2 years, respectively, and to continue to grow. During the 1990s, the population older than 85 years was the fastest growing group at 38% growth. This older age group is the largest consumer of health care services.[1–7]

In 2005, only 5% of the population older than 75 years had no health visits. Of people with 10 or more visits, 30% were in this age group, although the group constitutes only 10% of the population.

In 2007, it was estimated that the average age of patients starting renal replacement therapy (hemodialysis or peritoneal dialysis) in the United States was 62.3 years for men and 63.4 years for women, and this continues to be on an increasing trend. Twenty percent of all patients treated for end-stage kidney disease (ESKD) are older than 75 years, and about 50% of all patients on hemodialysis are older than 65 years.

The prevalence of the most common diseases causing ESKD, diabetes mellitus and hypertension, also increases substantially with aging; in 1999, the United States Renal Data System (USRDS) records show that the peak incident counts of treated ESKD occur in the 70- to 79-year age group at 15,000 patients per year. Peak incident rates of treated ESKD occur in the 70- to 79-year age group at 1543 per million population.

These trends are not entirely unexpected, considering the aging population, increased life expectancy brought about by advances in medical technology, concomitant decrease in renal function with age (ie, from age 40 onwards, creatinine clearance decreases at a rate of 0.87 mL/min/y), and the elderly's increased access to care.

With the current projected increase in the number of elderly patients, it is estimated that there will be a corresponding increase in the number of elderly patients requiring renal replacement therapy. In 1999, in recognition of the above trends, Luke and Beck coined the term "gerontologizing nephrology."

At that time, it was estimated that approximately 3 million Americans were older than 85 years, and this number is estimated to increase to 10 to 50 million by 2050. Nursing home beds were predicted to increase from 1.5 million in 1993 to 5 million

Clin Geriatr Med 25 (2009) xi–xiii
doi:10.1016/j.cger.2009.07.009
0749-0690/09/$ – see front matter © 2009 Elsevier Inc. All rights reserved.
geriatric.theclinics.com

in 2040. The percentage of health care expenditure in the United States going to those older than 65 years is likely to increase from 38% in 1999 to 75% by 2030. In 1999, the annual incidence of end-stage renal disease (ESRD) increased at a rate of 6% to 7% annually.

Chronic kidney disease (CKD) and ESKD are huge financial burdens to our medical system. In 2005, Medicare costs for CKD and ESKD were $42 billion and $20 billion, respectively. The cost of ESKD was one-half that of CKD, although only a very small percentage of patients with CKD progress to ESKD. According to the National Health and Nutrition Examination Survey (NHANES) data, about 11% of the United States population has CKD, whereas less than 0.2% of the United States population has ESKD. Despite this low prevalence, ESKD was responsible for 6.4% of the entire Medicare budget. The annual per person cost for dialysis alone exceeded $65,000 in 2005. If all medical care is included, this figure is even higher. For the 70- to 79-year age group, the per person annual cost of dialysis is more than $69,000, and in the 80+ year group, it is more than $74,000.

At present, 26 million Americans (13% of the United States adult population) suffer from CKD. Studies predict that these numbers will rise further due to other confounding risk factors: high obesity rates (one-third of all adults), diabetes and hypertension, and the aging of the baby boom generation (because age is considered as another risk factor for CKD).

When discussing dialysis, patients and families need to understand that, although renal replacement therapy does prolong life, life expectancy is very limited in the older population. Average 1-year survival for a 70- to 79-year-old is 70%, and 60% for an 80-year-old. By 2 years, survival drops to 52.7% and 39.7%, respectively.

These changing demographics mandate advances in our general understanding of geriatrics and nephrology as subspecialties.

In 2008, the Accreditation Council for Graduate Medical Education (ACGME) mandated that fellows in training should receive formal training in geriatric nephrology, but nearly 25% of United States institutions with ACGME-accredited nephrology training programs did not have comparable training programs in geriatrics.

Recognizing the importance of this issue to physician training and patient care, the American Society of Nephrology (ASN) convened the ASN Geriatrics Task Force. Co-chaired by Drs Dimitrios G. Oreopoulos and Jocelyn Wiggins, the task force designed and developed the ASN Geriatrics Nephrology Online Curriculum with generous financial support from the Association of Specialty Professors (ASP).

The curriculum was based on the ACGME's 6 core competencies (patient care, medical knowledge, practice-based learning and improvement, interpersonal and communication skills, professionalism, and systems-based practice).

As guest editor of this issue of *Clinics in Geriatric Medicine* focusing on renal diseases, I and the other contributors attempt to address some of these aspects of caring for aging patients with kidney disease, including assessing glomerular filtration rate in the elderly, drug dosing and renal toxicity, management of ESRD in elderly patients, and end-of-life decision making.

This issue is meant to supplement the aforementioned curriculum. In this issue, I am honored and privileged by renowned mentors and colleagues who have all agreed to contribute well-written articles that give the readers a true perspective of the blend between geriatrics and nephrology. In addition, we also have an article addressing issues on renal transplantation, a still-evolving field, especially as it applies to the geriatric population.

I am hopeful that primary care physicians (internists and family practitioners), geriatricians, nephrologists, and nurse practitioners and social workers who are involved with care of the elderly will find this issue quite informative and useful to their daily practices.

Edgar V. Lerma, MD
Department of Medicine
Division of Nephrology
University of Illinois at Chicago College of Medicine
3543 Wisconsin Avenue
Berwyn, IL 60402, USA

E-mail address:
edgarvlermamd@pol.net

REFERENCES

1. Lindeman RD, Tobin J, Shock NW. Longitudinal studies on the rate of decline in renal function with age. J Am Geriatr Soc 1985;33:278–85.
2. Luke RG, Beck LH. Gerontologizing nephrology. J Am Soc Nephrol 1999;10: 1824–7.
3. Oreopoulos DG, Wiggins J. Geriatric nephrology has come of age: at last. Washington, DC: American Society of Nephrology. Online Geriatric Nephrology Curriculum. Available at: http://www.asn-online.org/education_and_meetings/geriatrics/. Accessed July 2009.
4. Sclanger L. Kidney senescence. Washington, DC: American Society of Nephrology. Online Geriatric Nephrology Curriculum. Available at: http://www.asn-online.org/education_and_meetings/geriatrics/. Accessed July 2009.
5. Wiggins J, Patel C. The coming pandemic of CKD/ESKD and the aging population. Washington, DC: American Society of Nephrology. Online Geriatric Nephrology Curriculum. Available at: http://www.asn-online.org/education_and_meetings/geriatrics/. Accessed July 2009.
6. Wiggins J. Why do we need a geriatric nephrology curriculum? Washington, DC: American Society of Nephrology. Online Geriatric Nephrology Curriculum. Available at: http://www.asn-online.org/education_and_meetings/geriatrics/. Accessed July 2009.
7. US Renal Data System. USRDS 2007 Annual Data Report: Atlas of chronic kidney disease and end-stage renal disease in the United States. Bethesda, MD, National Institutes of Health, National Institute of Diabetes and Digestive and Kidney Diseases, 2007.

Geriatric Nephrology: Old or New Subspecialty

Lynn E. Schlanger, MD[a,b,]*, James Lynch Bailey, MD[b],
Jeff M. Sands, MD, PhD[b]

KEYWORDS

- Elderly acute kidney injury • Kidney disease
- End-stage renal disease • Renal transplant
- Geriatric nephrology

As a result of an increase in life expectancy and improvement in medical technology, the elderly population, those 65 years or greater, is expected to double to 71 million by 2030.[1,2] A similar trend is predicted worldwide with a near doubling of the elderly population from 6.9% (550 million) to 12% (973 million) by 2030.[1,3] The greatest growth rate is anticipated among octogenarians. It is estimated that 144 million or 26% of Europe's population will be more than 80 years old by 2050;[4] 19.5 million people will be more than 80 years old in the United States by 2030.[1] As the population ages, the prevalence and incidence of chronic kidney disease with its associated co-morbidities is predicted to increase.[5–10]

In the mid 1960s and early 1970s, there was a growing awareness of the projected increase in the number of elderly and the very elderly people in the United States and the necessity to address the associated medical, socioeconomic, psychological, and functional needs of this group.[11] In 1968 the American Board of Internal Medicine approved geriatrics as a medicine subspecialty. By 1982 Mount Sinai Hospital established the first department of geriatrics in the United States.[11] Geriatric fellowship programs followed.[11]

Unfortunately, academic geriatricians comprise only 1% of medical graduates making it difficult to care for this age group adequately.[12] As a response, the American Boards of Internal Medicine and Family Practice reduced the requirements for completion of the geriatric fellowship to 1 year.[13] Although the number of geriatricians has increased to 920 this number is still insufficient to meet the demand for academic geriatricians, projected to be more than 1400.[13] Because there are so few academic

[a] Medical Division, VAMC at Atlanta, 1670 Clairmont Road, Decatur, GA 30033, USA
[b] Renal Division, Emory University School of Medicine, Emory University, WMB, 1639 Peirce Drive, Suite 338, Atlanta, GA 30322, USA
* Corresponding author. Medical Division, VAMC at Atlanta, 1670 Clairmont Road, Decatur, GA 30033.
E-mail address: lynn.schlanger@va.gov (L.E. Schlanger).

Clin Geriatr Med 25 (2009) 311–324
doi:10.1016/j.cger.2009.04.002
0749-0690/09/$ – see front matter. Published by Elsevier Inc.

geriatric.theclinics.com

geriatricians, time dedicated to research and teaching has necessarily been compromised. The task of caring for these individuals is even more daunting as the population ages because the medical complexity, associated comorbidities, physical restraints, socioeconomic and psychological issues also increase.

The International Association of Gerontology and Geriatrics and the European Union of Medical Specialties (Europe Section) studied the changing emphasis in gerontology in various teaching institutions in Europe and noted that from 1991 and in 2006, a greater emphasis was placed on geriatric education at all levels of medical education.[4]

In 1993 the Institute of Medicine in the Unites States recognized the need for geriatric education within the various medical subspecialties and funding for this initiative was provided a year later by the John A. Hartford Foundation (JAHF).[14,15] A portion of the funding provided to the American Geriatric Society established the "Integrating Geriatrics into the Subspecialties of Internal Medicine Program,"[14,15] which involved internal medicine subspecialty leaders and academic geriatricians in this initiative[14,16] at geriatric educational retreats. In 1998 the Nephrology Geriatric Retreat took place in Alberta, Canada.[14]

The goals of the John A. Hartford Foundation and the American Geriatric Society were to increase the awareness of geriatrics as a subspecialty, improve geriatric education, focus on research pertinent to geriatric problems, recruit junior and midlevel faculty with an interest in geriatrics, disseminate information at national and regional subspecialty meetings, incorporate geriatric questions on the American Board of Internal Medicine examination, and develop a geriatric curriculum for the designated subspecialty.[14–16] In 2004, the program leaders of the Association of Specialty Professors and of the Integrating Geriatrics into the Subspecialties of Internal Medicine surveyed the various societies of subspecialties to determine the impact of the geriatric educational retreats on integrating the education of geriatrics within the various subspecialties.[14] They evaluated five areas including: (1) annual subspecialty meeting; (2) subspecialty journals; (3) societal organizational structure; (4) continuing medical education (CME); and (5) recertification. The American Society of Nephrology was shown to have developed educational activities at annual meetings, a geriatric core curriculum,[17] and made available geriatric CME. However, the number of journal articles related to geriatrics had not increased from 1995 to 2004. As a response to this concern, the American Society of Nephrology increased funding for junior faculty with interest in gerontology through the T. Franklin Williams Career Development Award.

Geriatric nephrology is a branch of internal medicine and geriatric medicine that deals with diseases of the kidney.[18] Although it is a new subspecialty, a book was written on the subject as early as 1986.[19] Over time there has been an increased emphasis on the blending of nephrology and the geriatrics subspecialties, which has culminated in the publication of more nephrology-related research articles designated solely to the elderly and the very elderly. A fellowship course at the American Society of Nephrology meeting in geriatric nephrology is now offered and the faculties at some universities have dual fellowships in these areas.

At least 50% of the nephrologists' patient population are geriatrics with a high percentage of these patients diagnosed with chronic kidney disease and end-stage kidney disease.[20,21] Moreover, nephrologists deal with acute medical renal issues and long-term preventive care whenever they follow the guidelines set forth by K/DOQI.[22] Similarly, geriatricians have to deal with long-term care, assess daily life activities, and address socioeconomic and psychological issues of their patients and family members. As our population ages nephrologists must become more knowledgeable in renal-related medical issues that afflict the elderly and the very elderly population. Both of these areas have been outlined in the Geriatric Curriculum by Dr Wiggins in 2005.[17]

There has been a paradigm shift in the way in which the elderly and the very elderly are viewed by society. This is evident by the increase in the number of living and deceased donor renal transplants in older recipient patients, by the increase in the number of renal biopsies performed on very elderly persons, by the use of extended donor criteria for kidney transplantation, and by the application of medical intervention according to the patient's biologic age rather than the chronologic age. This article examines the areas of research that encompass geriatric nephrology and clinic observations applicable to the care of the geriatric population.

KIDNEY SENESCENCE

As an organ ages, it undergoes physiologic and histologic changes that correlate with changes in function. The kidney is no exception to the aging process. A variety of cross-sectional and longitudinal studies have looked at the natural progression of kidney function as it ages.[23,24] A linear relationship between aging and a decline in renal function was noted by Lindeman,[24] but elderly persons who have no underlying disease or stress have adequate renal reserve.[25–27] The Baltimore Longitudinal study (BLS), which studied a cohort of individuals from 1958 until 1981, found the overall rate of decline in creatinine clearance was 0.87 cm^3/min/y beginning at age 40 years. There was a greater loss of function when the mean arterial pressure was greater than 107.[28] However, a third of the individuals in the BLS had no decline in renal function as measured by creatinine clearance,[24] suggesting that processes related to aging do not occur uniformly in humans and that decisions regarding medical treatment must be individualized.

With aging some common histologic findings are seen. These include glomerulosclerosis, which mainly involves the superficial cortex, thickening of the glomerular basement membrane, interstitial fibrosis, tubular dilatation, and mesangial expansion with obliteration of capillary loops.[29–31] Cortical sclerosis increases with age from 5% at age 40 years to 10% by age 80 years.[30] Sclerotic changes in the adjacent arterioles suggest that there may be a hemodynamic role in the aging process.[32] The glomerular filtration rate and renal blood flow decreased with age in healthy volunteers. The effective renal blood flow declines from 647 mL/min/1.73 mm^2 in young adults to 339 mL/min/1.73 mm^2 in the elderly group.[26]

ACUTE KIDNEY INJURY

Because of the functional changes mentioned earlier and higher incidences of diabetes mellitus and atherosclerosis, as well as inaccurate estimates of glomerular filtration rate, the elderly are more prone to acute kidney injury (AKI) in the setting of exposure to nephrotoxins, volume depletion, or hemodynamic instability.[26,33–35] The most common causes of AKI in elderly persons are prerenal failure secondary to loss of renal tubular concentrating ability, loss of thirst sensation, and toxicity related to prescribed medications.[25,33] A prospective study that evaluated the prevalence and outcome of AKI in the elderly and very elderly[35] found that 30% of the patients with AKI were very elderly, greater than 80 years old, even though they made up only 10% of hospital admissions.[36] The most common cause of AKI in elderly hospitalized patients was prerenal failure secondary to dehydration. The various causes for acute tubular necrosis or indication for dialysis did not differ among the different age groups. However, the recovery of renal function in elderly patients was less than the younger cohort and the recovery time was longer.[36] Similar results were found in a retrospective study from India in which the major cause of acute kidney injury was medically related in 80% of the cases with 50% of the cases of acute kidney injury resulting from prerenal causes.[35]

In a meta-analysis of 17 observational cohort studies, kidney function in the elderly patients tended to recover either during hospitalization or following discharge.[37] Recovery was less likely in those older than 65 years.[37] The reason for differences in the rates of recovery was not determined in this study. Those elderly patients placed on continuous replacement therapy faired better than those placed on intermittent hemodialysis.[37]

The long-term mortality in those individuals with acute kidney injury requiring renal replacement therapy was evaluated by Schiffl in a prospective observational study.[38] The major cause of AKI was ischemia (60%) followed by acute tubular injury (33%). Forty-seven percent died during hospitalization; only 25% had survived by the end of the 5-year study. Higher mortality was seen in the elderly.[38] Independent risk factors for a decrease in long-term survival were presence of pre-existing comorbidities, surgical admission, and partial recovery from acute renal failure.[38]

Using Medicare Beneficiary claim data and the US Renal Data System (USRDS) registry, Ishani looked at the outcome of the elderly who developed AKI during their hospitalization.[39] Of the 3.1% of the elderly discharged with a diagnosis of AKI, 25.2% developed end-stage kidney disease (ESKD). The adjusted hazard ratio for developing ESKD from AKI was 13.00, from CKD was 8.43, and from AKI superimposed on CKD was 41.19.[39] The 2-year mortality was higher in those with AKI superimposed on CKD than when either AKI or CKD was present alone, 64.3% versus 53.4% versus 26.9%.respectively.[39] This study highlights the importance of avoiding acute kidney injury in the elderly.

GLOMERULONEPHRITIS

Over the past few decades there has been a change in attitude in the renal community on the use of the renal biopsy in the elderly person because studies show that there is no increased risk from the procedure. Moreover, many of the pathologic findings are treatable and progression to chronic kidney disease can be avoided.[40–42] This is important because chronic kidney disease is associated with increased cardiovascular risk and an increase in mortality.[9,10] In the past, the likelihood of performing a kidney biopsy on an elderly person was low because the prevailing view was that the finding of glomerulonephritis was uncommon.[40,42] In a study from 1949,[40] no cases of acute glomerulonephritis were noted in those more than 60 years old. In the 1960s, there were case reports and articles published showing elderly and very elderly persons who developed treatable types of glomerulonephritis.[42] In 1966,[40] Lee reported on seven biopsies performed in patients more than 50 years old (ranging from 53 to 78 years old) who presented with AKI. Active glomerulonephritis was present in all seven biopsies.

In 1990, Preston reported that the number of kidney biopsies in the elderly increased (mean age 70.5 ± 4.5 years old) in his series of 1334 patients. Approximately 3% of the renal biopsies were performed in the very elderly population.[43] The most common reason for performing a kidney biopsy was proteinuria (41%). Glomerular disease was the major histologic finding (75.4%) with membranous glomerulonephritis being the most common (15%) followed by crescentic glomerulonephritis (13.55%). Crescentic glomerulonephritis accounted for 50% of the cases of acute kidney injury and 35% of the cases of subacute kidney injury.[43]

There has been limited information on the prevalence of renal disease in the very elderly (80 years of age or older). Recently, a retrospective study reviewing renal biopsies from 2001 to 2003 compared the very elderly with other age groups.[44] A total of 3227 individuals underwent a kidney biopsy. One hundred and two renal biopsies were from the very elderly and comprised 3.2% of all biopsies. An elderly cohort ranging from age 66 to 79 years had 433 renal biopsies, which comprised 13.4% of all the renal biopsies. The most common indications for performing a renal biopsy in the very elderly group were as follows: acute kidney injury (23%), nephrotic syndrome (33%), and acute glomerulonephritis (20%). Pauci-immune crescentic glomerulonephritis was the most common diagnosis (19%). At least 40% of the renal biopsies performed revealed pathologic findings that were potentially treatable and suggested that kidney biopsies were beneficial in the very elderly. Complications were low (2%).[44]

CHRONIC KIDNEY DISEASE

There has been a tremendous increase in the number of elderly patients with chronic kidney disease, especially with stages III and IV kidney disease, end-stage kidney disease, and renal transplant recipients. The prevalence of predialysis chronic kidney disease (CKD) in the United States was evaluated from the National Health and Nutrition Examination Survey (NHANES) during two time periods stretching from 1988 until 1994 and from 1999 until 2004.[6] Over these time periods the prevalence of CKD I to IV in noninstitutionalized adults increased from 10% to 13%.[6] The CKD III estimated prevalence increased from 5.4 to 7%, whereas the estimated prevalence of CKD stage IV increased from 0.21% to 0.35%. The greatest prevalence was in those individuals more than 70 year of age. Similarly, the greatest increase in individuals with CKD III was noted in the group more than 70 years of age.[6] This increase in prevalence of CKD III was partly explained by the increase in diabetes, hypertension, body mass index, and age, which are all known risk factors for CKD.[6]

Cardiovascular disease is a common cause of death in CKD and ESRD[5,9,10,45] and generally increases with the severity of CKD.[9,10] Although the adjusted risk of cardiovascular death was not greatly increased in the elderly with an estimated GFR between 50 and 59 $cm^3/min/1.73$ mm^2 when compared with a cohort with an estimated GFR more than 60 $cm^3/min/1.73$ mm^2,[10] the adjusted risk of death increased significantly with a further decline in the estimated GFR. The absolute death rate from cardiovascular causes is highest in the elderly and very elderly but there has been a decline in this trend over the past decade; this decline has been attributed to better preventive care.[5]

The Kidney Early Evaluation Program (KEEP) and NHANES studies found that risk factors for chronic kidney disease were age, hypertension, diabetes, obesity, smoking, and cardiovascular disease.[46] Similarly, the elderly populations with CKD IV have a higher percentage of diabetes, hypertension, and cardiovascular disease compared with a similar population without severe chronic kidney disease.[5] Similar data collected from the Cardiovascular Health Study showed a threefold increase in cardiovascular death with elevated creatinine levels and increased mortality with age.[9] The prevention of CKD in the elderly or very elderly, either by avoidance of AKI, treatment of GN, or aggressive treatment of comorbidities associated with both age and CKD, may decrease overall mortality.

END-STAGE RENAL DISEASE

Before 1972, there were limited resources for the initiation of chronic hemodialysis, and patients greater than 45 years old or diabetics were excluded from consideration.[47,48] It was not until Congress passed an amendment to the Social Security Act in 1972 that federal funding provided for ESKD care.[47–49] Presently, more than

4000 per million population in the United States are on dialysis. It is estimated that there will be 610,000 people on dialysis in 2010[5] secondary to the increase in the elderly and very elderly population, the more liberal criteria for initiating renal replacement therapy, and improved technology. This far exceeds estimates made at the time federal funding was initiated in the 1970s. Linked to this increase in chronic kidney disease has been an ever greater increase in health care costs that can be directly attributed to associated comorbidities. In 2006 there was a fourfold increase in the annual Medicare cost in the elderly population with CKD compared with the elderly population without CKD.[5] In 2004 spending for ESKD accounted for 6.7% of the total Medicare expenditure.[50] The Medicare expenditure is expected to continue to accrue as the prevalence of CKD and ESKD in the elderly and very elderly population increases. Questions of cost/benefit are certain to arise.

Data from the USRDS registry from 2008 showed that the highest incidence rate for ESKD was in the population exceeding 74 years of age with an incidence of 1744 per million population (pmp).[5] Individuals between the ages of 66 and 74 years had the second highest incidence of ESKD with a rate of 1452 pmp, whereas those individuals between 45 until 65 years had an incidence of ESKD of 625 pmp.[5] These findings were similar in developed countries with the exception of New Zealand, which had a decline in ESKD incident rate.[5] This was probably due to the banning of phenacetin in the 1980s.

Areas well known to geriatricians and gerontologists have recently been the focus of clinical research in dialysis patients. These studies have confirmed that there is an increase in fragility, an increase in syncope, and a decrease in memory in the elderly population, which may be further aggravated by dialytic therapy.[51] Ultimately, mortality and well-being are affected.[52,53] More than 50% of older dialysis patients need some supervision at home or assistance with at least one activity at home.[51,54,55] In ESKD, the decrease in life expectancy of the very elderly ranges from 8.9 to 24 months[48,49] and the quality of life is also a concern.[54-56] Cook and Jassal performed a cross-sectional study evaluating how well elderly hemodialysis patients were able to perform basic activities of daily living (ADL) or instrumental activities of daily living (IADL). This is of interest because disability and functional dependence have been shown to be related to poor outcome.[55] The ADL are consider to be self-care tasks such as bathing, grooming, dressing, toileting, eating, transferring, and ambulation.[55] The IADL are household management tasks including shopping, housecleaning, laundry, meal preparation, transportation, telephone use, and management of medicine and finances.[55] The ability to perform ADLs or IADLs or functionality score as measured in 162 hemodialysis patients more than 65 years of age was low.[55] Seventy-five percent were unable to rise from a chair without using an arm or requiring some assistance, 68% were not able to tandem walk, and 75% were unable to perform a task for more than 10 seconds. Only 5% were totally independent. Most cohorts had some decline in independence and 52% had low performances on IADL and ADL.[55] These studies underscore the importance of nephrologists recognizing and preventing further decline in functional dependencies. Intervention may improve overall outcome.

Declines in functional independency have been reported during hospital stays that ultimately require extended stay at rehabilitation centers or nursing homes.[57] Lo observed changes in the elderly patients' basic daily living activities before hospitalization and following discharge.[57] At admission only 8/35 patients were independent but all deteriorated in their ability to perform basic activities of daily living 1 week after discharge except in their ability to use the telephone and manage financial affairs.[57]

The Toronto Rehabilitation Institute in partnership with the Toronto University Health Network developed an in-patient hemodialysis rehabilitation unit for the elderly with functional limitations.[51] Most patients who were transferred to this facility after acute hospitalization were unable to ambulate. The units were established to permit short daily dialysis on the premises with integration of multidisciplinary care. Sixty-nine percent of these patients went home within 50 days suggesting there may be a benefit to a geriatric nephrology rehabilitation unit.[51,56]

In ESKD patients, the incidence of dementia and cognitive impairment is twice that of the general population.[58,59] A longitudinal and cross-sectional study evaluated cognitive impairment and possible mediators of cognitive impairment using the Modified Mini Mental Status (3MS) in an elderly cohort.[58] Dementia was defined by a score less than 80 and a higher incidence of dementia was found in the elderly, particularly those with CKD.[58]

Murray performed a cross-sectional study of those 55 years of age or higher on renal replacement therapy and compared them with age-matched controls.[59] Cognitive impairment was found to be more severe in the dialysis patients than in age-matched controls, 33.7% versus 11.9%, respectively.[59] Adjusted logistic regression showed that hemodialysis and age were independent risk factors for a severe decline in cognitive skills.[59]

Dementia diagnosed before initiating renal replacement therapy has been associated with a decrease in life expectancy compared with a cohort without dementia.[60] Those with dementia were older and lived on average 1.1 years, whereas the cohort without dementia lived on average 2.7 years.[60] Dementia was shown to be an independent risk factor for death in dialysis (adjusted hazard ratio 1.9, 95% confidence interval 1.77 to 1.98, $P < .001$). Risk factors associated with dementia were age, inability to ambulate, diabetes, vascular disease, congestive heart failure, and cancer.[60] Recommendations by the Renal Physicians Association and the American Society of Nephrology Practice guidelines for the initiation and withdrawal of patients on dialysis suggest consideration for a limited trial of dialysis in patients with dementia.[60,61]

Kutner evaluated the occurrence of depression and measured life satisfaction in a longitudinal prospective study[62] for the elderly on renal replacement therapy compared with age-matched controls. A quarter of the elderly on dialysis and the respective age-matched controls lived alone. There was significant functional impairment at baseline and at the 3-year follow-up in the dialysis group.[62] Although a direct relationship between greater functional impairment and depression was found, life satisfaction was no different in the two groups at the 3-year follow-up. Kutner concluded that the elderly appeared to adjust better to chronic dialysis treatment than younger dialysis patients.[62]

The fifth leading cause of death in the elderly person is unintentional trauma with falls being most common.[55] In elderly patients on hemodialysis, falls were significant predictors of mortality.[51] In general, the elderly are prone to fall because of underlying fragility, and functional dependencies. In dialysis patients, the risk is compounded by fluid shifts, polypharmacy, dysautonomia, and diabetes mellitus.[51,55,63] In a cross-sectional study, a third of elderly patients on hemodialysis reported falling once in 12 months; 4% had sustained a fracture or head injury.[54] Does fluctuation in the volume status with dialysis cause hemodynamic instability? To answer this question a survey was sent to patients aged 70 years or older on hemodialysis.[63] Of the 47 patients interviewed, nine had no symptoms, 34 reported episodes of dizziness, 15 reported episodes of presyncope and syncope, and 13 experienced unexplained falls in the 12 months preceding the study.[63] Twenty-three patients had blood pressure recorded before and after dialysis and autonomic insufficiency was tested in 10 patients.[63] Eight out of 23 patients had orthostatic blood pressure readings before dialysis and 16 out of 23 patients had postdialysis orthostasis, which correlated with symptoms in 12 out of the 16 patients.[63] All 10 patients who underwent auto-nomic testing were found to have autonomic insufficiency.[63]

In addition to falls, elderly dialysis patients have an increased incidence of bone fractures that is independent from renal bone disease.[64] In a study of those ESKD patients less than 70 years of age who were either on the transplant waiting list or transplanted from 1990 to 2001,[64] the total number of hip fractures was 971 during the 314,767 person-years of follow-up.[64] Risks factors for bone fracture were female gender, white race, increasing age, and time on dialysis before being placed on the renal transplant list. Age was the strongest risk factor for hip fracture even after adjust-ment for race, diabetes nephropathy, time on dialysis, and gender. There was a 3.27-fold greater risk in those aged 56 to 70 years compared with those less than 40 years of age.[64] For those who had received a transplant, there was an initial in-crease in the risk of fracture in the first 128 days post-transplant; the risk then declined afterwards.[64]

The life expectancy for very elderly patients on hemodialysis is poor. In the United States, the survival time is 15.6 months for those from 80 to 84 years of age, 11.6 months for those 85 to 89 years of age, and only 8.4 months for those 90 years of age or older.[65] The overall 1-year survival rate in the very elderly is 54%. The elderly have a higher mortality rate within the first 3 months of dialysis (20%) than the general dialysis population does during the first year of dialysis (16%).[65]

The factors influencing the decision to initiative hemodialysis and survival in octoge-narians were evaluated in a 12-year retrospective study.[53] Reasons why octogenar-ians were not offered dialysis included social issues, late referral, poor Karnofsky score, and diabetes mellitus.[53] The median survival for those offered dialysis was 28.9 months, which was longer than those octogenarians who went without dialytic intervention (8.9 months).[53] The 12- and 24-month survival for patients receiving dial-ysis was 73.6% and 60%, respectively, compared with 29% and 15%, respectively, in patients treated conservatively.[53] Independent risk factors for dying within 1 year on dialysis were poor nutritional status, late referral, and decreased functional depen-dence.[53] After 1 year on dialysis the presence of peripheral vascular disease and other comorbidities largely determined the risk of death.[53] The decision to initiate dialysis n very elderly patients requires involvement of the patient and family members to discuss overall benefit, resources, and quality of life.[53]

Similar results have been found in the United Kingdom. A retrospective study looked at dialysis outcomes in three different age groups: those 75 years of age or older, those 65 to 74 years of age and those less than 65 years of age.[48] Peritoneal dialysis was the dialytic modality of choice for 52%. At 3 years, only 5% of the very elderly patients, 22% of the elderly patients, and 64% of the adult patients had survived.[48] Life expectancy was decreased for all ages compared with the general population. The very elderly patients had increased comorbidities with 46% having two or more, including hypertension and cardiovascular disease.[48] The cause of death in the very elderly patients was elective withdrawal in 38%, infection in 22%, and a cardiovascular event in 24%.[48]

Because of the high mortality rates in elderly ESKD patients, a prospective, multi-center, randomized control study comparing the usefulness of a low-protein diet versus dialysis was performed.[66] The primary outcome was mortality.[66] The 1-year observed survival with intention to treat was no different between the two groups: 83.7% versus 87.3% (log rank test for noninferiority, $P < .001$) with a mean time of 10.7 months on the low-protein diet.[66] The two common reasons for initiating dialysis were hyperkalemia and hypervolemia. The study suggested that the use of a low-protein diet was safe and effective in appropriate patients and might postpone the need to initiate dialysis for a year.[66] The study suggested that a restricted renal diet might be an alternative option in a select group of patients who were not considered to be candidates for dialysis or who refused to consider dialysis.

The decrease in survival for elderly and very elderly patients on dialysis may be related to late referrals to the nephrologist, a factor that has been shown to have a negative impact on outcome.[48,67] Late referrals were more likely to be seen in very elderly patients (P = .007) with a median of 3.5 weeks before initiating dialysis in those 75 years of age or older compared with 20.5 weeks for those less than 75 years of age.[67] The survival at 88.5 weeks was 53.25% for the very elderly patients compared with 76.5% in the younger group.[67] Zhoa found that late referrals were directly related to the distance to the office, age, female gender, underlying diseases, number in primary care population, and underlying comorbidities.[8]

The decision to initiate dialysis often becomes an ethical issue in elderly and very elderly patients because of their poor outcome on renal replacement therapy, which is worsened by the number of comorbidities. In a recent survey, most geriatric fellows interviewed reported that they felt comfortable addressing end-of-life issues with their patients.[68] In contrast, the renal fellows reported that they did not believe that they were trained sufficiently to handle such issues.[69] In a survey sent out to second-year renal fellows in 2003 to determine their experience with palliative care,[69] Holley found that only 26% were more comfortable in handling palliative care issues. Moreover, the renal fellows reported that more instruction was offered when they consulted palliative care. Although the same fellows reported receiving feedback 92% of the time from their nephrology attending whenever they performed a renal biopsy, they received feedback less than 25% of the time on palliative care issues. Less than 30% reported receiving any formal training on end-of-life care, however, more than 50% felt this was an important enough issue that needed to be incorporated into their formal training.[69]

In a small study, Somogyi-Zalud observed that those more than 80 years of age who were hospitalized preferred comfort measures and avoidance of pain.[70] However, they underwent many invasive procedures including dialysis during their hospital stay and their wishes were often not followed.[70] This study suggests that education in palliative care should be part of a resident's or fellow's education; it should also include instruction on dietary intervention for those patients not initiated on dialysis, subcutaneous injections, and appropriate renal adjustment of medications.

TRANSPLANT

Before 1997, persons with end-stage renal failure 80 years of age or older were not placed on the renal transplant waiting list and did not receive a renal transplant. As the number of elderly persons increases, those requiring renal replacement therapy or the need for renal transplant has increased. The rate of renal transplantation has increased extremely slowly over the past decade[5] and the pool for kidney transplants is insufficient to meet the demand. The expanded donor criteria were developed to accommodate this shortage of deceased kidney donors and expand the recipient population. The expanded donor criterion (ECD) was defined by the United Network for Organ Sharing (UNOS) in 2002. The definition of ECD included harvesting a kidney from those greater than or equal to 60 years of age or older than 50 years of age with two of the following criteria: hypertension; serum creatinine greater than 1.5 mg/dL; or death from cerebrovascular disease.[71,72] There is a 70% higher risk of graft failure with these criteria than with a non-ECD renal transplant.[72] Combined observational studies comparing ECD and standard donor criteria (SCD) transplants found a decrease in the waiting time with the use of ECD, an increase in the number of transplants, and a decrease in mortality associated with transplantation, compared with dialysis.[73] It has been suggested that the ECD is not appropriate in recipients less than 40 years of age, or for a re-transplant, but it may be appropriate in those older than 40 years of age with diabetes and persons on the waiting list for more than 4 years.[72,73]

The number of very elderly people placed on the waiting list has increased over the past decade.[71] The elderly who were on the ESKD waiting list increased from 1992 to 2004, increasing from 3.4% to 13.8%, respectively.[5,50] Data from the USRDS registry showed that from 1994 to 2000 only 0.3% of deceased donor organs were allocated to those more than 75 years of age.[74] At 5 years, the death censored graft survival in the very elderly population was 72% and patient survival was 59.9% for living related donor transplant, 40.35% for deceased donor transplant, 29.7% on the waiting list, and 12.5% remaining on dialysis.[74] The very elderly recipients had better survival rates after receiving a kidney transplant than those who remained on the transplant wait list[72,73] or on dialysis.[72]

Gill studied elderly transplant recipients more than 60 years of age who had received kidney transplants from four donor groups: old living donor, young living donor, standard donor criteria, and extended donor criteria.[75] The overall 4-year graft and patient survival was 77.5% and 82.4% for old living donor graft, which was similar to the standard criteria graft kidneys. The extended donor criteria graft survival was 57.1% and recipient survival was 67.5%.[75] There was longer graft delay and graft rejection in extended donor criteria recipients.[75] Kidney transplant from an older living person seems to be a viable option with excellent results. It does not take away from the donor pool for younger dialysis patients and it increases the number of kidney transplants that are available for the elderly recipient.[75]

In a retrospective study, Stratta reviewed the patient and graft outcomes in 144 kidney transplant recipients.[71] Thirty-seven recipients were 60 years of age or older and 107 were between 19 and 59 years of age. Most of the extended donor criteria kidneys were transplanted in the older group and most of the younger transplant group received standard criteria donor kidneys. The extended criteria donor recipients were selected by age, HLA matching, low panel reactive antigen, primary transplant, and compatible body mass index. By using these selection criteria, there was no significant difference in patient or graft survival in the two age groups at 27 months.[71] Similar findings were found with a good outcome in very elderly donors and elderly recipients when the donors had no comorbidities, and a Cock-Croft-Gault clearance greater than 80 cm^3/min.[76] There was an overall benefit of renal transplant in the older recipients despite an increased risk of infections secondary to immunosuppression.[77]

The outcome with renal transplant is better than other renal modalities for a selected group of elderly and very elderly. The increased use of extended donor criteria and old living donors will increase the donor pool for elderly and very elderly renal transplant recipients, and not impinge on the number of donors available for the younger patients.

SUMMARY

In the 1980s geriatric nephrology was introduced as a subspecialty in anticipation of the increased number of elderly and very elderly people during the 21st century. Many of the goals set forth by the JAHF/AGS have been accomplished. There has been more clinical research dedicated to geriatric nephrology, education on the subspecialty has been implemented at national and university level, and funds for career development have been instituted over the past two decades. Our treatment of the elderly and very elderly patients seems to be more focused on their biologic age rather than chronologic age; they undergo diagnostic tests such as kidney biopsies and are candidates for kidney transplant. Although great strides have been made in the assimilation of geriatrics into nephrology more has to be done.

REFERENCES

1. Centers for Disease Control and Prevention. Public health and aging: trend in aging – United States and worldwide. MMWR Morb Mortal Wkly Rep 2003;52: 101–6.
2. Stevens LA, Coresh J, Levey AS. CKD in the elderly – old questions and new challenges: World Kidney Day 2008. Am J Kidney Dis 2008;51(3):353–7.
3. Hallan SI, Coresh J, Astor BC, et al. International comparison of the relationship of chronic kidney disease prevalence and ESRD risk. J Am Soc Nephrol 2006;17(8): 2275–84.
4. Michel JP, Huber P, Cruz-Jentoft AJ. Representative of each surveyed country. Europe-wide survey of teaching in geriatric medicine. J Am Geriatr Soc 2008; 56(8):1536–42.
5. US renal data system: USRDS 2006 annual data report, ii. Bethesda (MD): The National Institutes of Health, National Institute of Diabetes and Digestive and Kidney Diseases; 2006. p. 192–212.
6. Coresh J, Selvin E, Stevens LA, et al. Prevalence of chronic kidney disease in the United States. JAMA 2007;298(17):2038–47.
7. Oreopoulos G, Dimkovic N. Geriatric nephrology is coming of age. J Am Soc Nephrol 2003;14(4):1099–101.
8. Zhoa Y, Brooks JM, Flanigan JM, et al. Physicians access and early nephrology care in elderly patients with end-stage renal disease. Kidney Int 2008;74(12): 1596–602.
9. Fried LF, Shlipak MG, Crump C, et al. Renal insufficiency as a predictor of cardiovascular outcomes and mortality in elderly individuals. J Am Coll Cardiol 2003; 41(3):1364–72.
10. O'Hare AM, Bertenthal D, Convinsky KE, et al. Mortality risk stratification in chronic kidney disease: one size for all ages? J Am Soc Nephrol 2006;17(3): 846–53.
11. Libow LS. Commentary: the first geriatric residency-fellowship in the United States. J Gerontol A Biol Sci Med Sci 2004;59(11):1165–6.
12. Hazzard WR. Capturing the power of the academic medicine to enhance health and healthcare of the elderly in the USA. Geriatr Gerontol Int 2004;4:5–14.
13. Boult C, Christmas C, Durso S. Perspective: transforming chronic care for older persons. Acad Med 2008;83(7):627–31.
14. Sonu IS, High KP, Clayton CP, et al. An evaluation of geriatrics activities within internal medicine subspecialties. Am J Med 2006;119(11):995–1000.
15. Hazzard WR, Woolard N, Regenstreiff D, et al. Integrating geriatrics into the subspecialties of internal medicine: the Hartford Foundation/American Geriatrics Society/Wake Forest University Bowman Gray School of Medicine initiative. J Am Geriatr Soc 1997;45(5):638–40.
16. Joiner KA, Haponik E, High KP. Integrating geriatric and subspecialty internal medicine; results of a survey on patient care practices, training, attitudes, and research. Am J Med 2002;112(3):249–54.
17. Wiggins J. Geriatrics. Am J Kidney Dis 2005;46(1):147–58.

18. Musso CG. Geriatric nephrology and the "nephrogeriatric giants". Int Urol Nephrol 2002;34(2):255–6.
19. Michelis MF, Davis BB, Preuss HG. Geriatric nephrology. New York: Field, Rich and Associates, Inc.; 1986. p. 1–166.
20. Keith DS, Nichols GA, Gullion CM, et al. Longitudinal follow-up and outcomes among a population with chronic kidney disease in a large managed care organization. Arch Intern Med 2004;164(6):659–63.
21. Hunsicker LG. The consequences and costs of chronic kidney disease before ESRD. J Am Soc Nephrol 2004;15(5):1363–4.
22. National Kidney Foundation. K/DOQI clinical practice guidelines for chronic kidney disease: evaluation, classification, and stratification. Am J Kidney Dis 2002;39:S1–266.
23. Baggio B, Budakovic A, Perissinotto E, et al. ILSA Working Group. Atherosclerotic risk factors and renal function in the elderly: the role of hyperfibrinogenaemia and smoking. Results from the Italian Longitudinal Study on Ageing (ILSA). Nephrol Dial Transplant 2005;20(1):114–23.
24. Lindeman RD, Tobin J, Shock NW. Longitudinal studies on the rate of decline in renal function with age. J Am Geriatr Soc 1985;33(4):278–85.
25. Fehrman- Ekholm I, Skeppholm L. Renal function in the elderly (>70 years old) measured by means of iohexol clearance, serum creatinine, serum urea and estimated clearance. Scand J Urol Nephrol 2004;38(1):73–7.
26. Fliser D, Zeler M, Nowack R, et al. Renal functional reserve in healthy elderly subjects. J Am Soc Nephrol 1993;3(7):1371–7.
27. Hemmelgarn R, Zhang J, Manns BJ, et al. Progression of kidney dysfunction in the community-dwelling elderly. Kidney Int 2006;69:2155–61.
28. Lindeman RD, Tobin JD, Shock NW. Association between blood pressure and the rate of decline in renal function with age. Kidney Int 1984;26(6):861–8.
29. Anderson S, Brenner BM. Effect of aging on the renal glomerulus. Am J Med 1986;80(5):436–42.
30. Lamb EJ, O'Riordan SE, Delaney MP. Kidney function in older people: pathology, assessment, and management. Clin Chim Acta 2003;334(1–2):24–40.
31. Thomas SE, Anderson S, Gordon K, et al. Tubulointerstitial disease in aging: evidence for underlying peritubular capillary damage, a potential role for renal ischemia. J Am Soc Nephrol 1998;9(2):231–42.
32. Kasiske BL. Relationship between vascular disease and age-associated changes in the human kidney. Kidney Int 1987;31(5):1153–9.
33. Pascual J, Liano F, Ortuno J. The elderly patient with acute renal failure. J Am Soc Nephrol 1995;6(2):144–53.
34. Abuelo JG. Normotensive ischemic acute renal failure. N Engl J Med 2007;357(8):797–805.
35. Arora P, Kher V, Kohli HS, et al. Acute renal failure in the elderly: experience from a single centre in India. Nephrol Dial Transplant 1993;8(9):827–30.
36. Pascual J, Liano F. Causes and prognosis of acute renal failure in the very old. Madrid Acute Renal Failure Study Group. J Am Geriatr Soc 1998;46(6):721–5.
37. Schmitt R, Coca S, Kanbay M, et al. Recovery of kidney function after acute kidney injury in the elderly: a systematic review and meta-analysis. Am J Kidney Dis 2008;52(2):262–71.
38. Schiffl H, Fischer F. Five-year outcome of severe acute kidney injury requiring renal replacement therapy. Nephrol Dial Transplant 2008;23(7):2235–41.
39. Ishani A, Xue JL, Himmelfarb J, et al. Acute injury increases risk of ESRD among elderly. J Am Soc Nephrol 2009;20(1):223–8.

40. Lee HA, Stirling G, Sharptone P. Acute glomerulonephritis in middle-aged and elderly patients. BMJ 1966;2:1361–3.
41. Kaplan-Pavlovčič S, Cerk K, Kveder R, et al. Clinical prospective factors in renal outcome in anti-neutrophil cytoplasmic antibodies in elderly patients. Nephrol Dial Transplant 2003;18(5):V5–7.
42. Samiy AH, Field RA, Merrill JP. Acute glomerulonephritis in elderly patients: report of seven cases over sixty years of age. Ann Intern Med 1961;54(1):603–9.
43. Preston RA, Stemmer CL, Materson BJ, et al. Renal biopsy in the patients 65 years of age or older; analysis of the results of 334 biopsies. J Am Geriatr Soc 1990;38(6):669–74.
44. Nair R, Bell JM, Walker PD. Renal biopsy in patients aged 80 years and older. Am J Kidney Dis 2004;44(4):618–26.
45. Culleton BF, Larson MG, Evans JC, et al. Prevalence and correlates of elevated serum creatinine levels: the Framingham Heart Study. Arch Intern Med 1999; 159(15):1785–90.
46. Whaley-Connell AT, Sowers JR, Stevens LA, et al. CKD in the United States: Kidney Early Evaluation Program (KEEP) and National Health and Nutrition Examination Survey (NHANES) 1999–2004. Am J Kidney Dis 2008;51(4):S13–20.
47. Himmelfarb J, Berns A, Wesson D. Cost, quality and value: the changing political economy of dialysis care. J Am Soc Nephrol 2007;18(7):2021–7.
48. Munshi SK, Vijayakumar N, Taub NA, et al. Outcome of renal replacement therapy in the very elderly. Nephrol Dial Transplant 2001;16(1):128–33.
49. Krishnan M, Lok CE, Jassal SV. Epidemiology and demographic aspect of treated end-stage renal disease in the elderly. Semin Dial 2002;15(2):79–83.
50. Foley RN, Collins AJ. End-stage renal disease in the United States; an update from United States Renal Data System. J Am Soc Nephrol 2007;18(10): 2644–8.
51. Li M, Porter E, Lam R, et al. Quality improvement through the introduction of interdisciplinary geriatric hemodialysis rehabilitation care. Am J Kidney Dis 2007; 50(1):90–107.
52. Johansen KL, Chertow GM, Jin C, et al. Significance of frailty among dialysis patients. J Am Soc Nephrol 2007;18(11):2960–7.
53. Joly D, Anglicheau D, Alberti C, et al. Octogenarians reaching end stage renal disease: cohort study of decision-making and clinical outcomes. J Am Soc Nephrol 2003;14(4):1012–21.
54. Cook WL, Jassal SV. Prevalence of falls among seniors maintained on hemodialysis. Int Urol Nephrol 2005;37(3):649–52.
55. Cook W, Jassal SV. Functional dependencies among the elderly on hemodialysis. Kidney Int 2008;73(11):1289–95.
56. Jassal SV, Chiu E, Li M. Geriatric hemodialysis rehabilitation care. Adv Chronic Kidney Dis 2008;15(2):115–22.
57. Lo D, Chiu E, Jassal SV. A prospective pilot study to measure changes in functional status associated with hospitalization in the elderly dialysis-dependent patients. Am J Kidney Dis 2008;52(5):956–61.
58. Kurella MT, Chertow GM, Fried LF, et al. Chronic kidney disease and cognitive impairment in the elderly: the health, aging, abdomen body composition study. J Am Soc Nephrol 2005;16(7):2127–33.
59. Murray AM, Tupper DE, Knopman DS, et al. Cognitive impairment in hemodialysis patients is common. Neurology 2006;67(2):216–23.
60. Rakowski D, Caillard S, Agodoa LY, et al. Dementia as a predictor of mortality in dialysis patients. Clin J Am Soc Nephrol 2006;1(5):1000–5.

61. Moss AH. Shared decision making in dialysis: the new RPA/ASN guidelines on appropriate initiation and withdrawal of treatment. Am J Kidney Dis 2001;37(5): 1081–91.
62. Kutner NG, Jassal SV. Quality of life and rehabilitation of the elderly dialysis patients. Semin Dial 2002;15(2):107–12.
63. Roberts RG, Kenny RA, Brierley EJ. Are elderly hemodialysis patients at risk of falls and postural hypotension? Int Urol Nephrol 2003;35(3):415–21.
64. Ball AM, Gillen DL, Sherrard D, et al. Risk of hip fracture among dialysis and renal transplant recipients. JAMA 2002;288(23):3014–8.
65. Kurella TM, Wadley V, Yaffe K, et al. Kidney function and cognitive impairment in US adults: the Reasons for Geographic and Racial Differences in Stroke (RE-GARDS) study. Am J Kidney Dis 2008;52(2):227–34.
66. Brunori G, Viola BF, Parrinello G, et al. Efficacy and safety of a very-low protein diet when postponing dialysis in the elderly: a prospective randomized multi-center controlled study. Am J Kidney Dis 2007;49(5):569–80.
67. Schwenger V, Christian M, Hofmann A, et al. Late referral – a major cause of poor outcome in the very elderly dialysis patient. Nephrol Dial Transplant 2006;31(4): 962–7.
68. Pan CX, Carmody S, Leipzig RM, et al. There is hope for the future: national survey results reveal that geriatric medicine fellows are well-educated in end-of-life care. J Am Geriatr Soc 2005;53(4):705–10.
69. Holley JL, Carmody SS, Moss AH, et al. The need for end-of-life training in nephrology: national survey results of nephrology fellows. Am J Kidney Dis 2003;42(4):813–20.
70. Somogyi-Zalud E, Zhong Z, Hamel MB, et al. The use of life-sustaining treatments in hospitalized persons aged 80 and older. J Am Geriatr Soc 2002;50(5):930–4.
71. Stratta RJ, Sundberg AK, Rohr MS, et al. Optimal use of older donors and recipients in kidney transplantation. Surgery 2006;139(3):324–33.
72. Merion RM, Ashby VB, Wolfe RA, et al. Deceased-donor characteristics and the survival benefit of kidney transplantation. JAMA 2005;294(21):2726–33.
73. Pascual J, Zamora J, Pirsch JD. A systemic review of kidney transplantation from expanded criteria donors. Am J Kidney Dis 2008;52(3):553–86.
74. Macrae J, Friedman AL, Friedman EA, et al. Live and deceased donor kidney transplantation in patients aged 75 years and older in the United States. Int Urol Nephrol 2005;37(3):641–8.
75. Gill J, Bunnapradist S, Danovitch GM, et al. Outcome of kidney transplantation from older living donors to older recipient. Am J Kidney Dis 2008;52(3):541–52.
76. Geissing M, Fuler TF, Friedersdorff F, et al. Outcomes of transplanting deceased-donor kidneys between elderly donor and recipients. J Am Soc Nephrol 2009; 20(1):37–40.
77. Meier-Kriesche H, Ojo AO, Hanson JA, et al. Exponentially increase risk of infectious deaths in older renal transplant recipients. Kidney Int 2001;59(4):1539–43.

Anatomic and Physiologic Changes of the Aging Kidney

Edgar V. Lerma, MD

KEYWORDS

- Glomerulosclerosis • Tubulointerstitial • Hyalinosis
- Juxtamedullary • Microalbuminuria • Natriuresis
- Osmoregulation • Nocturia

ANATOMIC CHANGES

The human kidney reaches a maximum size of approximately 400 g (roughly corresponding to 12 cm in length) in the fourth decade of life. After this, there is a natural decline in kidney size, amounting to an approximately 10% decrease in renal mass for every 10 years thereafter, with a tendency for such decrease to be greater in men as opposed to women. This decrease is also associated with progressive cortical thinning and loss in the number of functioning nephrons. Renal biopsies show progressive focal and segmental glomerulosclerosis, tubulointerstitial fibrosis, and arteriolar hyalinosis.

Glomerular Changes

Several ultrastructural changes have been observed and described in the glomerulus with aging. Preserved glomeruli often show an increase in overall tuft cross-sectional area and a thickened glomerular basement membrane; this is consistent with glomerular hypertrophy.[1] Most characteristic is the development of focal and segmental or, rarely, global glomerulosclerosis. Whereas the prevalence of glomerulosclerosis is less than 5% of glomeruli at age 0 years, this increases to 10% to 30% of glomeruli by the eighth decade.[2] In aging mice and rats, which show similar histologic changes, a strong relationship between the glomerular hypertrophy and glomerulosclerosis has been shown,[3] consistent with the hypothesis that glomerular hypertrophy may predispose to the development of glomerulosclerosis.[4] Glomerulosclerosis is associated with mesangial matrix expansion and a progressive loss of capillary loops. Periglomerular fibrosis is often prominent, and there may be so-called atubular glomeruli, in which the exit from the Bowman capsule to the proximal tubular lumen is blocked by fibrosis.

Division of Nephrology, University of Illinois at Chicago College of Medicine/Associates in Nephrology, SC, 3543 Wisconsin Avenue, Berwyn, IL 60402, USA
E-mail address: edgarvlermamd@pol.net

Clin Geriatr Med 25 (2009) 325–329
doi:10.1016/j.cger.2009.06.007
0749-0690/09/$ – see front matter © 2009 Published by Elsevier Inc.

Tubular and Interstitial Changes

Tubulointerstitial injury mostly involves the outer medulla and medullary rays, with typical features: tubular dilatation and atrophy, mononuclear cell infiltration, and interstitial fibrosis. Many tubules express osteopontin, which is a marker of tubular injury and a known chemotactic protein. The infiltrating interstitial cells consist of macrophages and myofibroblasts, and the fibrosis is due in part to the deposition of types I and III collagen,[5] which seems to be mediated by the local expression of transforming growth factor-β.[6] Some tubules (especially of the distal tubule and collecting duct) may develop small diverticuli; it has been suggested that these diverticuli play a role in the development of upper urinary tract infections (pyelonephritis) by harboring bacteria, thereby predisposing to recurrent infection.[7] Still others suggest that such outpouchings may be indications of early kidney cyst formations.

Vascular Changes

Arterioles often develop hyalinosis with aging. Hyalinosis is defined as thickening of the arteriole; such an increase in the ratio of the thickness of the media to the luminal diameter is common with aging but is observed almost exclusively in individuals with hypertension.[7] The arcuate arteries become more angulated and irregular with aging, and there is increased tortuosity and spiraling of the interlobar vessels. These changes occur independently of hypertension but are augmented in its presence. With aging, some afferent arterioles, particularly of juxtamedullary glomeruli, develop vascular shunts to the efferent arterioles, thereby bypassing glomeruli, leading to "aglomerular arterioles."[8] Studies in rats have also demonstrated focal losses of glomerular capillary loops and peritubular capillaries, consistent with a state of impaired angiogenesis.[9] Such changes have been attributed to decreased concentration of the vascular endothelial growth factor (proangiogenic) and increased expression of thrombospondin-1 (antiangiogenic), as demonstrated in rats.

FUNCTIONAL CHANGES
Glomerular Filtration Rate

Serum creatinine is a relatively unreliable indicator of renal function in the aging population. This is because creatinine generation reflects muscle mass, and muscle mass decreases with aging. Normally, males excrete 20 to 25 mg/kg body weight of creatinine in the urine each day, and women excrete 15 to 20 mg/kg body weight of creatinine. However, after the age of 60 years, there is a progressive decrease in urinary creatinine excretion, resulting in excretion rates lower than these ranges.[10]

When accurate creatinine clearances are performed, there is clear evidence for a reduction in renal function with age. In one study, the mean creatinine clearance fell from 140 mL/min/1.73 m^2 at age 25 years to 34 to 97 mL/min/1.73 m^2 at age 75 to 84 years.[11] Serum creatinine was not different between these groups due to the loss of muscle mass that occurs with aging. The decrease in renal function has been corroborated by inulin clearance studies, which show a progressive decrease in glomerular filtration rate (GFR) after the age of 40 years, with a relatively greater decline in men.[12]

Formulas such as the Modification of Diet in Renal Disease (MDRD) equation or the Cockcroft-Gault formula take into account changes with age. Both have a tendency to underestimate true GFR in the aging (>65 years) population when compared with standard techniques such as technetium-labeled diethylene-triamine-pentacetate (^{99m}Tc-DTPA). However, the MDRD appears to be more accurate (−11.3 vs −3.7 mL/min/1.73 m^2 comparing the Cockcroft-Gault to MDRD formula).[13,14]

In addition to the decrease in GFR with aging, there may be a reduction in "renal reserve." Usually, GFR increases with a protein load or with feeding. Some studies suggest that aging humans show a normal increase in GFR after amino acid infusion. However, a more profound challenge was performed in aging rats; in this study, aging rats showed a markedly blunted increase in GFR with feeding.[15]

Not all individuals show a decrease in GFR with aging. In particular, in as many as one-third of subjects who remain normotensive, there is no decrease in creatinine clearance with age.[7]

Renal Plasma Flow

There is also a decrease in renal plasma flow (RPF) with aging. RPF measured by p-aminohippurate clearances decrease from a mean of 650 mL/min in the fourth decade to 290 mL/min by the ninth decade, and this is associated with increasing renal vascular resistance.[12] The fall in RPF tends to be greater in men than in women and is also greater in elderly subjects who have hypertension.[16] Because RPF decreases relatively more than GFR, filtration fraction (defined as GFR/RPF) increases with age.

The decrease in RPF does not simply reflect a decrease in renal mass. Studies using a xenon washout technique demonstrated that there is a true reduction in renal blood flow when factored for renal mass.[17] The decrease in renal blood flow especially involves the cortex, and blood flow to the medulla is relatively preserved.

Capillary Permeability and Proteinuria

The prevalence of microalbuminuria (urinary albumin levels of 30 to 300 mg/day) and albuminuria increase progressively in the US population after the age of 40 years. The increased prevalence is most marked in subjects with diabetes and hypertension, but it is also observed in patients lacking these risk factors.[18] The prevalence of microalbuminuria and albuminuria are higher in blacks, Mexican Americans, and those with elevated serum creatinine.[18] This is clinically relevant because microalbuminuria has been found to be an independent risk factor for cardiovascular events (such as carotid disease and left ventricular hypertrophy) and cardiovascular mortality.

Sodium Balance and Hypertension

Sodium balance is also altered in aging. There is evidence for impaired sodium excretion of a salt load[19] and defective conservation in the setting of sodium restriction.[20] Proximal sodium reabsorption (reflected by lithium clearances) is increased in aging, whereas distal sodium reabsorption may be reduced.[21] Studies in rats suggest that the pressure natriuresis is impaired in aging.[22] Because the diet of most individuals in developed countries contains excess sodium (8–10 g salt/d), there is a tendency in the elderly population for total body sodium excess.

The relative defect in sodium excretion and increased total body sodium may be a predisposing factor for the development of hypertension. Blood pressure increases with age. After the age of 60 years, most of the population has hypertension.[23] The majority (>85%) of hypertension in the aging population is sodium-sensitive, in that restricting sodium will result in a significant fall (>10 mm Hg) in mean arterial pressure.[24] Populations that ingest low sodium diets, such as the Yanomamo Indians of Southern Venezuela, do not show an increase in blood pressure with age.[25] Other mechanisms may also be involved in aging-associated hypertension, including loss of vascular compliance due to collagen deposition in the larger arterial vessels. Endothelial dysfunction, perhaps mediated by oxidative stress, has been shown to be increased in the aging population, and may contribute to the development of increased blood pressure.

The observation that aging-associated renal and vascular changes may be responsible for the high frequency of hypertension in the population likely explains why correction of secondary forms of hypertension (such as primary aldosteronism, Cushing syndrome, renovascular hypertension, and hypothyroidism) is more effective at curing hypertension in younger patients. In one study, diastolic blood pressure fell to less than 90 mm Hg in 24 of 25 subjects under the age of 40 years after treating the mechanism responsible for the secondary hypertension, but the blood pressure fell only in 38 of 61 subjects over the age of 40 years.[26]

Osmoregulation and Water Handling

There is also impaired water handling with aging. Both concentration and dilution are affected, and nocturia is common. There is a reduced maximal urinary osmolality and thirst response to hyperosmolality, which may be predisposing factors for the development of dehydration. Subjects respond to antidiuretic hormone (vasopressin) with an increase in urine osmolarity, but it is blunted compared with younger subjects. Total body water also decreases with age. Conversely, there is slower excretion of a water load, leading to an increased predisposition to hyponatremia.

Other Tubular Defects and Electrolyte Problems

Potassium excretion is impaired and is likely due to decreased tubular mass. Hyperkalemia occurs more frequently in elderly subjects treated with drugs that interfere with potassium excretion (such as potassium sparing diuretics) than in younger people. Other predispositions to hyperkalemia in the elderly include decreased GFR and lower basal levels of aldosterone. Hypokalemia is also common due to renal or extrarenal losses. Acid-base disturbances may result from the impaired distal tubular acidification that occurs with aging; aging subjects do not excrete an acid load as effectively as younger subjects.

Hypercalcemia occurs in 2% to 3% of institutionalized elderly patients. Causes are multifactorial and include malignant tumors, hyperparathyroidism, immobilization, and thiazide diuretic use. Hypocalcemia is less common and is observed mainly in patients with chronic renal failure, chronic malabsorption, and severe malnutrition. Aging is associated with increased parathyroid hormone levels (which correlate inversely with GFR) and a decrease in serum calcitriol and phosphate levels.[21] Hypomagnesemia may be present in as many as 7% to 10% of elderly patients admitted to the hospital; most commonly this is the result of malnutrition, laxatives, or diuretic use. Hypermagnesemia is less common and is found primarily in patients with chronic renal failure or who are taking large doses of magnesium-containing antacids. Gout (and an elevation in serum uric acid levels) is also more common in the aging population.

REFERENCES

1. McLachlan MS. The aging kidney. Lancet 1978;2:143–5.
2. Kaplan C, Pasternack B, Shah H, et al. Age-related incidence of sclerotic glomeruli in human kidneys. Am J Pathol 1975;80:227–34.
3. Ferder L, Inserra F, Romano L, et al. Decreased glomerulosclerosis in aging by angiotensin-converting enzyme inhibitors. J Am Soc Nephrol 1994;5:1147–52.
4. Fogo AB. Glomerular hypertension, abnormal glomerular growth, and progression of renal diseases. Kidney Int 2000;57:S15–21.
5. Thomas SE, Anderson S, Gordon KL, et al. Tubulointerstitial disease in aging: evidence for underlying peritubular capillary damage. A potential role for renal ischemia. J Am Soc Nephrol 1998;9:231–42.

6. Ruiz-Torres MP, Bosch RJ, O'Valle F, et al. Age-related increase in expression of TGF- β1 in the rat kidney: relationship to morphologic changes. J Am Soc Nephrol 1998;9:782–91, 485–508.
7. Lindeman RD, Goldman R. Anatomic and physiologic age changes in the kidney. Exp Gerontol 1986;21:379–406.
8. Takazakura E, Sawabu N, Handa A, et al. Intrarenal vascular changes with age and disease. Kidney Int 1972;2:224–30.
9. Kang DH, Anderson S, Kim Y-G, et al. Impaired angiogenesis in the aging kidney: vascular endothelial growth factor and thrombospondin-1 renal disease. Am J Kidney Dis 2001;37:601–11.
10. Epstein M. Aging and the kidney. J Am Soc Nephrol 1996;7:1106–22.
11. Rowe JW, Andres R, Tobin J, et al. The effect of age on creatinine clearance in man: a cross-sectional and longitudinal study. J Gerontol 1976;31:155–63.
12. Wesson LG Jr. Renal hemodynamics in physiological states. Physiology of the human kidney. New York: Grune and Stratton; 1969. p. 96–108.
13. Harmoinen A, Lehtimaki T, Korpela M, et al. Diagnostic accuracies of plasma creatinine, cystatin c, and glomerular filtration rate calculated by the Cockcroft-Gault and Levey (MDRD) formulas. Clin Chem 2003;49:1223–5.
14. Verhave JC, Fesler P, Ribstein J, et al. Estimation of renal subjects with normal serum creatinine levels: influence of age and body mass index. Am J Kidney Dis 2005;46(2):233–41.
15. Corman BS, Chami-Khazraji J, Schaeverbeke J, et al. Effect of feeding on glomerular filtration rate and proteinuria in conscious aging rats. Am J Physiol Renal Physiol 1988;255:F250–6.
16. Baylis C. Changes in renal hemodynamics and structure in the aging kidney; sexual dimorphism and the nitric oxide system. Exp Gerontol 2005;40(4):271–8.
17. Hollenberg NK, Adams DF, Solomon HS, et al. Senescence and the renal vasculature in normal man. J Lab Clin Med 1976;87:411–7.
18. Jones CA, Francis ME, Eberhardt MS, et al. Microalbuminuria in the US population: third National Health and Nutrition Examination Survey. Am J Kidney Dis 2002;39:445–9.
19. Luft FC, Grim CE, Gineberg N, et al. Effects of volume expansion and contraction in normotensive whites, blacks, and subjects of different ages. Circulation 1979;59:643–50.
20. Epstein M, Hollenberg NK. Age as a determinant of renal sodium conservation in normal man. J Lab Clin Med 1976;87:411–7.
21. Filser D, Franek E, Joest M, et al. Renal function in the elderly: impact of hypertension and cardiac function. Kidney Int 1997;51:1196–204.
22. Baylis C, Corma B. The aging kidney: insights from experimental studies. J Am Soc Nephrol 1998;9:699–799.
23. Burt VL, Wheeton P, Roccella EJ, et al. Prevalence of hypertension in the US adult population. Results from the Third National Health and Nutrition Examination Survey, 1988–1991. Hypertension 1995;25:305–13.
24. Weinberger MH, Fineberg NS. Sodium and volume sensitivity of blood pressure. Age and pressure change over time. Hypertension 1991;18:67–71.
25. Oliver WB, Cohen EL, Neel JV. Blood pressure, sodium intake, and sodium related hormones in the Yanomamo Indians, a 'no-salt' culture. Circulation 1975;52:146–51.
26. Streeten DHP, Andersen GP, Wagnerr S. Effect of age on response of secondary hypertension to specific treatment. Am J Hypertens 1990;3:360–5.

Acute Kidney Injury in the Elderly

Khaled Abdel-Kader, MD[a], Paul M. Palevsky, MD[a,b],*

KEYWORDS

• Acute kidney injury • Acute renal failure • Elderly • Geriatric

Acute renal failure (ARF) is the rapid loss of kidney function, occurring over hours or days and resulting in the accumulation of metabolic waste products and the dysregulation of extracellular volume and electrolyte homeostasis. ARF is common, especially among the elderly ($\geq$65 years). It has been estimated to occur during 2% to 7% of all hospital admissions[1–3] and at even higher rates in elderly patients.[4–7] Until recently there was no generally accepted operational definition of ARF. As a result reported incidence rates varied greatly due to differences in the definitions used and the clinical settings studied. Despite this, acute kidney disease has consistently been associated with increased morbidity and mortality,[8–16] and multiple studies and a recent meta-analysis have demonstrated worse outcomes in the elderly.[17–23] In light of recent findings that have established an association between even small (0.3 mg/dL) increases in serum creatinine and adverse outcomes,[24–26] the descriptive terminology of acute kidney disease has been modified to recognize the importance of even modest decrements in kidney function.[27,28] In this article, the term acute kidney injury (AKI) is used to refer to any sudden reduction in kidney function and the term ARF is restricted to severe organ dysfunction, typically necessitating dialysis or other supportive interventions.

DEFINITION AND INCIDENCE

The definition of AKI in published studies has varied widely and this lack of standardization has been an impediment to a clear understanding of its epidemiology.[29] In 2002, the Acute Dialysis Quality Initiative (ADQI) group proposed the Risk, Injury, Failure, Loss, End-stage renal disease (RIFLE) criteria for diagnosis and stratification.[30] The RIFLE criteria (**Table 1**) use increasing degrees of renal dysfunction (defined based on relative increases in serum creatinine from baseline or duration

a Renal-Electrolyte Division, Department of Medicine, University of Pittsburgh School of Medicine, A 919 Scaife Hall, 3550 Terrace Street, Pittsburgh, PA 15261, USA
b Renal Section, VA Pittsburgh Healthcare System, Room 7E123 (111F-U), University Drive, Pittsburgh, PA 15240, USA
* Corresponding author. Renal Section, Room 7E123 (111F-U), VA Pittsburgh Healthcare System, University Drive, Pittsburgh, PA 15240.
E-mail address: palevsky@pitt.edu (P.M. Palevsky).

Clin Geriatr Med 25 (2009) 331–358
doi:10.1016/j.cger.2009.04.001
0749-0690/09/$ – see front matter. Published by Elsevier Inc.
geriatric.theclinics.com

Table 1
Acute kidney injury staging criteria

Stage	Creatinine Criteria	Urine Output Criteria
RIFLE criteria		
Risk	Creatinine increase of 1.5–2 times baseline value	<0.5 mL/kg/h × 6 h
Injury	Creatinine increase of 2–3 times baseline value	<0.5 mL/kg/h × 12 h
Failure	Creatinine increase of ≥3 times baseline value or a creatinine value >4 mg/dL with an acute increase of ≥0.5 mg/dL[a]	<0.3 mL/kg/h × 24 h or anuria × 12 h
Loss	Persistent acute renal failure (complete loss of kidney function) for >4 weeks	
End-stage kidney disease	Persistent acute renal failure (complete loss of kidney function) for >3 months	
AKIN criteria[b]		
1	Creatinine increase of 1.5–2 times baseline value or increase in creatinine of ≥0.3[a] mg/dL	<0.5 mL/kg/h × 6 h
2	Creatinine increase of 2–3 times baseline value	<0.5 mL/kg/h × 12 h
3	Creatinine increase of ≥3 times baseline value or a creatinine value >4 mg/dL with an acute increase of ≥0.5 mg/dL[a]	<0.3 mL/kg/h × 24 h or anuria × 12 h

[a] To convert creatinine from mg/dL to μmol/L, multiply by 88.4.
[b] Reduction in renal function must occur within 48 hours.

and severity of oliguria) and clinical outcome criteria (persistent ARF) to classify AKI.[30] Multiple studies have now demonstrated a clear association between RIFLE stage and clinical outcomes across patient care settings.[31–39] More recently, the Acute Kidney Injury Network (AKIN), convened by an international consortium of renal and critical care societies, proposed several refinements to the RIFLE criteria (**Table 1**).[28] Modifications to the definition of AKI included the addition of an absolute increase in serum creatinine of ≥ 0.3 mg/dL and the specification that the decline in kidney function occur within a 48-hour period. The AKIN workgroup also advocated for the use of the term "acute kidney injury" with the goal of enhancing future patient outcomes by fully capturing the broad range of acute renal dysfunction.[28] The use of the term "kidney" in place of "renal" may also assist in patient communication. The AKIN workgroup also proposed that the more traditional term "acute renal failure" be restricted to the severe state of complete organ dysfunction. This new terminology emphasizes that regardless of the cause, AKI is characterized by functional or morphologic alterations in the kidney.[40]

Despite these recent advances in defining AKI, limitations remain. The RIFLE and AKIN criteria are predominantly based on changes in serum creatinine concentration. Although creatinine remains the best clinical marker of kidney function, there are multiple limitations to its use as a marker of kidney function, especially in the nonsteady states that characterize AKI. Elevations in creatinine are often delayed in relation to the onset of AKI,[41,42] and serum creatinine levels are influenced by factors other than kidney function including muscle mass, volume of distribution, catabolic state, and medications.[43] For example, in the elderly or chronically infirm patient with reduced muscle mass, elevations in creatinine following even severe episodes of AKI may be modest. In addition, alterations in volume status can also affect creatinine values. Volume expansion in the setting of AKI can diminish the associated increase in serum creatinine or even result in a stable or decreased concentration as a result of hemodilution despite the decline in kidney function.[25] Due in part to these shortcomings, there has been recent emphasis on identifying and validating one or more biomarkers to assist in the early diagnosis of AKI and the differentiation between functional and structural kidney injury. Although multiple candidates have been identified,[44,45] none have been adequately validated, and their use in clinical practice cannot be recommended.

Not surprisingly in the absence of a well-accepted definition of AKI, researchers have used varying criteria. This, coupled with diverse clinical study settings and varying methods of ascertainment of AKI, has made it difficult to reliably characterize the epidemiology of AKI. Using the 5% random sample of Medicare Beneficiaries from 2000 and identifying AKI based on International Classification of Diseases Ninth Revision (ICD-9) coding, one recent study reported an incidence rate of AKI of 3.1% in a cohort of more than 233,000 patients surviving to hospital discharge.[18] In an analysis of data from the 5% Medicare Beneficiary Sample over the period 1992 to 2001, the AKI incidence rate based on ICD-9 coding was 2.4% in a sample that included more than 5 million hospital discharges.[46] There was a progressive increase in the incidence of AKI over these 10 years, rising from 1.5% of hospital discharges in 1992 to 3.6% in 2001.[46] Similar increases in the incidence of AKI in hospitalized patients have also been reported by other researchers.[7,47]

However, these findings are likely to underestimate the true incidence of AKI in hospitalized patients due to the limited sensitivity of ICD-9 coding.[29,46,48] Studies that have examined the accuracy of ICD-9 codes for AKI have demonstrated that although they are greater than 97% specific, their sensitivity is only approximately 20% to 35%,[3,48] suggesting that these studies underestimate the true incidence of

AKI. Despite these limitations, similar findings have also been noted in two often-cited studies conducted at two urban tertiary care medical centers in the United States 17 years apart. AKI, as judged by a graded scheme of creatinine elevation, occurred in 4.9% of approximately 2200 hospitalized patients in 1979 and 7.0% of approximately 4600 hospitalized patients in 1996.[1,7] These findings are also generally consistent with a community-based study using the Kaiser-Permanente of Northern California database that evaluated the period from 1996 to 2003 and found an overall incidence of AKI not requiring dialysis of 384.1 per 100,000 person-years and of AKI requiring dialysis of 24.4 per 100,000 person years, with a progressive increase over the study period.[49]

In addition to the rising incidence of AKI, the median age of patients with AKI also seems to be increasing.[20,50] This in part reflects improvements in life expectancy with a resultant aging population.[17,50,51] Indeed, recent estimates show that significant proportions of the United States and western European population are greater than 65 years of age (eg, approximately 17.5% of the Italian population, 16% of the British population, 16% of the Spanish population, and 12.5% of the United States population).[39,50] The elderly also represent the fastest growing age group in the western world with more than 395 million people expected to be over the age of 60 years by the year 2050.[51]

Multiple studies have demonstrated that the elderly are more susceptible to developing AKI.[4,17,50,52–55] In a Spanish hospital cohort, the incidence of AKI was 3.5 times higher in patients older than 70 years than in their younger counterparts.[4] A subsequent study in the same population and setting revealed that patients greater than 80 years were five times more likely to develop AKI than the general population.[52] In an Italian hospital cohort, the elderly (≥65 years) had 10 times the incidence rate of AKI compared with those less than 65 years of age.[50] In the Medicare 5% Beneficiary Sample, the incidence of AKI progressively increased with age from 1.9% in those younger than 65 years compared with 2.9% in those older than 85 years.[46] Similarly, in the Kaiser-Permanente of Northern California community-based cohort, the incidence rate of AKI not requiring dialysis increased from 78 per 100,000 person-years in patients younger than 50 years to 3545 per 100,000 person-years in those 80 years or older. The increased incidence of AKI in the elderly is believed to be multifactorial, attributable in part to anatomic and physiologic changes in the aging kidney, to an increased burden of comorbidities impacting kidney function, to more frequent exposure to medications and interventions that alter renal hemodynamics or are nephrotoxic, and to alterations in drug metabolism and clearance associated with aging.[6,17,43]

THE AGING KIDNEY

The kidney undergoes several important age-dependent changes (**Box 1**). Renal mass decreases with aging, reaching approximately 75% to 80% of young adulthood weight by the age of 80 to 90 years.[56–58] At age 70 years, the kidneys have lost between 30% and 50% of their cortical glomeruli due to ischemic changes, and a significant number of the remaining glomeruli manifest some degree of sclerosis.[59–62] Some have posited that the glomerulosclerosis of aging is dependent on subclinical injury to the kidney from comorbidities, including hypertension and vascular disease.[63] Other morphologic changes that occur with aging include a reduction in the number and size of tubules, increasing tubulointerstitial fibrosis, a decrease in glomerular filtering surface area due to an increasing proportion of mesangial cells, thickening of glomerular and tubular basement membranes, arteriosclerosis (even in

---

Box 1
Anatomic and physiologic changes in the aging kidney

Anatomic

Loss of renal mass

Glomerular drop out and glomerulosclerosis

Diminished glomerular filtering surface area

Decreased tubular size and number

Increased tubulointerstitial fibrosis

Thickened glomerular and tubular basement membranes

Decreased afferent arteriolar luminal area

Increased arteriosclerosis

Physiologic

Decreased renal blood flow

Decreased glomerular filtration rate

Diminished urinary concentrating and diluting capacity

Diminished capacity for sodium conservation

Decreased plasma renin and aldosterone levels

Decreased prostaglandin production

Increased vasoconstrictive response to stimuli (eg, volume depletion)

---

healthy nonhypertensive elderly patients), and decreased afferent arteriolar luminal area.[64–67]

The structural changes that occur with aging contribute to functional alterations (see **Box 1**). The most salient of these include a reduction in renal blood flow (RBF) of up to 50% from age 20 to age 80 years[68,69] and a progressive decline in glomerular filtration rate (GFR).[70,71] Based on longitudinal studies of healthy patients without hypertension, diabetes, heart disease, or clinically apparent atherosclerosis, a progressive decline in GFR of 0.75 mL/min/1.73 m^2 per year was observed after the age of 30 years. However, approximately 30% of patients did not manifest this age-related decline in GFR, making it unclear whether genetic, dietary, metabolic, or other factors contribute to this process. The decrease in RBF and GFR represent a loss of renal functional reserve in the elderly and contribute to an increased risk for development of AKI.[65]

Other important renal physiologic changes noted in the elderly are the loss of urinary concentrating and diluting ability, diminished sodium conservation, decreased plasma renin and aldosterone levels, decreased prostaglandin production, and an enhanced response to vasoconstrictive stimuli.[57,58,64,71–80] These changes have significant clinical implications. The reduced capacity to retain salt and water increases the propensity to develop volume depletion and dehydration.[6] The presence of an increased renal vasoconstrictive response and decreased production of vasodilatory prostaglandins may heighten sensitivity to pathologic stressors (eg, blood loss) and medications (eg, nonsteroidal antiinflammatory drugs).

These changes partially explain the susceptibility of the elderly to AKI.[72] In addition, the aged have a higher prevalence of systemic diseases that contribute to their predisposition to developing AKI including diabetes mellitus (DM), hypertension (HTN), cardiovascular and peripheral vascular disease, congestive heart failure (CHF), benign prostatic hypertrophy (BPH), and malignancies such as prostate cancer and multiple myeloma. Further, treatment of these and a myriad of other disorders in the elderly leads to greater exposure to potentially nephrotoxic medications. In addition, changes in volume of distribution of these medications and decreased renal and hepatic clearance may increase the risk of nephrotoxicity. Nonetheless, the kidneys of the healthy elderly patient are able to compensate and maintain homeostasis under normal conditions despite these age-related alterations. However, in the setting of significant renal stressors, renal adaptive capacity is limited and AKI may result.[6,72]

CAUSES OF ACUTE KIDNEY INJURY

Although there may be significant pathophysiologic overlap, the clinical assessment of AKI generally begins with categorization into prerenal, intrinsic, and postrenal causes. This classification has significant clinical usefulness, however, there may not be a clear demarcation between prerenal and intrinsic causes of AKI and the elderly frequently have multiple contributing causes.[81,82]

Prerenal AKI

Prerenal azotemia is defined as a functional decline in glomerular filtration associated with renal underperfusion and is a leading cause of AKI in the general and geriatric populations.[12,52,83] Although classically associated with hypovolemia and resulting from failure of normal adaptive responses to maintain GFR, prerenal AKI also commonly develops in the setting of effective intravascular volume depletion associated with congestive heart failure (cardiorenal syndrome) and liver disease.

The normal adaptive response to volume depletion includes activation of the renin–angiotensin–aldosterone axis (RAAS), upregulation of the sympathetic nervous system, and stimulation of vasopressin secretion. Activation of the RAAS increases angiotensin II levels. Angiotensin II, a potent vasoconstrictor, acts on the afferent (preglomerular) and efferent (postglomerular) arterioles; however its afferent vasoconstrictive effects are normally balanced by secretion of vasodilatory prostaglandins. The net effect is predominant efferent arteriolar vasoconstriction. Whereas the overall increase in arteriolar resistance results in a decrease in renal blood flow, the predominance of postglomerular vasoconstriction allows restoration of a near-normal intraglomerular pressure and maintenance of GFR, albeit at the expense of an increased filtration fraction (the ratio between GFR and renal plasma flow). Changes in intrarenal hemodynamics and upregulation of angiotensin II, aldosterone, vasopressin, and the sympathetic nervous system modulate renal tubular function increasing sodium, water, and urea conservation.

Prerenal AKI ensues if the decrease in renal perfusion exceeds the ability of these counterregulatory systems to maintain a near-normal GFR Nonetheless, the adaptive responses maximizing reabsorption of sodium, water, and urea continue to operate, leading to a reduced urine volume, decreased urine sodium concentration, and increased urine osmolality. Hence, the features of prerenal AKI are (**Table 2**): low urine sodium concentration (U_{Na} <20 meq/L), low fractional excretion of sodium (F_ENa <1%), low fractional excretion of urea (F_EUrea <35%), high urine osmolality (U_{Osm} >500 mosm/kg), and an elevated blood urea nitrogen (BUN)/serum creatinine ratio (>20:1).

In the elderly, these indices may be less useful due to age-associated defects in sodium and water conservation.[84] Urine sodium may be greater than 20 mEq/L and U_{Osm} less than 500 mosm/kg despite effective intravascular volume depletion. In addition, an inability to maximally concentrate the urine may result in prerenal AKI with

Table 2
Comparison of laboratory findings in prerenal AKI and acute tubular necrosis

Laboratory Measure	Prerenal	Intrinsic
BUN/creatinine	>20:1	<15:1
Urine osmolality (mosm/kg)	>500	<350
Urine sodium (meq/L)	<20	>40
Fractional excretion of sodium (%)	<1	>2
Fractional excretion urea (%)	<35	>50
Urine microscopy	Nonspecific, may include hyaline casts	Renal tubular epithelial cells or casts, granular casts ("muddy brown")

urine volumes in excess of 500 mL/d. Similarly, diuretics, which may also predispose to prerenal AKI, may diminish the usefulness of these indices through their effects on renal salt and water handling. Because the hallmark of prerenal azotemia is the rapid restoration of renal function following normalization of kidney perfusion, a therapeutic trial of intravenous fluids may be required to confirm the cause if diagnostic indices are ambiguous or inconsistent with the clinical setting.

Although frequently regarded as benign, prerenal AKI is associated with an increased mortality risk,[7] most likely related to underlying comorbidities that contribute to its development. Prerenal states are a significant risk factor for the development of intrinsic AKI. Pre-existing prerenal states increase the risk of ischemic and nephrotoxic insults. In addition, prolonged or severe renal hypoperfusion that is initially manifest as functional prerenal AKI may develop into intrinsic AKI (ie, ischemic acute tubular necrosis) with structural injury to the renal tubules.

Causes of prerenal AKI (**Box 2**) include states of true volume depletion and conditions in which decreased effective arterial blood volume causes renal underperfusion. Common causes of true volume depletion include vomiting and diarrhea, blood loss due to hemorrhage, third-spacing of fluids following surgery or pancreatitis and increased renal losses associated with diuretics. Elderly patients may be at increased risk for true volume depletion due to changes in body composition with aging, leading to decreased total body water as a fraction of body weight, and from an increased burden of comorbid disease. Treatment of prerenal AKI associated with true volume depletion requires volume resuscitation with isotonic crystalloid. Prerenal AKI arises from decreased effective arterial blood volume in CHF, cirrhosis, and in select patients with nephrotic syndrome, often exacerbated by diuretic therapy. Treatment in these situations will usually require volume resuscitation or treatment of the underlying disease process.

Medication use may also play a significant role in the development of prerenal AKI. Diuretic use exacerbates the underlying predisposition to volume depletion and may contribute in up to 25% to 40% of cases of prerenal AKI in elderly patients.[85] Medications that alter renal hemodynamics also contribute to the development of prerenal AKI. Nonsteroidal antiinflammatory drugs (NSAIDs), which are used by approximately 10% to 25% of the elderly,[86–89] inhibit production of vasodilatory prostaglandins. NSAID use has been associated with a threefold higher risk of AKI in the general population,[90] and an absolute risk of prerenal AKI of 13% in a nursing home cohort (mean age 87 years).[91] The simultaneous presence of chronic kidney disease, CHF, DM, HTN, diuretic or angiotensin-converting enzyme inhibitor (ACEI) use further increases

---

Box 2
Causes of prerenal acute kidney injury

True volume depletion

    Blood loss

    Insensible losses

    Adrenal insufficiency

    Gastrointestinal losses

        Vomiting

        Diarrhea

    Genitourinary losses

        Diuretics

        Osmotic diuresis (hyperglycemia)

    Third-spacing

Decreased effective arterial blood volume

    Heart failure

    Cirrhosis

    Nephrotic syndrome

Medications

    Nonsteroidal antiinflammatory drugs

    ACEI/ARB

    Calcineurin inhibitors

Hypercalcemia

---

this risk.[90–92] The elderly are believed to have a higher baseline risk of AKI from NSAID use due to prolonged NSAID half-life, decreased body mass, and the age-related physiologic changes (previously outlined) that make them more reliant on prostaglandin-dependent afferent arteriolar vasodilation.[55,93] Judicious use of these medications and close patient follow-up are recommended in the aged, especially in those with reduced GFR. If prerenal AKI occurs, timely discontinuation of NSAIDs and volume repletion may help restore renal function before the onset of ischemic acute tubular necrosis (ATN). Patient education is also warranted given the wide availability of NSAIDs without prescription and findings that suggest many patients would be willing to switch to other safer, albeit less effective, analgesics.[94]

Two other classes of agents frequently used by the elderly that carry a significant risk of prerenal AKI are angiotensin-converting enzyme inhibitors (ACEI) and angiotensin receptor blockers (ARB).[85] The use of these medications has increased in the setting of CHF and HTN. Risk factors associated with the development of AKI due to ACEI or ARB include volume depletion, underlying chronic kidney disease, bilateral renal artery stenosis (or unilateral renal artery stenosis with a solitary kidney), CHF, and concomitant diuretic use.[55] Although these agents are not contraindicated in the elderly, they must be used with caution. Follow-up serum chemistries should be obtained 1 to 2 weeks after initiating or increasing the dose of these medications to monitor for AKI or hyperkalemia. A creatinine increase of greater than 30% from baseline should prompt discontinuation or dose reduction of the medication.[95] Although evaluation for renal artery stenosis may be considered,[95] most cases of AKI induced by ACEI or ARB are not associated with renal artery stenosis.[96] Prompt volume repletion and cessation of the medication usually restore kidney function.

Intrinsic AKI

Intrinsic AKI is differentiated from prerenal states by the presence of structural injury to the kidneys that persists after withdrawal of the inciting factors. It is useful to categorize the causes of intrinsic AKI based on the histologic compartment of the kidney that is predominantly injured as follows: primary damage to the tubular epithelium (acute tubular necrosis, ATN); inflammatory diseases of the interstitium (acute interstitial nephritis, AIN); glomerular disease (acute or rapidly progressive glomerulonephritis); and acute vascular disorders. Their treatment and outcomes differ significantly.

Acute tubular necrosis

ATN is the most common form of intrinsic AKI. It accounts for nearly half of all cases of AKI in hospitalized patients[12,52,97] and is the predominant cause of AKI in critical illness.[98] Although ATN is classified as ischemic or nephrotoxic, these causes frequently coexist and many cases are multifactorial. Ischemic ATN may develop in approximately 50% of critically ill patients.[9,99] Septic ATN, although previously considered a subset of ischemic ATN, has a more complex pathophysiology than exclusive renal ischemia.[99] Sepsis has been linked to 30% of ATN cases in the elderly[100–102] and endotoxemia-triggered renal vasoconstriction may heighten the elderly patient's susceptibility to ATN.[64] Recent studies also indicate that endotoxemia may independently activate inflammatory mediators and incite endothelial damage that potentiates the renal injury due to hypoperfusion.[99,103–105] Prerenal AKI can lead to ischemic ATN if volume repletion is delayed and this progression seems to be more common in the aged.[83] Surgical interventions are associated with almost one third of cases of ischemic ATN in the elderly with cardiac surgery and aortic aneurysm repair as the most common precipitants.[21,106] Perioperative hypotension, blood loss, gastrointestinal drainage, and preoperative cardiac complications account for many of these cases of ATN.[4,5]

The development of ischemic ATN involves multiple pathways including ischemia-reperfusion injury to the tubular epithelial cells, endothelial injury with disruption of microvascular flow, and activation of inflammatory pathways.[107–113] Clinically, ischemic ATN can follow a highly variable course, however, four characteristic stages have been identified: initiation, extension, maintenance, and recovery.[107,111]

In the initiation phase, ischemia-reperfusion injury causes a loss of tubular epithelial cell polarity, cellular detachment, and triggers apoptosis and necrosis.[114,115] The combination of renal vasoconstriction, sloughed tubular debris forming obstructing intratubular casts, and back leak of glomerular filtrate across the denuded epithelial surface leads to a loss of renal function.[114] Clinically, BUN and creatinine levels increase. Urine output can vary; although oliguria or anuria may be present, some patients remain nonoliguric throughout their course. The initiation phase rapidly transitions into the extension phase. Although the inciting insult may have resolved, this phase is characterized by continued renal ischemia and hypoxia that is mediated by microvascular endothelial injury and inflammatory processes.[107] In the maintenance phase, renal function remains suppressed despite resolution of renal ischemia. During this stage, endothelial cells and tubular epithelial cells have an opportunity to repair, proliferate, and redifferentiate to help restore previous structure and function.[114,116] However, superimposed insults including recurrent hypotension, nephrotoxin administration, and intravascular volume depletion may prolong this phase and delay recovery. The maintenance phase is followed by recovery of kidney function. In the recovery phase, urine output may increase briskly as persistent tubular dysfunction results in impaired salt and water homeostasis despite recovery of GFR, necessitating careful monitoring of volume and electrolyte status.

Risk factors for ischemic ATN include pre-existing chronic kidney disease, diabetes, atherosclerosis, active malignancy, and low serum albumin[117]; conditions that are more prevalent among the elderly. Patients with impaired renal autoregulation are also at increased risk for developing ATN even in the absence of frank hypotension. Impaired renal autoregulation is generally seen in patients with advanced age, hypertension, atherosclerosis, chronic kidney disease, or renal artery stenosis.[118]

The treatment of ATN is primarily supportive, as no specific therapeutic interventions have been found to hasten recovery of kidney function. In elderly patients with ATN, careful attention must be paid to medication dosing, using pharmacokinetic monitoring to minimize the risk of drug toxicity. Although dopamine has been tried as a therapeutic agent, based on its renal vasodilatory properties, it has not been demonstrated to provide clinical benefit, is associated with an increased risk of cardiac arrhythmias, and has no role in the treatment of ATN.[119,120] The role of diuretic therapy in established ATN is less clear. Although nonoliguric ATN is associated with a better prognosis, use of diuretics to convert patients from oliguric to nonoliguric ATN is not associated with improved outcomes. Rather, diuretic response identifies a subset of patients with a better prognosis. Nevertheless, diuretics may be helpful in volume management, although high doses of loop diuretics ($\geq$160 mg of furosemide) are often required. If the patient fails to respond, further doses are generally not helpful or indicated. Initiation of renal replacement therapy, if otherwise indicated, should not be deferred for a trial of diuretics, as doing so may be associated with worsened outcomes.[121,122]

Nephrotoxic ATN results from direct tubular injury from endogenous or exogenous renal toxins. Myoglobin, hemoglobin, and light chains are frequently encountered endogenous substances associated with tubular toxicity. Heme-pigment nephrotoxicity can be seen in the setting of severe hemolysis or rhabdomyolysis. The AKI seen in myeloma kidney is in part attributable to the renal toxicity of light chains. Antibiotics, particularly aminoglycosides and amphotericin B, and chemotherapeutic agents such as cisplatin remain important causative agents of nephrotoxic ATN in the elderly. Age is a well-described risk factor for the development of aminoglycoside nephrotoxicity.[123] The often inappropriate dosing of medications as the result of overestimation of the level of renal function and loss of lean body mass place the elderly at increased risk of nephrotoxicity from other medications as well.[55]

Contrast-induced nephropathy (CIN) is a major cause of AKI in hospitalized elderly patients.[82,124] Older adults may also have an elevated risk of developing contrast-induced nephropathy due to a higher prevalence of chronic kidney disease,[125,126] an important risk factor for contrast nephropathy.[127–129] However, age per se has not been consistently identified as an independent predictor of contrast nephropathy. Other risk factors include diabetic nephropathy, volume depletion, volume of contrast administered, and use of high osmolar (compared with low or iso-osmolar) contrast agents.[127–129] Clinically, CIN is characterized by an acute increase in creatinine levels within 24 to 48 hours after contrast administration, which subsequently peaks after 3 to 5 days followed by a return to baseline within 7 to 10 days. The patient usually remains nonoliguric and the urinary sediment may reveal granular casts and renal tubular epithelial cells.

The primary means of preventing CIN is avoidance of the unnecessary administration of contrast to high-risk patients. If contrast administration is indicated, a low osmolarity or iso-osmolar agent should be used and the volume of contrast administered should be minimized. The primary intervention for prevention of CIN is adequate administration of isotonic intravenous fluids before and following contrast administration.[130–132] The optimal regimen for fluid administration is uncertain, however the use of at least 1 mL/kg of isotonic saline for 4 to 12 hours pre- and postprocedure are generally recommended.[133] Although several studies have suggested added benefit with the use of sodium bicarbonate rather than saline,[134] the actual benefit is uncertain.[135,136] The role of the antioxidant N-acetylcysteine in preventing CIN remains unclear. Multiple large studies have yielded conflicting results and multiple meta-analyses have similarly produced contradictory findings.[137–143] Based on these inconsistent results, it seems unlikely that N-acetylcysteine exerts a large protective effect. However, given the safety profile and minimal cost of oral N-acetylcysteine as well as the significant morbidity associated with CIN, its continued use is not inappropriate.

Acute interstitial nephritis

Acute interstitial nephritis (AIN) is a less common cause of intrinsic AKI accounting for less than 5% of cases, although the reported incidence in biopsy series of unexplained AKI is much higher at approximately 20% to 25%.[144,145] Pathologically, AIN is characterized by an acute lymphocytic infiltrate of the renal interstitium, often with accompanying eosinophils. Although the classic presentation consists of AKI accompanied by the triad of fever, rash, and eosinophilia, the complete triad is observed only in approximately 15% of patients.[146,147] Typical urinary abnormalities include sterile pyuria, white blood cell casts, hematuria, and subnephrotic proteinuria. Although eosinophiluria has been considered a hallmark finding it is not specific,[148–150] as it may be seen in pyelonephritis, prostatitis, cystitis, and atheroembolic disease. Although the diagnosis is often made on the basis of the clinical presentation, renal biopsy may be necessary to confirm the diagnosis.

Hypersensitivity to medications is the most frequent cause of AIN, accounting for 60% to 70% of cases.[146,147] Antibiotics, particularly penicillins, cephalosporins, and sulfonamides, are the most commonly implicated drugs. The onset of AIN is usually within 3 weeks of initiation of the inciting medication although this is highly variable. Infections are the second leading cause, followed by systemic collagen vascular diseases. AIN seems to be more common in the elderly, perhaps related to the more frequent use of prescription and over-the-counter medications, including NSAIDs.[146]

Treatment consists of discontinuation of the offending agent or treatment of the underlying infection or systemic disorder. Renal recovery is variable and often takes days to weeks. The role of corticosteroids is controversial although they have been used in small uncontrolled trials to accelerate kidney recovery.[151] Although it has been suggested that early initiation of corticosteroids is associated with more complete recovery of kidney function,[152] results have not been consistent[153] and have not been validated in randomized studies.

The presentation and course of NSAID-induced AIN differ considerably from other forms of medication-induced AIN. The onset of NSAID-induced AKI is often delayed months after the initiation of the medication and classic hypersensitivity symptoms are seldom present.[154] Frequently, the patient exhibits nephrotic range proteinuria and minimal change disease or membranous nephropathy is commonly found on kidney biopsy.[154,155] Prompt cessation of NSAID use is required and renal recovery, including resolution of proteinuria, usually occurs within 2 months.[154]

Acute renal vascular disease

Vascular diseases associated with AKI can be divided into large-vessel or small-vessel processes. The large-vessel processes that can produce AKI include renal artery thromboembolism, renal artery dissection, and renal vein thrombosis. Their incidence in the elderly may be increased.[97] Although all of these may cause renal infarction, AKI will only result if the lesions are bilateral, occur unilaterally in a solitary kidney, or occur in a patient with significant pre-existing chronic kidney disease. Clinically, these disorders present with sudden flank pain, hematuria, and oligoanuria, depending on severity, and are associated with elevation in serum lactate dehydrogenase (LDH). Risk factors include trauma, nephrotic syndrome, and atrial fibrillation. Confirmation of the diagnosis requires imaging with contrast-enhanced CT scan, magnetic resonance imaging (MRI), radionuclide renal scan, or angiography to demonstrate the vascular lesion or renal perfusion defect. The lesions are typically not amenable to fibrinolytic therapy or interventional approaches, and therapy usually consists of anticoagulation and supportive care.

Small-vessel involvement with atheroembolic disease is more common. Atheroembolic disease is largely a disorder of the elderly, with a mean age of 71 years in one series,[156] and is associated with diffuse atherosclerosis. Although atheroembolism can occur spontaneously, it is more commonly triggered by vascular surgery or angiographic procedures, anticoagulation, or thrombolytic agents. Destabilized atheromatous plaques shower cholesterol crystals into the small arteries of the skin, central nervous system, extremities, gastrointestinal system, and kidneys; the kidneys are frequently involved due to the high renal blood flow. The cholesterol emboli are usually nonobstructing; however, they incite a vigorous inflammatory response that eventually occludes the vascular lumen. Although the presentation may occur immediately after vascular surgery or angiography, patients often present days to weeks after the procedure with worsening renal function, livedo reticularis, and ischemic necrosis of the toes. Eosinophilia, eosinophiluria, proteinuria, and hypocomplementemia are often documented. The renal course is highly variable but often manifests as subacute kidney injury with a progressive or stuttering deterioration in renal function over a period of days to weeks. Although atheroembolic disease carries a poor prognosis, renal functional recovery can occur.[157] There is no specific treatment for atheroembolic disease. Care is supportive including nutritional support, especially if there is concomitant gastrointestinal involvement, and aggressive management of hyperlipidemia. Anticoagulation is contraindicated as it may precipitate further cholesterol embolization.

Acute glomerulonephritis

AKI can also develop from acute or rapidly progressive glomerulonephritis. Timely diagnosis and treatment of these conditions is critical to preserve renal function and avoid life-threatening complications. Diffuse proliferative forms of glomerulonephritis can be associated with infections and generally carry a good prognosis in the elderly and in the young.[158–161] Rapidly progressive (crescentic) glomerulonephritis is a fulminant presentation of glomerular disease that will lead to renal failure over days to weeks if left untreated. Evidence suggests that rapidly progressive glomerulonephritis may be more common among the elderly and carries a poorer prognosis.[158,159,162–166] Clinically, patients often present with AKI, hypertension, hematuria, and proteinuria. Characteristically, the urinary sediment demonstrates dysmorphic red blood cells and red blood cell casts. Serologic studies including complement levels, antinuclear antibodies (ANA), antineutrophil cytoplasmic antibodies (ANCA), antiglomerular basement membrane antibodies, cryoglobulin levels, and hepatitis B and C antibodies can be useful in suggesting the cause, although kidney biopsy is nearly universally required for specific diagnosis. Treatment, including high-dose glucocorticoids, immunosuppressive therapy and plasmapheresis, will be dependent on the specific cause. Despite the potential for treatment associated toxicities, case series have demonstrated that elderly patients with limited comorbidities may tolerate and respond well to therapy.[167]

Postrenal AKI

Postrenal or obstructive AKI is more common in the aged than in the young,[52] accounting for 9% to 30% of cases.[54,97,100,168] Postrenal AKI can be categorized as affecting either the upper urinary tract (proximal to the bladder) or lower urinary tract (obstruction occurring at the bladder outlet or urethra). Obstruction of the lower tract will affect both kidneys and diminish renal function. In contrast, unilateral upper tract obstructing processes may cause renal colic and unilateral hydronephrosis, but will not cause deterioration in renal function if the contralateral kidney can compensate. However, if the obstruction is bilateral, is of a unilateral functioning kidney, or if there is significant underlying chronic kidney disease, upper tract obstruction can also cause AKI.

The most frequent causes of postrenal AKI (**Box 3**) in the elderly include benign prostatic hypertrophy (BPH) or prostate cancer, retroperitoneal adenopathy or malignancies, pelvic neoplasms, and neurogenic bladder. Although BPH and prostate cancer are common in older men, they cause obstruction in only a minority of cases. In elderly women, pelvic and retroperitoneal malignancies are the most frequent causes of postrenal AKI.[6]

Postrenal AKI may present with either complete or partial obstruction. Complete obstruction is characterized by anuria. The patient may also report flank and abdominal pain or suprapubic fullness. In contrast, the patient with partial obstruction may remain completely asymptomatic or may report similar pain symptoms, as well as voiding complaints including frequency, urgency, hesitancy, hematuria, and nocturia. Urine output can be variable, ranging from oliguria to polyuria, or fluctuating between the two.

Due to its increased incidence in the elderly and varying presentation, the clinician must maintain a high index of suspicion for postrenal AKI. The diagnosis should especially be considered in patients with BPH or lower urinary tract symptoms, diabetes, kidney stones, abdominal or pelvic malignancies, surgeries or radiation, retroperitoneal adenopathy or neoplasms, and medication use associated with urinary retention. Lower tract obstruction is diagnosed by confirmation of urinary retention using ultrasonographic bladder scans or placement of a bladder catheter. An elevated residual bladder volume (>100–150 mL) after voiding is highly suggestive of postrenal AKI, although, some elderly patients may suffer from chronic urinary retention with elevation in the postvoid residual bladder volume in the absence of kidney dysfunction.[169,170] Radiographic workup for upper tract obstruction usually begins with ultrasound imaging, which is sensitive and specific in detecting obstruction.[171] However, ultrasonography may appear normal in patients presenting with early obstruction or with retroperitoneal processes encasing the kidneys and ureters, preventing ureteral dilation.[172] CT can be valuable in determining the cause and level of obstruction if ultrasound fails to identify the lesion. Together, ultrasound, abdominal plain films, and CT scanning are diagnostic in most cases.[173,174] Intravenous

Box 3
Causes of postrenal acute kidney injury

Upper tract obstruction

Nephrolithiasis

Blood clots

Papillary tissue

Pelvic neoplasms

Endometriosis

Retroperitoneal processes

    Neoplasms

    Adenopathy

    Fibrosis

    Hematoma

Gastrointestinal neoplasms

Radiation treatment

Lower tract obstruction

Urethral strictures

Nephrolithiasis

Blood clots

Phimosis/paraphimosis

Prostatic processes

    Benign hypertrophy

    Carcinoma

    Calculi

Bladder processes

    Carcinoma

    Calculi

Neurogenic bladder

pyelography has been supplanted by CT imaging and is now only rarely required. Antegrade or retrograde pyelography, however, can be valuable in identifying the site and cause of obstruction, and provides an opportunity for therapeutic intervention. Laboratory findings are nonspecific in postrenal AKI often mimicking prerenal AKI in the early phase and intrinsic AKI later.[175,176]

Treatment of postrenal AKI consists of the rapid detection and relief of obstruction. This can be accomplished by placement of a bladder catheter in lower tract disease or ureteral stents or percutaneous nephrostomy tubes for upper tract disease. A brisk postobstructive diuresis frequently ensues due to water and sodium reabsorptive deficits as well as an osmotic diuresis attributable to previously retained solutes including urea.[64] Careful monitoring of the patient's volume status and electrolytes is essential to avoid the development of volume depletion or serious electrolyte disturbances. Although use of intravenous fluids may be required, it is important to avoid overly aggressive fluid replacement that can drive further diuresis. If the obstruction has been quickly diagnosed and reversed, renal function will improve. However, in patients with a longer duration and higher grade of obstruction, renal functional recovery may be delayed, incomplete, or absent.[177] Brisk urine output following correction of the obstruction does not always correlate with renal recovery and hence close laboratory monitoring remains necessary.

DIAGNOSTIC APPROACH TO THE PATIENT WITH AKI

A detailed history and physical examination is critical in differentiating the causes of AKI. Questions identifying previously mentioned symptoms or risk factors for hypovolemia, obstruction, ATN, AIN, heme-pigment nephropathy, myeloma, and atheroembolic disease are part of the requisite thorough history. An examination must also include careful assessment of volume status, evidence of systemic vasculitis, atheroembolic disease, extrarenal manifestations of systemic diseases, and signs of uremia. Initial diagnostic studies (**Table 3**) should include a urinalysis including urine sediment examination, urine chemistries (urine sodium and creatinine), a bedside postvoid bladder sonogram or placement of a bladder catheter to rule out lower urinary tract obstruction, and renal ultrasound. The urinary sediment examination remains important as the presence of cellular elements and casts may confirm the previous clinical impression or force the clinician to re-examine the original working diagnosis. If the cause of AKI remains unclear following a careful history, physical examination, and laboratory workup, or if the workup suggests the presence of acute glomerular disease, consideration of a kidney biopsy is warranted. A kidney biopsy is a low-risk procedure that is well tolerated by patients, even among the elderly. Approximately 30% of diagnoses were altered in one case series of kidney biopsies for AKI in older adults (age >60 years).[145]

TREATMENT

The therapeutic modalities available for specific causes of AKI have been reviewed under each cause. All patients with significant AKI also require attentive management of volume, electrolyte and acid-base status, and nutrition. Prompt reversal of fluid deficits is critical in preventing further exacerbation of AKI. Once deficits have been corrected, the clinician must continue to carefully assess volume status to ensure the patient does not develop excessive volume expansion that may lead to pulmonary edema. Sodium and fluid restriction may be necessary. Similarly, electrolytes should be monitored closely. Potassium, phosphorus, and magnesium intake can be restricted as appropriate and phosphate binders may be necessary to treat hyperphosphatemia. Although mild hypocalcemia and hyperuricemia may be seen, if asymptomatic, these often do not require correction. If significant acidosis develops (pH <7.2), supplemental bicarbonate may be provided to maintain pH within a safe range. In addition, medication doses should be adjusted for the impairment in kidney function. Serum creatinine values may not adequately reflect the true level of kidney function, and drug levels should be monitored, if possible. Nutritional support must not be overlooked as nutritional status is an important predictor of prognosis in AKI,[178] and the elderly are particularly at risk for developing malnutrition.

In addition to the supportive measures discussed earlier, renal replacement therapy (RRT) may be required in cases of severe AKI. Indications for RRT in the setting of AKI include hyperkalemia, volume overload, especially if associated with pulmonary edema, severe acidosis, or overt uremia. However, RRT is frequently started prophylactically, before the development of these complications. To date, studies have been

Table 3
Urinary findings in acute kidney injury

Test	Associated Disorders	Miscellaneous Notes
Urine Sodium		
<20 meq/L	Prerenal, hepatorenal syndrome, postrenal	Rhabdomyolysis can be associated with low urine sodium but usually with superimposed intravascular volume depletion
>40 meq/L	ATN, AIN, postrenal	Postrenal AKI can mimic either prerenal AKI or ATN in its urinary findings
Fractional excretion of sodium		
<1%	Prerenal, hepatorenal, acute glomerulonephritis, rhabdomyolysis, postrenal	
>2%	ATN, AIN, postrenal	
Urine specific gravity		
≥1.020	Prerenal, hepatorenal, contrast nephropathy, postrenal	Contrast agents with increased osmolality will increase the urinary specific gravity
1.010	ATN, AIN, postrenal	
Urine dipstick		
Proteinuria	Glomerulonephritis, AIN, renal artery thromboembolism, renal vein thrombosis, atheroembolic disease, TTP/HUS, malignant hypertension, pyelonephritis/urinary tract infection	

Blood	Glomerulonephritis, AIN, renal artery thromboembolism, renal vein thrombosis, atheroembolic disease, TTP/HUS, malignant hypertension, rhabdomyolysis, postrenal	Rhabdomyolysis will generate a positive dipstick response for heme but microscopy usually reveals no red blood cells. Postrenal AKI may be associated with hematuria depending on the cause
Urine sediment		
WBCs	AIN, pyelonephritis/urinary tract infection, atheroembolic disease, glomerulonephritis	AIN, atheroembolic disease, and pyelonephritis may all be associated with eosinophiluria
RBCs	glomerulonephritis, AIN, renal artery thromboembolism, renal vein thrombosis, atheroembolic disease, TTP/HUS, malignant hypertension, postrenal	
RBC casts	glomerulonephritis, malignant hypertension	
WBC casts	AIN, pyelonephritis, rarely atheroembolic disease	
Granular casts	ATN, occasionally seen in a variety of other causes	Marked hyperbilirubinemia may be associated with casts that appear granular

unable to delineate the ideal timing for initiation of RRT.[179-181] Options for RRT include conventional intermittent hemodialysis, peritoneal dialysis, the various modalities of continuous renal replacement therapy including continuous hemodialysis and continuous hemofiltration, and the newer hybrid therapies, such as sustained low-efficiency dialysis. Recent studies indicate that the specific modality of RRT does not affect outcomes,[182-184] and that the resources and expertise available at the local institution should guide the choice of dialysis modality. A recent, large, multi-center randomized trial demonstrated that in the setting of critical illness, higher intensities of RRT did not improve morbidity or mortality over more conventionally dosed RRT.[185] In older adults with AKI, age alone should not be a contraindication to RRT as many elderly patients with AKI will recover renal function and do well.[6]

PROGNOSIS

AKI has been consistently associated with increased morbidity and mortality, although outcomes seem to be improving.[8-16,47,186] Most patients with AKI recover renal function. Yet, one recent study revealed that among surviving intensive care unit patients with AKI, only approximately 55% recovered completely.[187] Growing evidence also indicates that AKI is a significant risk factor for chronic kidney disease and dialysis dependence in the elderly,[4,17,18,54,168,188] with a recent meta-analysis revealing that 31% of elderly patients failed to recover renal function after an episode of AKI compared with 26% of younger patients.[17] In one recent analysis following multivariate adjustment, the risk of end-stage renal disease was 13 times higher in hospitalized elderly patients with AKI than in elderly patients without AKI.[18] In that study, the risk of new dialysis dependence in elderly AKI patients steadily increased from 1% at 30 days following discharge to 7% at 2 years.[18] This risk was further elevated in the presence of pre-existing chronic kidney disease.[18] These findings imply that hospitalized elderly patients with AKI require close follow-up of their renal function on discharge, as a significant proportion will have residual functional defects and many may eventually require RRT. The same study also documented an absolute 2-year mortality risk increase of 29% for elderly patients with AKI compared with their elderly counterparts without AKI.[18] These findings are consistent with other recent studies that have demonstrated an increased mortality in older patients with AKI.[187,189] Hence, AKI should not be viewed as a self-limited disease process from which most patients eventually recover but rather as a significant risk factor for long-term morbidity and mortality following hospital discharge.

SUMMARY

The incidence of AKI is increasing, especially among the elderly. Anatomic and physiologic changes related to aging, coupled with increased comorbidities, elevate the risk of developing AKI in older adults. A multitude of causes may contribute to AKI and a careful assessment aided by serum, urinary, and radiologic tests will often arrive at the appropriate diagnosis. Studies reveal that the elderly suffer higher morbidity and mortality from AKI. However, reasonable outcomes are obtained in most elderly patients with AKI and age alone should not be a criterion for withholding supportive therapies. A standardized staging system for AKI coupled with a growing knowledge of its pathophysiology may allow for the identification of future treatments and consequent improvements in outcomes in the coming years.

ACKNOWLEDGMENT

This work was supported by a Ruth L. Kirschstein National Research Service Award Institutional Research Training Grants, T32-DK061296 (Abdel-Kader).

REFERENCES

1. Hou SH, Bushinsky DA, Wish JB, et al. Hospital-acquired renal insufficiency: a prospective study. Am J Med 1983;74(2):243–8.
2. Shusterman N, Strom BL, Murray TG, et al. Risk factors and outcome of hospital-acquired acute renal failure. Clinical epidemiologic study. Am J Med 1987;83(1): 65–71.
3. Liangos O, Wald R, O'Bell JW, et al. Epidemiology and outcomes of acute renal failure in hospitalized patients: a national survey. Clin J Am Soc Nephrol 2006; 1(1):43–51.
4. Pascual J, Orofino L, Liano F, et al. Incidence and prognosis of acute renal failure in older patients. J Am Geriatr Soc 1990;38(1):25–30.
5. Rosenfeld JB, Shohat J, Grosskopf I, et al. Acute renal failure: a disease of the elderly? Adv Nephrol Necker Hosp 1987;16:159–67.
6. Pascual J, Liano F, Ortuno J. The elderly patient with acute renal failure. J Am Soc Nephrol Aug 1995;6(2):144–53.
7. Nash K, Hafeez A, Hou S. Hospital-acquired renal insufficiency. Am J Kidney Dis 2002;39(5):930–6.
8. Barretti P, Soares VA. Acute renal failure: clinical outcome and causes of death. Ren Fail 1997;19(2):253–7.
9. Brivet FG, Kleinknecht DJ, Loirat P, et al. Acute renal failure in intensive care units – causes, outcome, and prognostic factors of hospital mortality; a prospective, multicenter study. French Study Group on Acute Renal Failure. Crit Care Med 1996;24(2):192–8.
10. Groeneveld AB, Tran DD, van der Meulen J, et al. Acute renal failure in the medical intensive care unit: predisposing, complicating factors and outcome. Nephron 1991;59(4):602–10.
11. Levy EM, Viscoli CM, Horwitz RI. The effect of acute renal failure on mortality. A cohort analysis. JAMA 1996;275(19):1489–94.
12. Liano F, Pascual J. Epidemiology of acute renal failure: a prospective, multi-center, community-based study. Madrid Acute Renal Failure Study Group. Kidney Int 1996;50(3):811–8.
13. Lombardi R, Zampedri L, Rodriguez I, et al. Prognosis in acute renal failure of septic origin: a multivariate analysis. Ren Fail 1998;20(5):725–32.
14. Mangano CM, Diamondstone LS, Ramsay JG, et al. Renal dysfunction after myocardial revascularization: risk factors, adverse outcomes, and hospital resource utilization. The Multicenter Study of Perioperative Ischemia Research Group. Ann Intern Med 1998;128(3):194–203.
15. Neveu H, Kleinknecht D, Brivet F, et al. Prognostic factors in acute renal failure due to sepsis. Results of a prospective multicentre study. The French Study Group on Acute Renal Failure. Nephrol Dial Transplant 1996;11(2):293–9.
16. Vivino G, Antonelli M, Moro ML, et al. Risk factors for acute renal failure in trauma patients. Intensive Care Med 1998;24(8):808–14.
17. Schmitt R, Coca S, Kanbay M, et al. Recovery of kidney function after acute kidney injury in the elderly: a systematic review and meta-analysis. Am J Kidney Dis 2008;52(2):262–71.

18. Ishani A, Xue JL, Himmelfarb J, et al. Acute kidney injury increases risk of ESRD among elderly. J Am Soc Nephrol 2009;20(1):223–8.

19. Guly UM, Turney JH. Post-traumatic acute renal failure, 1956–1988. Clin Nephrol 1990;34(2):79–83.

20. Turney JH, Marshall DH, Brownjohn AM, et al. The evolution of acute renal failure, 1956–1988. Q J Med 1990;74(273):83–104.

21. Gornick CC Jr, Kjellstrand CM. Acute renal failure complicating aortic aneurysm surgery. Nephron 1983;35(3):145–57.

22. Berisa F, Beaman M, Adu D, et al. Prognostic factors in acute renal failure following aortic aneurysm surgery. Q J Med 1990;76(279):689–98.

23. Bullock ML, Umen AJ, Finkelstein M, et al. The assessment of risk factors in 462 patients with acute renal failure. Am J Kidney Dis 1985;5(2):97–103.

24. Chertow GM, Burdick E, Honour M, et al. Acute kidney injury, mortality, length of stay, and costs in hospitalized patients. J Am Soc Nephrol 2005;16(11):3365–70.

25. Lassnigg A, Schmidlin D, Mouhieddine M, et al. Minimal changes of serum creatinine predict prognosis in patients after cardiothoracic surgery: a prospective cohort study. J Am Soc Nephrol 2004;15(6):1597–605.

26. Praught ML, Shlipak MG. Are small changes in serum creatinine an important risk factor? Curr Opin Nephrol Hypertens 2005;14(3):265–70.

27. Mehta RL, Chertow GM. Acute renal failure definitions and classification: time for change? J Am Soc Nephrol 2003;14(8):2178–87.

28. Mehta RL, Kellum JA, Shah SV, et al. Acute Kidney Injury Network: report of an initiative to improve outcomes in acute kidney injury. Crit Care 2007;11(2):R31.

29. Himmelfarb J, Ikizler TA. Acute kidney injury: changing lexicography, definitions, and epidemiology. Kidney Int 2007;71(10):971–6.

30. Bellomo R, Ronco C, Kellum JA, et al. Acute renal failure – definition, outcome measures, animal models, fluid therapy and information technology needs: the Second International Consensus Conference of the Acute Dialysis Quality Initiative (ADQI) Group. Crit Care 2004;8(4):R204–12.

31. Uchino S, Bellomo R, Goldsmith D, et al. An assessment of the RIFLE criteria for acute renal failure in hospitalized patients. Crit Care Med 2006;34(7):1913–7.

32. Hoste EA, Clermont G, Kersten A, et al. RIFLE criteria for acute kidney injury are associated with hospital mortality in critically ill patients: a cohort analysis. Crit Care 2006;10(3):R73.

33. Bell M, Liljestam E, Granath F, et al. Optimal follow-up time after continuous renal replacement therapy in actual renal failure patients stratified with the RIFLE criteria. Nephrol Dial Transplant 2005;20(2):354–60.

34. Abosaif NY, Tolba YA, Heap M, et al. The outcome of acute renal failure in the intensive care unit according to RIFLE: model application, sensitivity, and predictability. Am J Kidney Dis 2005;46(6):1038–48.

35. Kuitunen A, Vento A, Suojaranta-Ylinen R, et al. Acute renal failure after cardiac surgery: evaluation of the RIFLE classification. Ann Thorac Surg 2006;81(2):542–6.

36. Lopes JA, Jorge S, Silva S, et al. An assessment of the RIFLE criteria for acute renal failure following myeloablative autologous and allogeneic haematopoietic cell transplantation. Bone Marrow Transplant 2006;38(5):395 [letter].

37. Lopes JA, Jorge S, Neves FC, et al. An assessment of the RIFLE criteria for acute renal failure in severely burned patients. Nephrol Dial Transplant 2007;22(1):285 [letter].

38. Cruz DN, Bolgan I, Perazella MA, et al. North East Italian Prospective Hospital Renal Outcome Survey on Acute Kidney Injury (NEiPHROS-AKI): targeting the problem with the RIFLE Criteria. Clin J Am Soc Nephrol 2007;2(3):418–25.

39. Ali T, Khan I, Simpson W, et al. Incidence and outcomes in acute kidney injury: a comprehensive population-based study. J Am Soc Nephrol 2007;18(4):1292-8.
40. Khalil P, Murty P, Palevsky PM. The patient with acute kidney injury. Prim Care 2008;35(2):239-64, vi.
41. Moran SM, Myers BD. Course of acute renal failure studied by a model of creatinine kinetics. Kidney Int 1985;27(6):928-37.
42. Perrone RD, Madias NE, Levey AS. Serum creatinine as an index of renal function: new insights into old concepts. Clin Chem 1992;38(10):1933-53.
43. Cheung CM, Ponnusamy A, Anderton JG. Management of acute renal failure in the elderly patient: a clinician's guide. Drugs Aging 2008;25(6):455-76.
44. Coca SG, Yalavarthy R, Concato J, et al. Biomarkers for the diagnosis and risk stratification of acute kidney injury: a systematic review. Kidney Int 2008;73(9): 1008-16.
45. Waikar SS, Bonventre JV. Biomarkers for the diagnosis of acute kidney injury. Nephron Clin Pract 2008;109(4):c192-7.
46. Xue JL, Daniels F, Star RA, et al. Incidence and mortality of acute renal failure in Medicare beneficiaries, 1992 to 2001. J Am Soc Nephrol 2006;17(4):1135-42.
47. Waikar SS, Curhan GC, Wald R, et al. Declining mortality in patients with acute renal failure, 1988 to 2002. J Am Soc Nephrol 2006;17(4):1143-50.
48. Waikar SS, Wald R, Chertow GM, et al. Validity of International Classification of Diseases, Ninth Revision, Clinical Modification Codes for Acute Renal Failure. J Am Soc Nephrol 2006;17(6):1688-94.
49. Hsu CY, McCulloch CE, Fan D, et al. Community-based incidence of acute renal failure. Kidney Int 2007;72(2):208-12.
50. Baraldi A, Ballestri M, Rapana R, et al. Acute renal failure of medical type in an elderly population. Nephrol Dial Transplant 1998;13(Suppl 7):25-9.
51. Van Den Noortgate N, Mouton V, Lamot C, et al. Outcome in a post-cardiac surgery population with acute renal failure requiring dialysis: does age make a difference? Nephrol Dial Transplant 2003;18(4):732-6.
52. Pascual J, Liano F. Causes and prognosis of acute renal failure in the very old. Madrid Acute Renal Failure Study Group. J Am Geriatr Soc 1998;46(6):721-5.
53. de Mendonca A, Vincent JL, Suter PM, et al. Acute renal failure in the ICU: risk factors and outcome evaluated by the SOFA score. Intensive Care Med 2000; 26(7):915-21.
54. Feest TG, Round A, Hamad S. Incidence of severe acute renal failure in adults: results of a community based study. BMJ 1993;306(6876):481-3.
55. Jerkic M, Vojvodic S, Lopez-Novoa JM. The mechanism of increased renal susceptibility to toxic substances in the elderly. Part I. The role of increased vasoconstriction. Int Urol Nephrol 2001;32(4):539-47.
56. Lindeman RD. Overview: renal physiology and pathophysiology of aging. Am J Kidney Dis 1990;16(4):275-82.
57. Lindeman RD, Goldman R. Anatomic and physiologic age changes in the kidney. Exp Gerontol 1986;21(4-5):379-406.
58. Tauchi H, Tsuboi K, Okutomi J. Age changes in the human kidney of the different races. Gerontologia 1971;17(2):87-97.
59. Frocht A, Fillit H. Renal disease in the geriatric patient. J Am Geriatr Soc 1984; 32(1):28-43.
60. Goyal VK. Changes with age in the human kidney. Exp Gerontol 1982;17(5): 321-31.
61. Kaplan C, Pasternack B, Shah H, et al. Age-related incidence of sclerotic glomeruli in human kidneys. Am J Pathol 1975;80(2):227-34.

62. McLachlan MS, Guthrie JC, Anderson CK, et al. Vascular and glomerular changes in the ageing kidney. J Pathol 1977;121(2):65–78.

63. Fliser D. Ren sanus in corpore sano: the myth of the inexorable decline of renal function with senescence. Nephrol Dial Transplant 2005;20(3):482–5.

64. Brenner BM, Rector FC. Brenner & Rector's the kidney. 8th edition. Philadelphia: Saunders Elsevier; 2008.

65. Esposito C, Plati A, Mazzullo T, et al. Renal function and functional reserve in healthy elderly individuals. J Nephrol 2007;20(5):617–25.

66. Abrass CK, Adcox MJ, Raugi GJ. Aging-associated changes in renal extracellular matrix. Am J Pathol 1995;146(3):742–52.

67. Hoy WE, Douglas-Denton RN, Hughson MD, et al. A stereological study of glomerular number and volume: preliminary findings in a multiracial study of kidneys at autopsy. Kidney Int Suppl Feb 2003;(83):S31–7.

68. Hollenberg NK, Adams DF, Solomon HS, et al. Senescence and the renal vasculature in normal man. Circ Res 1974;34(3):309–16.

69. Fliser D, Zeier M, Nowack R, et al. Renal functional reserve in healthy elderly subjects. J Am Soc Nephrol 1993;3(7):1371–7.

70. Lindeman RD, Tobin J, Shock NW. Longitudinal studies on the rate of decline in renal function with age. J Am Geriatr Soc 1985;33(4):278–85.

71. Rowe JW, Andres R, Tobin JD, et al. The effect of age on creatinine clearance in men: a cross-sectional and longitudinal study. J Gerontol 1976;31(2):155–63.

72. Ungar A, Castellani S, Di Serio C, et al. Changes in renal autacoids and hemodynamics associated with aging and isolated systolic hypertension. Prostaglandins Other Lipid Mediat 2000;62(2):117–33.

73. Fliser D, Franek E, Joest M, et al. Renal function in the elderly: impact of hypertension and cardiac function. Kidney Int 1997;51(4):1196–204.

74. Crane MG, Harris JJ. Effect of aging on renin activity and aldosterone excretion. J Lab Clin Med 1976;87(6):947–59.

75. Epstein M, Hollenberg NK. Age as a determinant of renal sodium conservation in normal man. J Lab Clin Med 1976;87(3):411–7.

76. Flood C, Gherondache C, Pincus G, et al. The metabolism and secretion of aldosterone in elderly subjects. J Clin Invest 1967;46(6):960–6.

77. Macias Nunez JF, Garcia Iglesias C, Bondia Roman A, et al. Renal handling of sodium in old people: a functional study. Age Ageing 1978;7(3):178–81.

78. Macias Nunez JF, Garcia Iglesias C, Tabernero Romo JM, et al. Renal management of sodium under indomethacin and aldosterone in the elderly. Age Ageing 1980;9(3):165–72.

79. Rowe JW, Shock NW, DeFronzo RA. The influence of age on the renal response to water deprivation in man. Nephron 1976;17(4):270–8.

80. Castellani S, Ungar A, Cantini C, et al. Excessive vasoconstriction after stress by the aging kidney: inadequate prostaglandin modulation of increased endothelin activity. J Lab Clin Med 1998;132(3):186–94.

81. Davidman M, Olson P, Kohen J, et al. Iatrogenic renal disease. Arch Intern Med 1991;151(9):1809–12.

82. Kohli HS, Bhaskaran MC, Muthukumar T, et al. Treatment-related acute renal failure in the elderly: a hospital-based prospective study. Nephrol Dial Transplant 2000;15(2):212–7.

83. Macias-Nunez JF, Lopez-Novoa JM, Martinez-Maldonado M. Acute renal failure in the aged. Semin Nephrol 1996;16(4):330–8.

84. Lash JP, Gardner C. Effects of aging and drugs on normal renal function. Coron Artery Dis 1997;8(8-9):489–94.

85. van Kraaij DJ, Jansen RW, Gribnau FW, et al. Diuretic therapy in elderly heart failure patients with and without left ventricular systolic dysfunction. Drugs Aging 2000;16(4):289–300.

86. Johnson AG, Simons LA, Simons J, et al. Non-steroidal anti-inflammatory drugs and hypertension in the elderly: a community-based cross-sectional study. Br J Clin Pharmacol 1993;35(5):455–9.

87. Jones AC, Berman P, Doherty M. Non-steroidal anti-inflammatory drug usage and requirement in elderly acute hospital admissions. Br J Rheumatol 1992; 31(1):45–8.

88. Motola D, Vaccheri A, Silvani MC, et al. Pattern of NSAID use in the Italian general population: a questionnaire-based survey. Eur J Clin Pharmacol 2004; 60(10):731–8.

89. Pilotto A, Franceschi M, Leandro G, et al. NSAID and aspirin use by the elderly in general practice: effect on gastrointestinal symptoms and therapies. Drugs Aging 2003;20(9):701–10.

90. Huerta C, Castellsague J, Varas-Lorenzo C, et al. Nonsteroidal anti-inflammatory drugs and risk of ARF in the general population. Am J Kidney Dis 2005;45(3):531–9.

91. Gurwitz JH, Avorn J, Ross-Degnan D, et al. Nonsteroidal anti-inflammatory drug-associated azotemia in the very old. JAMA 1990;264(4):471–5.

92. Adhiyaman V, Asghar M, Oke A, et al. Nephrotoxicity in the elderly due to co-prescription of angiotensin converting enzyme inhibitors and nonsteroidal anti-inflammatory drugs. J R Soc Med 2001;94(10):512–4.

93. Cuny G, Royer RJ, Mur JM, et al. Pharmacokinetics of salicylates in elderly. Gerontology 1979;25(1):49–55.

94. Fraenkel L, Wittink DR, Concato J, et al. Informed choice and the widespread use of antiinflammatory drugs. Arthritis Rheum 2004;51(2):210–4.

95. Ahmed A. Use of angiotensin-converting enzyme inhibitors in patients with heart failure and renal insufficiency: how concerned should we be by the rise in serum creatinine? J Am Geriatr Soc 2002;50(7):1297–300.

96. Bridoux F, Hazzan M, Pallot JL, et al. Acute renal failure after the use of angiotensin-converting-enzyme inhibitors in patients without renal artery stenosis. Nephrol Dial Transplant 1992;7(2):100–4.

97. Lameire N, Matthys E, Vanholder R, et al. Causes and prognosis of acute renal failure in elderly patients. Nephrol Dial Transplant 1987;2(5):316–22.

98. Liano F, Junco E, Pascual J, et al. The spectrum of acute renal failure in the intensive care unit compared with that seen in other settings. The Madrid Acute Renal Failure Study Group. Kidney Int Suppl 1998;66:S16–24.

99. Schrier RW, Wang W. Acute renal failure and sepsis. N Engl J Med 2004;351(2): 159–69.

100. Gentric A, Cledes J. Immediate and long-term prognosis in acute renal failure in the elderly. Nephrol Dial Transplant 1991;6(2):86–90.

101. Klouche K, Cristol JP, Kaaki M, et al. Prognosis of acute renal failure in the elderly. Nephrol Dial Transplant 1995;10(12):2240–3.

102. Santacruz F, Barreto S, Mayor MM, et al. Mortality in elderly patients with acute renal failure. Ren Fail 1996;18(4):601–5.

103. Linas SL, Whittenburg D, Parsons PE, et al. Mild renal ischemia activates primed neutrophils to cause acute renal failure. Kidney Int 1992;42(3):610–6.

104. Langenberg C, Bellomo R, May CN, et al. Renal vascular resistance in sepsis. Nephron Physiol 2006;104(1):1–11.

105. Langenberg C, Wan L, Egi M, et al. Renal blood flow in experimental septic acute renal failure. Kidney Int 2006;69(11):1996–2002.

106. Rosner MH, Okusa MD. Acute kidney injury associated with cardiac surgery. Clin J Am Soc Nephrol 2006;1(1):19–32.
107. Molitoris BA, Sutton TA. Endothelial injury and dysfunction: role in the extension phase of acute renal failure. Kidney Int 2004;66(2):496–9.
108. Rabb H. Immune modulation of acute kidney injury. J Am Soc Nephrol 2006; 17(3):604–6.
109. Friedewald JJ, Rabb H. Inflammatory cells in ischemic acute renal failure. Kidney Int 2004;66(2):486–91.
110. Rabb H, O'Meara YM, Maderna P, et al. Leukocytes, cell adhesion molecules and ischemic acute renal failure. Kidney Int 1997;51(5):1463–8.
111. Sutton TA, Fisher CJ, Molitoris BA. Microvascular endothelial injury and dysfunction during ischemic acute renal failure. Kidney Int 2002;62(5): 1539–49.
112. Rabb H, Daniels F, O'Donnell M, et al. Pathophysiological role of T lymphocytes in renal ischemia-reperfusion injury in mice. Am J Physiol Renal Physiol 2000; 279(3):F525–31.
113. Bonventre JV, Zuk A. Ischemic acute renal failure: an inflammatory disease? Kidney Int 2004;66(2):480–5.
114. Bonventre JV, Weinberg JM. Recent advances in the pathophysiology of ischemic acute renal failure. J Am Soc Nephrol 2003;14(8):2199–210.
115. Thadhani R, Pascual M, Bonventre JV. Acute renal failure. N Engl J Med 1996; 334(22):1448–60.
116. Humes HD, Liu S. Cellular and molecular basis of renal repair in acute renal failure. J Lab Clin Med 1994;124(6):749–54.
117. Chawla LS, Abell L, Mazhari R, et al. Identifying critically ill patients at high risk for developing acute renal failure: a pilot study. Kidney Int 2005;68(5): 2274–80.
118. Abuelo JG. Normotensive ischemic acute renal failure. N Engl J Med 2007; 357(8):797–805.
119. Bellomo R, Chapman M, Finfer S, et al. Low-dose dopamine in patients with early renal dysfunction: a placebo-controlled randomised trial. Australian and New Zealand Intensive Care Society (ANZICS) Clinical Trials Group. Lancet 2000;356(9248):2139–43.
120. Friedrich JO, Adhikari N, Herridge MS, et al. Meta-analysis: low-dose dopamine increases urine output but does not prevent renal dysfunction or death. Ann Intern Med 2005;142(7):510–24.
121. Mehta RL, Pascual MT, Soroko S, et al. Diuretics, mortality, and nonrecovery of renal function in acute renal failure. JAMA 2002;288(20):2547–53.
122. Uchino S, Doig GS, Bellomo R, et al. Diuretics and mortality in acute renal failure. Crit Care Med 2004;32(8):1669–77.
123. Moore RD, Smith CR, Lipsky JJ, et al. Risk factors for nephrotoxicity in patients treated with aminoglycosides. Ann Intern Med 1984;100(3):352–7.
124. Rich MW, Crecelius CA. Incidence, risk factors, and clinical course of acute renal insufficiency after cardiac catheterization in patients 70 years of age or older. A prospective study. Arch Intern Med 1990;150(6):1237–42.
125. Iseki K, Kinjo K, Iseki C, et al. Relationship between predicted creatinine clearance and proteinuria and the risk of developing ESRD in Okinawa, Japan. Am J Kidney Dis 2004;44(5):806–14.
126. Wetzels JF, Kiemeney LA, Swinkels DW, et al. Age- and gender-specific reference values of estimated GFR in Caucasians: the Nijmegen Biomedical Study. Kidney Int 2007;72(5):632–7.

127. Mehran R, Aymong ED, Nikolsky E, et al. A simple risk score for prediction of contrast-induced nephropathy after percutaneous coronary intervention: development and initial validation. J Am Coll Cardiol 2004;44(7):1393–9.
128. Barrett BJ. Contrast nephrotoxicity. J Am Soc Nephrol 1994;5(2):125–37.
129. Lautin EM, Freeman NJ, Schoenfeld AH, et al. Radiocontrast-associated renal dysfunction: incidence and risk factors. AJR Am J Roentgenol 1991;157(1): 49–58.
130. Lepor NE. A review of pharmacologic interventions to prevent contrast-induced nephropathy. Rev Cardiovasc Med 2003;4(Suppl 5):S34–42.
131. Masuda M, Yamada T, Mine T, et al. Comparison of usefulness of sodium bicarbonate versus sodium chloride to prevent contrast-induced nephropathy in patients undergoing an emergent coronary procedure. Am J Cardiol 2007; 100(5):781–6.
132. Solomon R, Deray G. How to prevent contrast-induced nephropathy and manage risk patients: practical recommendations. Kidney Int Suppl Apr 2006;(100):S51–3.
133. McCullough PA, Stacul F, Becker CR, et al. Contrast-Induced Nephropathy (CIN) Consensus Working Panel: executive summary. Rev Cardiovasc Med 2006;7(4):177–97.
134. Merten GJ, Burgess WP, Gray LV, et al. Prevention of contrast-induced nephropathy with sodium bicarbonate: a randomized controlled trial. JAMA 2004; 291(19):2328–34.
135. Joannidis M, Schmid M, Wiedermann CJ. Prevention of contrast media-induced nephropathy by isotonic sodium bicarbonate: a meta-analysis. Wien Klin Wochenschr 2008;120(23–24):742–8.
136. Navaneethan SD, Singh S, Appasamy S, et al. Sodium bicarbonate therapy for prevention of contrast-induced nephropathy: a systematic review and meta-analysis. Am J Kidney Dis 2009;53(4):617–27.
137. Kay J, Chow WH, Chan TM, et al. Acetylcysteine for prevention of acute deterioration of renal function following elective coronary angiography and intervention: a randomized controlled trial. JAMA 2003;289(5):553–8.
138. Shyu KG, Cheng JJ, Kuan P. Acetylcysteine protects against acute renal damage in patients with abnormal renal function undergoing a coronary procedure. J Am Coll Cardiol 2002;40(8):1383–8.
139. Tepel M, van der Giet M, Schwarzfeld C, et al. Prevention of radiographic-contrast-agent-induced reductions in renal function by acetylcysteine. N Engl J Med 2000;343(3):180–4.
140. Nallamothu BK, Shojania KG, Saint S, et al. Is acetylcysteine effective in preventing contrast-related nephropathy? A meta-analysis. Am J Med 2004; 117(12):938–47.
141. Marenzi G, Assanelli E, Marana I, et al. N-Acetylcysteine and contrast-induced nephropathy in primary angioplasty. N Engl J Med 2006;354(26): 2773–82.
142. Bagshaw SM, McAlister FA, Manns BJ, et al. Acetylcysteine in the prevention of contrast-induced nephropathy: a case study of the pitfalls in the evolution of evidence. Arch Intern Med 2006;166(2):161–6.
143. Birck R, Krzossok S, Markowetz F, et al. Acetylcysteine for prevention of contrast nephropathy: meta-analysis. Lancet 2003;362(9384):598–603.
144. Farrington K, Levison DA, Greenwood RN, et al. Renal biopsy in patients with unexplained renal impairment and normal kidney size. Q J Med 1989;70(263): 221–33.

145. Haas M, Spargo BH, Wit EJ, et al. Etiologies and outcome of acute renal insufficiency in older adults: a renal biopsy study of 259 cases. Am J Kidney Dis 2000;35(3):433–47.
146. Davison AM, Jones CH. Acute interstitial nephritis in the elderly: a report from the UK MRC Glomerulonephritis Register and a review of the literature. Nephrol Dial Transplant 1998;13(Suppl 7):12–6.
147. Baker RJ, Pusey CD. The changing profile of acute tubulointerstitial nephritis. Nephrol Dial Transplant 2004;19(1):8–11.
148. Corwin HL, Korbet SM, Schwartz MM. Clinical correlates of eosinophiluria. Arch Intern Med 1985;145(6):1097–9.
149. Nolan CR 3rd, Anger MS, Kelleher SP. Eosinophiluria – a new method of detection and definition of the clinical spectrum. N Engl J Med 1986; 315(24):1516–9.
150. Rossert J. Drug-induced acute interstitial nephritis. Kidney Int 2001;60(2): 804–17.
151. Galpin JE, Shinaberger JH, Stanley TM, et al. Acute interstitial nephritis due to methicillin. Am J Med 1978;65(5):756–65.
152. Gonzalez E, Gutierrez E, Galeano C, et al. Early steroid treatment improves the recovery of renal function in patients with drug-induced acute interstitial nephritis. Kidney Int 2008;73(8):940–6.
153. Clarkson MR, Giblin L, O'Connell FP, et al. Acute interstitial nephritis: clinical features and response to corticosteroid therapy. Nephrol Dial Transplant 2004; 19(11):2778–83.
154. Porile JL, Bakris GL, Garella S. Acute interstitial nephritis with glomerulopathy due to nonsteroidal anti-inflammatory agents: a review of its clinical spectrum and effects of steroid therapy. J Clin Pharmacol 1990;30(5):468–75.
155. Kleinknecht D. Interstitial nephritis, the nephrotic syndrome, and chronic renal failure secondary to nonsteroidal anti-inflammatory drugs. Semin Nephrol 1995;15(3):228–35.
156. Scolari F, Ravani P, Pola A, et al. Predictors of renal and patient outcomes in atheroembolic renal disease: a prospective study. J Am Soc Nephrol 2003; 14(6):1584–90.
157. Thadhani RI, Camargo CA Jr, Xavier RJ, et al. Atheroembolic renal failure after invasive procedures. Natural history based on 52 histologically proven cases. Medicine (Baltimore) 1995;74(6):350–8.
158. Montoliu J, Darnell A, Torras A, et al. Acute and rapidly progressive forms of glomerulonephritis in the elderly. J Am Geriatr Soc 1981;29(3):108–16.
159. Moorthy AV, Zimmerman SW. Renal disease in the elderly: clinicopathologic analysis of renal disease in 115 elderly patients. Clin Nephrol 1980;14(5): 223–9.
160. Arieff AI, Anderson RJ, Massry SG. Acute glomerulonephritis in the elderly. Geriatrics 1971;26(9):74–84.
161. Potvliege PR, De Roy G, Dupuis F. Necropsy study on glomerulonephritis in the elderly. J Clin Pathol 1975;28(11):891–8.
162. Modesto-Segonds A, Ah-Soune MF, Durand D, et al. Renal biopsy in the elderly. Am J Nephrol 1993;13(1):27–34.
163. Watts RA, Lane SE, Bentham G, et al. Epidemiology of systemic vasculitis: a ten-year study in the United Kingdom. Arthritis Rheum 2000;43(2):414–9.
164. Booth AD, Almond MK, Burns A, et al. Outcome of ANCA-associated renal vasculitis: a 5-year retrospective study. Am J Kidney Dis 2003;41(4): 776–84.

165. de Lind van Wijngaarden RA, Hauer HA, Wolterbeek R, et al. Clinical and histo-logic determinants of renal outcome in ANCA-associated vasculitis: a prospec-tive analysis of 100 patients with severe renal involvement. J Am Soc Nephrol 2006;17(8):2264–74.

166. Furci L, Medici G, Baraldi A, et al. Rapidly progressive glomerulonephritis in the elderly. Long-term results. Contrib Nephrol 1993;105:98–101.

167. Higgins RM, Goldsmith DJ, Connolly J, et al. Vasculitis and rapidly progressive glomerulonephritis in the elderly. Postgrad Med J 1996;72(843):41–4.

168. Arora P, Kher V, Kohli HS, et al. Acute renal failure in the elderly: experience from a single centre in India. Nephrol Dial Transplant 1993;8(9):827–30.

169. Kaplan SA, Wein AJ, Staskin DR, et al. Urinary retention and post-void residual urine in men: separating truth from tradition. J Urol 2008;180(1):47–54.

170. Kolman C, Girman CJ, Jacobsen SJ, et al. Distribution of post-void residual urine volume in randomly selected men. J Urol 1999;161(1):122–7.

171. Cronan JJ. Contemporary concepts in imaging urinary tract obstruction. Radiol Clin North Am 1991;29(3):527–42.

172. Naidich JB, Rackson ME, Mossey RT, et al. Nondilated obstructive uropathy: percutaneous nephrostomy performed to reverse renal failure. Radiology 1986;160(3):653–7.

173. Webb JA, Reznek RH, White FE, et al. Can ultrasound and computed tomog-raphy replace high-dose urography in patients with impaired renal function? Q J Med 1984;53(211):411–25.

174. Webb JA. Ultrasonography in the diagnosis of renal obstruction. BMJ 1990; 301(6758):944–6.

175. Gillenwater JY, Westervelt FB Jr, Vaughan ED Jr, et al. Renal function after release of chronic unilateral hydronephrosis in man. Kidney Int 1975;7(3):179–86.

176. Hoffman LM, Suki WN. Obstructive uropathy mimicking volume depletion. JAMA 1976;236(18):2096–7.

177. Sarmina I, Resnick MI. Obstructive uropathy in patients with benign prostatic hyperplasia. J Urol 1989;141(4):866–9.

178. Druml W. Nutritional management of acute renal failure. J Ren Nutr 2005;15(1): 63–70.

179. Palevsky PM. Renal replacement therapy I: indications and timing. Crit Care Clin 2005;21(2):347–56.

180. Palevsky PM. Clinical review: timing and dose of continuous renal replacement therapy in acute kidney injury. Crit Care 2007;11(6):232.

181. Rondon-Berrios H, Palevsky PM. Treatment of acute kidney injury: an update on the management of renal replacement therapy. Curr Opin Nephrol Hypertens 2007;16(2):64–70.

182. Augustine JJ, Sandy D, Seifert TH, et al. A randomized controlled trial comparing intermittent with continuous dialysis in patients with ARF. Am J Kidney Dis 2004;44(6):1000–7.

183. Mehta RL, McDonald B, Gabbai FB, et al. A randomized clinical trial of contin-uous versus intermittent dialysis for acute renal failure. Kidney Int 2001;60(3): 1154–63.

184. Vinsonneau C, Camus C, Combes A, et al. Continuous venovenous haemodia-filtration versus intermittent haemodialysis for acute renal failure in patients with multiple-organ dysfunction syndrome: a multicentre randomised trial. Lancet 2006;368(9533):379–85.

185. Palevsky PM, Zhang JH, O'Connor TZ, et al. Intensity of renal support in critically ill patients with acute kidney injury. N Engl J Med 2008;359(1):7–20.

186. Cruz DN, Ronco C. Acute kidney injury in the intensive care unit: current trends in incidence and outcome. Crit Care 2007;11(4):149.
187. Chertow GM, Soroko SH, Paganini EP, et al. Mortality after acute renal failure: models for prognostic stratification and risk adjustment. Kidney Int 2006; 70(6):1120–6.
188. Rodgers H, Staniland JR, Lipkin GW, et al. Acute renal failure: a study of elderly patients. Age Ageing 1990;19(1):36–42.
189. Liano F, Felipe C, Tenorio MT, et al. Long-term outcome of acute tubular necrosis: a contribution to its natural history. Kidney Int 2007;71(7):679–86.

Clinical Presentation of Renal Failure in the Aged: Chronic Renal Failure

Sarbjit Vanita Jassal, MB, MD(UK), FRCPC

KEYWORDS

- Elderly • Geriatric • Chronic kidney disease
- Dialysis • Renal function

Chronic kidney disease (CKD) is increasingly being recognized in elderly individuals across the world. An understanding of the methods used to estimate or to measure kidney function, the likelihood and factors associated with progressive decline in renal function, and the clinical syndromes associated with poor renal function are key topics for individuals working across many medical disciplines. This review aims to address some of the important aspects of CKD, and summarize some of the clinical and laboratory features associated with progressive disease.

DEFINITIONS, USEFULNESS, AND DEMOGRAPHICS OF CHRONIC KIDNEY DISEASE AND END-STAGE RENAL DISEASE
Dasefinitions and Staging of Chronic Kidney Disease

CKD is the term used to denote changes in the physiology and histology of the kidney that are potentially progressive and may lead to renal impairment. The term chronic is only applied after the functional or structural changes have been present for at least 3 months.[1] Using current standards, all individuals with low glomerular filtration rate (GFR), regardless of the cause, are considered to have CKD but not all individuals with CKD have evidence of decreased GFR. The latter include patients with, for example, glomerulonephritis who have an active urinary sediment but maintain a normal GFR. These individuals are at risk of renal damage and therefore are defined as having CKD.

A staging nomenclature, developed by the National Kidney Foundation (NKF), and adopted several years ago is often used in research and in clinical practice (**Table 1**).[1] This nomenclature encompasses a wide range of patients, such as those with newly diagnosed diabetes or offspring of parents with hereditary renal syndromes, who are

University Health Network, 8NU-857, 200 Elizabeth Street, Toronto, Ontario, M5G 2C4 Canada
E-mail address: vanita.jassal@uhn.on.ca

Clin Geriatr Med 25 (2009) 359–372
doi:10.1016/j.cger.2009.06.002   geriatric.theclinics.com

at risk of renal disease and therefore in need of regular follow-up screening (stages 0 and I) to those with established renal disease approaching or requiring renal replacement therapy (RRT) (stages IV and V). The use of this nomenclature, particularly in older individuals, is increasingly being questioned but to date it remains widely used.[2–7]

In many regions of the world laboratories automatically convert serum creatinine measurements, using mathematical formulae, into estimates of glomerular filtration rate (eGFR), and report these together with the absolute serum creatinine measurement.[8] Although still controversial, this practice has promoted the adoption of the staging system and increased awareness of CKD.[9–13] The widespread use of the NKF staging system has led to the development of national guidelines to help clinicians determine when and how to target different aspects of care and improve renal outcomes.

Why Stage Chronic Kidney Disease?

When initially introduced, the different stages of CKD were intended to remind clinicians of how individuals may transition through what was felt to be an essentially progressive disease.[1] The thought was that recognizing renal disease at an earlier stage might lead to better preventative care, with initial efforts being focused on preventing progression of renal disease, for example, using angiotensin-converting enzyme (ACE) inhibitors, whereas treatments in later stages were being focused on improved predialysis care. However, over the past decade, it has become increasingly clear that, at a population level, individuals with laboratory criteria for CKD stage III (or higher) have overall poor outcomes and that many individuals will not survive long enough to require dialysis initiation.[9–13] The presence of CKD, defined using estimated GFR, is associated with increased mortality risk (all-cause and cardiovascular causes), and prolonged hospitalization in younger and older individuals.[14,15] Age seems to play an important role although clearly the relationships are complicated, nonlinear and interdependent. Important factors modulating progression and risk of mortality include

Table 1		
Staging criteria for CKD and estimated prevalence in those more than 60 years of age		
Stage	Definition	Estimated % Proportion of Those Older Than 60 Years
0	Normal renal function, no histologic changes but patient at increased risk of CKD (examples include new onset diabetes; individuals from families with hereditary diseases such as polycystic kidney disease; patients with active nonrenal lupus syndromes)	
I	Kidney involvement or damage, normal or increased renal function as defined by an eGFR $\geq$ 90 mL/min	5.0 (4.1–6.1)
II	eGFR between 60 and 89 mL/min	12.8 (11.3–14.5)
III	eGFR between 30 and 59 mL/min	20.2 (18.6–22.0)
IV	eGFR between 15 and 29 mL/min	1.3 (1.0–1.7)[a]
V	eGFR <15 mL/min or on RRT	

[a] Reported as combined stages IV and V.

Data from K/DOQI clinical practice guidelines for chronic kidney disease: evaluation, classification, and stratification. Kidney disease outcome quality initiative. Am J Kidney Dis 2002;39(2 Suppl 2):S1–246.

the baseline eGFR, the rate of renal progression and age. When the data are considered, overall they suggest that the absolute risk of death may be higher in older individuals compared with younger individuals regardless of the stage of CKD, but that the relative risk for those with CKD compared with those without CKD is attenuated with increasing age (**Fig. 1**).

Methods Used to Measure Renal Function

The gold standard for measurement of renal function is to directly measure the GFR using a substance that is freely cleared, and neither secreted nor absorbed.[16] The most accepted measure, inulin clearance, is costly, time consuming, and impractical. Nuclear GFR scans or radioisotope clearance may be used when accurate readings are essential. In most cases indirect evaluation through the measurement of the excretion of endogenous substances, such as creatinine or cystatin C, is adequate. Serum creatinine remains the most common way of measuring renal function. Levels are affected by muscle mass, dietary protein intake, the tubular secretion of creatinine, and some commonly used medications (such as cimetidine, statins, and trimethoprim).[8] As the relationship between GFR and creatinine is nonlinear, changes in renal function may not result in higher serum creatinine levels until renal loss is large. Modest changes in renal function may go unnoticed if there is a concurrent decrease in the muscle mass to body weight ratio or a reduction in protein intake. Interlaboratory variations in serum creatinine results can be as high as 10% making it important to monitor patients at a single laboratory whenever possible.

Multiple mathematical formulae have been used to estimate either creatinine clearance (CrCl) or GFR from serum creatinine measurements.[17] The most known are the Cockcroft-Gault equation (CGE)[18] and the modification of diet in renal disease (MDRD) equations[19] although many formulae have been published. Although the use of various formulae help to identify physiologic from pathologic changes over time, it is important to remember that they cannot correct for interlaboratory variations.

The CGE, although well established, would be unlikely to meet today's research standards as a reliable method for renal evaluation. The formula was derived from

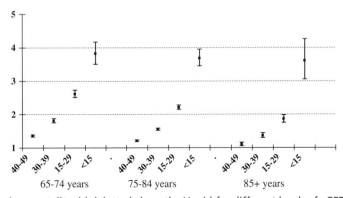

Fig. 1. Showing mortality risk (plotted along the Y axis) for different levels of eGFR. Data are shown for patients falling into three age groupings (65-74 years, 75-84 years, 85+ years). (*Data from* O'Hare AM, Bertenthal D, Covinsky KE, et al. Mortality risk stratification in chronic kidney disease: one size for all ages? J Am Soc Nephrol 2006;17(3):846–53.)

a small study population of primarily stable, hospitalized men.[18] CrCl calculated from 24-h urine collections was used as the gold standard for renal function and so the CGE reports renal function as a CrCl uncorrected for body size. Measured CrCl and the CGE overestimate GFR in individuals with mild to modest renal loss because the contribution of urinary creatinine due to tubular excretion of creatinine relative to that filtered is higher. CGE has been shown to underestimate renal function in hospitalized patients.[20] When originally reported the equation used the ideal body weight, derived from the height of the patient, to estimate muscle mass, however today most people use measured weight. Studies have shown that the accuracy of the CGE is modest and that only 75% of results decrease within 30 mL/min of the true GFR.[17,20]

The second commonly used formula is the MDRD equation.[19] This method has been widely adopted by laboratories as it includes age, gender, and serum creatinine (these variables are easily available to the laboratories). As a result, some laboratories report an estimate of GFR (with a correction factor for Blacks) together with the absolute value of serum creatinine. eGFR has been shown to be of value in those individuals with true GFR readings of 60 mL/min or less, whereby 90% of values lie within 30 mL/min/1.73 m^2.[20] In other populations (living donors with normal renal function, Asian patients, and malnourished patients) it may be inaccurate. Despite these precautions it is considered a useful method to monitor changes in renal function over time within an individual. Due to its imprecision it does not inform as to which patients require renal follow-up and additional criteria are being investigated. The combination of eGFR calculated using the MDRD formula and an assessment of urinary protein, or inclusion of cystatin C may be most useful.[21]

Cystatin C is a novel marker of renal function. It is an endogenous protein (cysteine proteinease inhibitor) that is produced by all nucleated cells and involved in immune responses to viruses and bacteria. Cystatin C is freely filtered at the glomerulus, reabsorbed, and then catabolized by the kidney. It was initially believed to be a better marker of renal function than serum creatinine, however recent studies have shown variations with age, race, and muscle mass, although these variations appear to a lesser extent than those seen with serum creatinine measurements.[8,22–24] Common causes of artificially elevated levels include hypothyroidism, steroid use, and rheumatoid arthritis; hyperthyroidism is associated with artificially low levels. Its application as a marker of kidney function in the older population is unknown. Cross-sectional studies using the National Health and Nutrition Examination Survey (NHANES) data suggest "abnormal" levels are seen in almost 50% of those aged 80 years or more, and although elevated levels do correlate with death and loss of physical function, the true clinical significance is unclear.[25] In addition to age, higher levels are seen in certain racial groups (eg, white non-Hispanic), hypertension, current smokers, those with lower levels of education, raised high-density lipoprotein levels, high C-reactive protein and triglyceride values, and in obese individuals. The diagnostic accuracy of serum cystatin, reported as the proportion of values that lie within 30% of iodine-125 iothalamate GFR measurements, increases from 81% to 89% if serum cystatin levels are incorporated into a mathematical formula based on serum creatinine, age, sex, and race.[26]

Demographics of CKD

Overall, a diagnosis of CKD, based on eGFR values, is more likely to be made in an older individual than a younger individual. Estimates of the prevalence of CKD vary between 20% and 40% depending on the populations under study.[27–34] Residents of nursing homes and those with established cardiovascular disease tend to have higher prevalence rates, whereas population data such as NHANES data suggest lower rates.[30,33] NHANES data estimate CKD to be present in around 11.2% of the overall population, increasing to a prevalence of 34.4% in those aged 60 years or more **(Table 1)**.[35] In absolute numbers this translates to more than 1500 persons per million in the age group between 70 and 79 years having risk of CKD. In contrast younger populations have significantly lower risk (eg, in those aged 30–50 years the prevalence is estimated between 200 and 400 persons per million at risk).

Prevalence rates for CKD tend to be based on cross-sectional population studies, whereby individuals are classified using a single creatinine measure. Not all individuals experience the same change in renal function over time (see later discussion). Cross-sectional studies, for example those including patients with an eGFR of 30 to 40 mL/min, will include two different populations of seniors, those in whom eGFR has been stable at a low level for some time, and those in whom eGFR has deteriorated recently. It is only the latter who likely have progressive CKD. It remains a bit of a quandary as to how best to distinguish these two populations, with some emerging data suggesting that incorporation of urinary albumen findings may reduce the need for unnecessary follow-up.

Comparisons of data from NHANES II and NHANES III suggest an increasing number of individuals have CKD in more recent years. Comparisons were made between populations studied in 1976 to 1980 and 1982 to 1984, respectively.[27,28,35] Despite a short period of time between these two studies, the data showed an increase in the percentage of patients who were defined as having CKD stage III of 42.6%. Over the same time the number of individuals with stage IV increased by 66.7% to 0.35% of the general population.[27] The apparent increase in prevalence was not fully accounted for demographic changes in the population (increased numbers of older individuals, higher rates of hypertension, and diabetes) suggesting a true change in the prevalence of CKD. A similar trend is also seen in the numbers of individuals either starting on dialysis or who undergo preemptive renal transplantation (collectively termed RRT). Dialysis and transplantation are clear, hard end points that incorporate information about renal dysfunction and symptoms. Worldwide dialysis registries have seen a rapid increase in the number of patients initiating dialysis when aged 75 years or more over the last decade.[36–41]

RENAL PROGRESSION
Estimating Renal Progression

Recent discussions around the use of the NKF staging system and progressive renal disease have addressed issues mostly relating to older patients.[5,10,11,42–44] Estimates from iothalamate GFR measurements suggest a reduction beginning from the age of about 20 to 30 years, by 4.6 mL/min per decade in men and by 7.1 mL/min in women.[45] Some investigators have suggested, based on these observations, that renal decline is a natural and not a pathologic phenomenon that occurs with age, and that caution must be used before declaring older patients as CKD patients.[5,7]

For practicing clinicians the most valuable advice is that elderly patients with mild to moderate CKD should all be evaluated for signs suggestive of renal progression. For those with a eGFR between 60 and 89 mL/min, and no evidence of proteinuria, hypertension, or systemic disease, evaluation at least yearly is advised. For those with lower baseline eGFR or in whom renal function declined recently, evaluation four to six times a year may be necessary. The most accurate and informative assessment of the rate of progression is a review of the previous clinical history.

Multiple cross-sectional studies have shown that, on average, renal function is lower in older individuals compared with younger individuals. Longitudinal studies have shown the mean rate of renal decline to be approximately 0.75 to 1.03 mL/min/y.[42,46] Rates are slower for those aged 20 to 39 years (estimated at 0.26 mL/min/y) and higher in older patients (1.51 mL/min/y in those aged 80 years or more).Yet others have estimated the rate of decline in renal function to lie between 0.8 and 2.7 mL/min/y depending on gender and the presence of diabetes.[5,10,11,42–44] This seems to be a simplification as it suggests that the relationship between renal function changes and age is predictable. However, many studies have shown that the rate of renal function decline varies widely between individuals and more recent data suggest that it may be dependent on the baseline function. In a study of veterans in the United States, O'Hare and colleagues[33] showed that renal function declined faster in those whose baseline renal function was greater than 45 mL/min, and that there was a slower decline for those with baseline eGFR levels less than 45 mL/min. Much of the data leads to similar conclusions, that renal decline is not an inevitable consequence of aging but is rather an individual characteristic, and that the most helpful clinical tool is knowledge of what the previous laboratory results were.

Factors Known to Accelerate Renal Decline

Diabetes, proteinuria, and poorly controlled hypertension are all strongly associated with more rapid progression of renal disease and therefore therapy is often directed at these issues (**Table 2**).[47] Clinical guidelines do not differentiate blood pressure targets based on age and targets of less than 125/75 mm Hg in those with proteinuria and 130/85 mm Hg in those with nonproteinuric renal disease are still recommended.[48] Consideration of symptomatic postural hypotension and a decrease in risk is important when managing elderly patients and further studies are warranted in this area.

Most literature would suggest that men have faster rates of renal progression than women. In elderly populations the gender effect has been less marked[49] and may in part be explained by apparent differences in the renin-angiotensin axis

Table 2
Treatments used to slow renal progression[48]

Treatment	Proteinuria or Diabetic Kidney Disease	Nondiabetic, Nonproteinuric Kidney Disease
Glycemic control	Prevents/delays onset. Presumed value in slowing progression of disease	—
ACE inhibitor or ARB therapy	Slows progression	Slows progression particularly if patients have baseline proteinuria
Strict BP control	Slows progression. Target <125/75 mm Hg	Slows progression 130/85 mm Hg if no proteinuria
Dietary restriction of protein	Poor evidence in support of slowed progression when ACE/ARB is being used. Of concern particularly in frail elderly individuals	Poor evidence in support of slowed progression. Of concern particularly in frail elderly individuals

Proteinuria is defined as less than 1 g protein loss/24-h urine.
Abbreviations: ACE, Angiotensin converting enzyme; ARB, Angiotensin receptor blockade; BP, Blood pressure.

responsiveness in the estrogen-producing phases of the menstrual cycle. It is therefore likely that at least some gender differences are mitigated with the postmenopausal state.

CLINICAL MANAGEMENT OF PROGRESSIVE RENAL DISEASE
Causes of Chronic Kidney Disease in Older Patients

It is often difficult to determine a single cause for CKD changes in older individuals. A review of systems to include questions relating to symptoms during urination, recent infections, or admissions, new arthritic or vasculitic symptoms, and recent medication changes is essential. A history of chronic disease such as heart failure, cirrhosis, or gastrointestinal upsets should be sought. As diabetes and hypertension are more commonly seen in older populations than younger, these may be nonspecific findings, although they are the commonest reported cause of end-stage renal disease (ESRD) in those older patients who start dialysis. Systemic vascular disease should alert a physician to the likelihood of intrarenal atherosclerotic disease.

As expected, ESRD secondary to inherited or congenital diseases are uncommon, and conditions such as vascular or hypertensive nephrosclerosis are most common. A high proportion of older individuals start dialysis with no known cause of ESRD.

The clinical workup should include at least one spot urine specimen for albumin/creatinine ratio, urine dipstick testing, and urine microscopy analysis (looking for red blood cells, white blood cells, or casts).[48] It is important to actively exclude uncommon but easily treatable conditions (such as plasma cell dyscrasias/myeloma); those which may present with subtle signs (such as obstructive uropathy) and drug-related kidney injury. These are all increasingly prevalent as individuals age. Patients may still void small amounts of urine even when they have obstructive uropathy, so all cases must be evaluated radiologically for features of hydronephrosis. Vasculitis and primary glomerulopathies are increasingly being recognized in elderly individuals and must be considered in the differential in any patient with an active urine sediment, systemic symptoms, or rash. Weakly positive antineutrophil cytoplasmic antibody (ANCA) levels are commonly seen with advanced age, and so correlation with urinary findings and, on occasion, a biopsy is required.

Clinical Manifestations of Chronic Kidney Disease and Management

In many cases patients are found to have CKD when their physician is alerted to an elevated serum creatinine level on routine screening. Patients may not have reported symptoms or have complained only of vague nonspecific changes in well-being. Less commonly, patients will complain of shortness of breath or edema in association with fluid overload, itching particularly at night or in hot or humid weather, or fatigue. Anorexia is an important symptom that may manifest as gradual weight loss or meat aversion. In elderly patients malnutrition is an important consideration as this may lead to reduced energy levels, poor functioning, and overall poor well-being.

Patients with mildly decreased GFR, low risk for progressive decline in GFR, and low risk for cardiovascular disease are often asymptomatic and have an overall good prognosis.[48] Referral to a nephrologist is not always warranted for those with eGFR levels ≥ 30 mL/min unless there are concerns about deterioration in renal function, systemic symptoms, proteinuria, or hematuria. Re-evaluation, from the renal perspective, is recommended at least once per year. Additional monitoring to endure adequate blood pressure control and avoidance of drugs or procedures

Table 3
Extrarenal symptoms and clinical syndromes associated with CKD

Symptoms	Laboratory and Clinical Manifestations	Management
Anemia	Prevalence of low hemoglobin (usually normochromic normocytic picture) is 5.2% and 44.1% in CKD III and IV, respectively. Assess iron stores (transferring saturation and ferritin); exclude occult blood loss; reticulocyte count ± red blood cell indices	Subcutaneous or intravenous administration of an erythropoietin stimulating agent when Hgb decrease to less than 10 g/dL. Collaborative care with nephrologist is required Target Hgb ranges from 10–12 g/dL with some variation between guidelines in different countries. Targets >12 g/dL not recommended
Bone disease	Decreased phosphate excretion and poor conversion of vitamin D3 to the active form leads to hyperphosphatemia, hypocalcemia and stimulation of parathormone axis. Skeletal resistance to the effects of PTH are seen. Disturbances may contribute to vascular calcification as well as disordered bone function Target phosphate levels ≤1.48 mmol/L in stage III and IV CKD. Monitor calcium, phosphate, the product of calcium and phosphate and PTH levels yearly in CKD III and at 3 monthly intervals in those with CKD IV. Guidelines suggest monitoring 25-hydroxyvitamin D and 1, 25-dihydroxyvitamin D levels	Dietary phosphate restriction (800–1000 mg/d) Use of phosphate binders (such as calcium carbonate) taken with phosphate containing foods) indicated if phosphate levels remain persistently high Use of phosphate binders (such as calcium carbonate) taken with phosphate containing foods) indicated if phosphate levels remain persistently high
Malnutrition	Gradual onset weight loss, anorexia or meat aversion is seen with progressive uremia Laboratory indices: low serum albumin, low cholesterol and triglyceride levels. The subjective global assessment score is a useful screening tool	Dietary supplementation and nutritional advice. Collaboration with a renal dietician advised to limit malnutrition. Care must be taken to limit concomitant phosphate and fluids in some cases Severe or persistent symptoms may inform decision of when to initiate dialysis therapy
Neuropathy	Complaints of paresthesia, sleep disturbances and restless legs. More common in stage IV and V; infrequent in stage III CKD. Evaluation should include electrolytes, nerve conduction studies and EEG/sleep studies if appropriate	Symptoms may be difficult to control. Pregabalin and gabapentin are sometimes effective

(continued on next page)

Table 3
(continued)

Symptoms	Laboratory and Clinical Manifestations	Management
Cognitive function	Prevalence of abnormal cognition estimated between 5%–10% in CKD III and 20%–25% in CKD IV. May impact on treatment adherence and ability to participate in self-management. Depression is common and patients need to be carefully assessed by an interested clinician. The KDQOL cognitive function subscale has been validated as a screening tool although other tools are also frequently in use	Cognitive rehabilitation Supportive care Currently no pharmacologic intervention

Abbreviations: EEG, Electroencephalogram; Hgb, Hemoglobin; KDQOL, Kidney Disease Quality of Life, PTH, Phosphate and parathyroid hormone.

Table 4
Bone abnormalities seen in association with renal dysfunction

Osteopenia and osteoporosis	Seem to increase in prevalence with worsening kidney function. Poor correlation between dual energy X-ray absorptiometry (DEXA) scans and fractures in CKD means further research in the area is required before recommendations for screening can be made
Hyperparathyroid bone disease Mild Moderate to severe Osteitis fibrosa cystica	Associated with increased osteoclastic activity and bone fragility. The initial changes are driven by high phosphate and low calcium levels (ie, secondary hyperparathyroidism); but as time and disease severity progresses may be associated with autonomous parathyroid adenomas (tertiary hyperparathyroidism). Severe cases lead to cystic lesions (osteitis fibrosa cystica) due to abnormal bone mineralization; these are easily seen on radiographs and are known as Brown's tumors
Mixed bone disease	Results from a mixture of hyperparathyroid bone disease and osteomalacia
Osteomalacia	Similar to classic changes associated with vitamin D deficiency; osteomalacia in association with renal bone disease is a disorder of abnormal mineralization
Adynamic bone disease	Believed to be associated with overzealous treatment of hyperparathyroidism; adynamic bone disease is associated with low bone turnover due to severely reduced osteoclastic and osteoblastic activity. Resultant bones are fragile
Aluminum bone disease	Less commonly seen in more recent times, aluminum bone disease is associated with deposits of aluminum in the cortex of bone. The resulting bones have abnormal mineralization and increased fragility

that may precipitate acute kidney injury is appropriate. Patients with moderately or severely decreased GFR (<30 mL/min) are at risk of cardiovascular disease and multisystem alterations in function (**Table 3**) and should be referred to a nephrologist working within a multidisciplinary team setting. These teams serve to mitigate renal deterioration whenever possible, and also to prepare the patient for dialysis if appropriate. Predialysis care has been shown to improve survival in multiple studies. CKD clinics screen for, and manage abnormalities of bone mineralization and hemoglobin maintenance. Alterations in bone mineral function are associated with accelerated cardiac disease due to widespread vascular calcification.

Patients with CKD often have multiple associated disorders that impact greatly on day-to-day living. Cardiac outcomes are poor, and seem unresponsive to traditional interventions.[50–53] In addition, individuals with CKD IV are at risk of chronic anemia,[54] bone disorders leading to high rates of falls and fractures,[1,48,55–59] malnutrition in association with high rates of frailty,[60–62] and cognitive abnormalities (see **Table 3; Table 4**).[63–66] Patients with CKD stage III and IV seem to be prone to infections and abnormal bleeding due to alterations in immune function and platelet dysfunction.

What is less appreciated is that geriatric syndromes and functional disabilities are particularly common in those on RRT,[55,67–71] and preliminary reports suggest that dialysis initiation does not improve functional outcomes. Despite improved survival, overall outcomes for many older individuals seem pessimistic. Death rates before the need for dialysis are high, and outcomes on dialysis humbling. More concerning are the data suggesting many of the interventions that one would expect to mitigate cardiac disease and mortality are ineffective.

SUMMARY AND FUTURE DIRECTIONS

Over the past decade our understanding of the prevalence and consequences of CKD have catapulted physicians into a new era. Multidisciplinary clinics designed to slow renal progression and prepare patients for dialysis are the norm; population screening has increased and targeted therapies to reduce morbidity and mortality associated with CKD has increased. However, our current understanding of CKD is limited by the inclusion of patients with stable, but low GFR, in current cross-sectional studies. Future aims should include improved understanding of how to better identify patients with progressive CKD; a multidimensional approach to the provision of medical care looking not only at survival but also disease burden, functionality, and independent living.

REFERENCES

1. National Kidney Foundation. K/DOQI clinical practice guidelines for chronic kidney disease: evaluation, classification, and stratification. Am J Kidney Dis 2002;39(2 Suppl 1):S1–266.
2. Locatelli F, Vecchio LD, Pozzoni P. The importance of early detection of chronic kidney disease. Nephrol Dial Transplant 2002;17(Suppl 11):2–7.
3. Rossert JA, Wauters JP. Recommendations for the screening and management of patients with chronic kidney disease. Nephrol Dial Transplant 2002;17(Suppl 1): 19–28.
4. Eknoyan G. Chronic kidney disease definition and classification: the quest for refinements. Kidney Int 2007;72(10):1183–5.
5. Eknoyan G. Chronic kidney disease definition and classification: no need for a rush to judgment. Kidney Int 2009;75(10):1015–8.

6. Winearls CG, Glassock RJ. Dissecting and refining the staging of chronic kidney disease. Kidney Int 2009;75(10):1009–14.

7. Glassock RJ, Winearls C. Screening for CKD with eGFR: doubts and dangers. Clin J Am Soc Nephrol 2008;3(5):1563–8.

8. Stevens LA, Coresh J, Greene T, et al. Assessing kidney function – measured and estimated glomerular filtration rate. N Engl J Med 2006;354(23):2473–83.

9. Mathew TH, Johnson DW, Jones GR. Chronic kidney disease and automatic reporting of estimated glomerular filtration rate: revised recommendations. Med J Aust 2007;187(8):459–63.

10. Rainey PM. Automatic reporting of estimated glomerular filtration rate – jumping the gun? Clin Chem 2006;52(12):2184–7.

11. Levey AS, Stevens LA, Hostetter T. Automatic reporting of estimated glomerular filtration rate – just what the doctor ordered. Clin Chem 2006;52(12):2188–93.

12. Anavekar N, Bais R, Carney S, et al. Chronic kidney disease and automatic reporting of estimated glomerular filtration rate: a position statement. Clin Biochem Rev 2005;26(3):81–6.

13. Mathew TH. Chronic kidney disease and automatic reporting of estimated glomerular filtration rate: a position statement. Med J Aust 2005;183(3):138–41.

14. Go AS, Chertow GM, Fan D, et al. Chronic kidney disease and the risks of death, cardiovascular events, and hospitalization. N Engl J Med 2004;351(13): 1296–305.

15. Keith DS, Nichols GA, Gullion CM, et al. Longitudinal follow-up and outcomes among a population with chronic kidney disease in a large managed care organization. Arch Intern Med 2004;164(6):659–63.

16. Wesson L. Physiology of the human kidney. New York: Grune & Stratton; 1969.

17. Bostom AG, Kronenberg F, Ritz E. Predictive performance of renal function equations for patients with chronic kidney disease and normal serum creatinine levels. J Am Soc Nephrol 2002;13(8):2140–4.

18. Cockcroft DW, Gault MH. Prediction of creatinine clearance from serum creatinine. Nephron 1976;16(1):31–41.

19. Levey AS, Bosch JP, Lewis JB, et al. A more accurate method to estimate glomerular filtration rate from serum creatinine: a new prediction equation. Modification of Diet in Renal Disease Study Group. Ann Intern Med 1999;130(6): 461–70.

20. Poggio ED, Wang X, Greene T, et al. Performance of the modification of diet in renal disease and Cockcroft–Gault equations in the estimation of GFR in health and in chronic kidney disease. J Am Soc Nephrol 2005;16(2):459–66.

21. Hallan SI, Ritz E, Lydersen S, et al. Combining GFR and albuminuria to classify CKD improves prediction of ESRD. J Am Soc Nephrol 2009;20(5):1069–77.

22. Oddoze C, Morange S, Portugal H, et al. Cystatin C is not more sensitive than creatinine for detecting early renal impairment in patients with diabetes. Am J Kidney Dis 2001;38(2):310–6.

23. Rigalleau V, Beauvieux MC, Le Moigne F, et al. Cystatin C improves the diagnosis and stratification of chronic kidney disease, and the estimation of glomerular filtration rate in diabetes. Diabetes Metab 2008;34(5):482–9.

24. Tidman M, Sjostrom P, Jones I. A comparison of GFR estimating formulae based upon S-cystatin C and S-creatinine and a combination of the two. Nephrol Dial Transplant 2008;23(1):154–60.

25. Kottgen A, Selvin E, Stevens LA, et al. Serum cystatin C in the United States: the Third National Health and Nutrition Examination Survey (NHANES III). Am J Kidney Dis 2008;51(3):385–94.

26. Stevens LA, Coresh J, Schmid CH, et al. Estimating GFR using serum cystatin C alone and in combination with serum creatinine: a pooled analysis of 3,418 individuals with CKD. Am J Kidney Dis 2008;51(3):395–406.
27. Coresh J, Selvin E, Stevens LA, et al. Prevalence of chronic kidney disease in the United States. JAMA 2007;298(17):2038–47.
28. Coresh J, Astor B, Greene T, et al. Prevalence of chronic kidney disease and decreased kidney function in the adult US population: Third National Health and Nutrition Examination Survey. Am J Kidney Dis 2003;41(1):1–12.
29. Fried LF, Shlipak MG, Stehman-Breen C, et al. Kidney function predicts the rate of bone loss in older individuals: the Cardiovascular Health Study. J Gerontol A Biol Sci Med Sci 2006;61(7):743–8.
30. Garg AX, Papaioannou A, Ferko N, et al. Estimating the prevalence of renal insufficiency in seniors requiring long-term care. Kidney Int 2004;65(2):649–53.
31. Maaravi Y, Bursztyn M, Hammerman-Rozenberg R, et al. Moderate renal insufficiency at 70 years predicts mortality. QJM 2006;99(2):97–102.
32. Maaravi Y, Burzstyn M, Stessman J. Underdiagnosis of impaired kidney function in older adults with normal serum creatinine. J Am Geriatr Soc 2008; 56(2):382.
33. O'Hare AM, Bertenthal D, Covinsky KE, et al. Mortality risk stratification in chronic kidney disease: one size for all ages? J Am Soc Nephrol 2006;17(3):846–53.
34. Shlipak MG, Fried LF, Stehman-Breen C, et al. Chronic renal insufficiency and cardiovascular events in the elderly: findings from the Cardiovascular Health Study. Am J Geriatr Cardiol 2004;13(2):81–90.
35. Jones CA, McQuillan GM, Kusek JW, et al. Serum creatinine levels in the US population: Third National Health and Nutrition Examination Survey. Am J Kidney Dis 1998;32(6):992–9.
36. Canadian Institute of Health Information, 2007, Annual Report–Treatment of End-Stage Renal Failure in Canada, 1996–2005 (Ottawa: CIHI, 2008).
37. The UK Renal Registry. UK renal registry. Available at: http://www.renal.org. Accessed May 15, 2009.
38. European renal registry. Available at: http://www.era-edta-reg.org/index.jsp. Accessed May 15, 2009.
39. Renal replacement therapy in Germany 2004–5. Available at: http://www.quasi-niere. de; 2006. Accessed September 15, 2007.
40. ANZDATA registry annual report. Available at: http://www.anzdata.org.au/ANZOD/ ANZODReport/anzodreport.htm#2008. Accessed December 3, 2008.
41. USRDS Annual Data Report. Available at: http://www.usrds.org/. Chapter 2 Incidence and Prevalence ESRD in patients 75 or over 76. Accessed December 12, 2008.
42. Eriksen BO, Ingebretsen OC. The progression of chronic kidney disease: a 10-year population-based study of the effects of gender and age. Kidney Int 2006;69(2):375–82.
43. Hemmelgarn BR, Zhang J, Manns BJ, et al. Progression of kidney dysfunction in the community-dwelling elderly. Kidney Int 2006;69(12):2155–61.
44. Shlipak MG, Katz R, Kestenbaum B, et al. Rate of kidney function decline in older adults: a comparison using creatinine and cystatin C. Am J Nephrol 2009;30(3): 171–8.
45. Wetzels JF, Kiemeney LA, Swinkels DW, et al. Age- and gender-specific reference values of estimated GFR in Caucasians: the Nijmegen Biomedical Study. Kidney Int 2007;72(5):632–7.

46. Lindeman RD, Tobin JD, Shock NW. Longitudinal studies on the rate of decline in renal function with age. J Am Geriatr Soc 1985;33:278–85.
47. Soares CM, Diniz JS, Lima EM, et al. Predictive factors of progression to chronic kidney disease stage 5 in a predialysis interdisciplinary programme. Nephrol Dial Transplant 2009;24(3):848–55.
48. NKF guidelines for management of CKD. Available at: http://www.kidney.org/professionals/kdoqi/guidelines_ckd/toc.htm. Accessed May 10, 2009.
49. Klag MJ, Whelton PK, Randall BL, et al. Blood pressure and end-stage renal disease in men. N Engl J Med 1996;334(1):13–8.
50. Singh AK, Szczech L, Tang KL, et al. Correction of anemia with epoetin alfa in chronic kidney disease. N Engl J Med 2006;355(20):2085–98.
51. Drueke TB, Locatelli F, Clyne N, et al. Normalization of hemoglobin level in patients with chronic kidney disease and anemia. N Engl J Med 2006;355(20):2071–84.
52. Fabbri G, Maggioni AP. Cardiovascular risk reduction: what do recent trials with rosuvastatin tell us? Adv Ther 2009;26:469–87.
53. Fellstrom BC, Jardine AG, Schmieder RE, et al. Rosuvastatin and cardiovascular events in patients undergoing hemodialysis. N Engl J Med 2009;360(14):1395–407.
54. Kovesdy CP, Trivedi BK, Kalantar-Zadeh K, et al. Association of anemia with outcomes in men with moderate and severe chronic kidney disease. Kidney Int 2006;69(3):560–4.
55. Cook WL, Tomlinson G, Donaldson M, et al. Falls and fall-related injuries in older dialysis patients. Clin J Am Soc Nephrol 2006;1:1197–204.
56. Jassal SV, Naglie G, Cook WL. Accidental falls almost double the mortality risk for older dialysis patients. J Am Soc Nephrol 2006;17:422A.
57. Alem AM, Sherrard DJ, Gillen DL, et al. Increased risk of hip fracture among patients with end-stage renal disease. Kidney Int 2000;58(1):396–9.
58. Coco M, Rush H. Increased incidence of hip fractures in dialysis patients with low serum parathyroid hormone. Am J Kidney Dis 2000;36(6):1115–21.
59. Stehman-Breen CO, Sherrard DJ, Alem AM, et al. Risk factors for hip fracture among patients with end-stage renal disease. Kidney Int 2000;58(5):2200–5.
60. Johansen KL, Kaysen GA, Young BS, et al. Longitudinal study of nutritional status, body composition, and physical function in hemodialysis patients. Am J Clin Nutr 2003;77(4):842–6.
61. Johansen KL, Chertow GM, Jin C, et al. Significance of frailty among dialysis patients. J Am Soc Nephrol 2007;18(11):2960–7.
62. Shlipak MG, Stehman-Breen C, Fried LF, et al. The presence of frailty in elderly persons with chronic renal insufficiency. Am J Kidney Dis 2004;43(5):861–7.
63. Kurella M, Chertow GM, Luan J, et al. Cognitive impairment in chronic kidney disease. J Am Geriatr Soc 2004;52(11):1863–9.
64. Kurella M, Chertow GM, Fried LF, et al. Chronic kidney disease and cognitive impairment in the elderly: the health, aging, and body composition study. J Am Soc Nephrol 2005;16(7):2127–33.
65. Kurella M, Yaffe K, Shlipak MG, et al. Chronic kidney disease and cognitive impairment in menopausal women. Am J Kidney Dis 2005;45(1):66–76.
66. Murray AM, Tupper DE, Knopman DS, et al. Cognitive impairment in hemodialysis patients is common. Neurology 2006;67(2):216–23.
67. Cook WL, Jassal SV. Functional dependencies among the elderly on hemodialysis. Kidney Int 2008;73:1289–95.

68. Jassal SV. How can the outcomes in elderly dialysis patients be improved? Semin Dial 2008, in press.
69. Li M, Tomlinson G, Naglie G, et al. Geriatric comorbidities, such as falls, confer an independent mortality risk to elderly dialysis patients. Nephrol Dial Transplant 2008;23(4):1396–400.
70. Lo D, Chiu E, Jassal SV. A prospective pilot study to measure changes in functional status associated with hospitalization in elderly dialysis-dependent patients. Am J Kidney Dis 2008;52(5):956–61.
71. Chiu E, Markowitz SN, Cook WL, et al. Visual impairment in elderly patients receiving long-term hemodialysis. Am J Kidney Dis 2008;52(6):1131–8.

Diabetic Nephropathy in the Elderly

Anthony J. Joseph, MD*, Eli A. Friedman, MD, MACP

KEYWORDS

• Diabetes • Nephropathy • Treatment • Elderly • Geriatric

DEFINITION AND EPIDEMIOLOGY

Diabetic nephropathy, a major microvascular and macrovascular complication of diabetes mellitus, is most often clinically defined by persistent proteinuria greater than 500 mg/24 h in at least three consecutive samples in an individual with diagnosed diabetes mellitus type 1 (T1-DM) or type 2 (T2-DM), and in more than 95% of those with background and proliferative diabetic retinopathy.[1] Registries in the United States, Japan, and most industrialized European nations show that the incidence and prevalence of treated end-stage renal disease attributed to diabetic nephropathy (ESRD-DM) have progressively increased, reaching pandemic proportions over the past 20 years. According to the 2008 report of the US Renal Data System (USRDS), diabetes in 2006 was listed as the leading cause of ESRD in North America, accounting for 44.4% of incident patients whose care was funded by the Centers for Medicare and Medicaid Services (CMS).[2] This upward trend derives directly from the incidence explosion in T2-DM coupled with an expanding prevalence based on increased survival of diabetic subjects and their greater acceptance of a dialysis program when ESRD develops. Individuals older than 65 years are disproportionately affected by diabetes and ESRD-DM. Analysis of nationally representative data collected in the 1999 to 2004 National Health and Nutrition Examination Survey (NHANES) reveals that diabetes has been diagnosed in 21.2% of adults aged 65 and older.[3] Growth in the prevalence of chronic kidney disease (CKD) based on an estimated glomerular filtration rate (GFR) of <60 mL/min/1.73 m^2 from 1988–1994 to 1999–2004 is evident among individuals aged 60 years and older, and among those with a diagnosis of diabetes.[4] Further to the point, in 2006 the adjusted point prevalence rates per million population of reported ESRD-DM for individuals aged 45 to 64 years was 1357.1, but 2806.8 for persons between 65 and 74 years of age, and 1772.1 for those 75 years or older.[2]

   Although diabetic renal disease represents a major health threat for the aging American population, CKD care in elderly subjects with diabetes is suboptimal. Patel and colleagues[5] reported that only 7.2% of 6033 veterans (mean age 66 ± 11 years)

Department of Medicine, Renal Division, Downstate Medical Center, 450 Clarkson Avenue, Box 52, Brooklyn, NY 11203, USA
* Corresponding author.
E-mail address: anjjoseph@netscape.net (A. Joseph).

Clin Geriatr Med 25 (2009) 373–389
doi:10.1016/j.cger.2009.06.005
0749-0690/09/$ – see front matter © 2009 Elsevier Inc. All rights reserved.

with diabetes and CKD underwent evaluation by a nephrologist during a 5-year study period. The lack of recognition of CKD may be due to an overestimation of kidney function by solely relying on serum creatinine level in elderly subjects.[6] The term of "concealed renal failure" has been applied to elderly patients with normal serum creatinine but decreasing GFR, a frequent component of aging.[6] Furthermore, clinical guidelines developed by the European Diabetes Working Party for Older People and the American Geriatrics Society Panel on Improving Care for Elders with Diabetes have not specifically focused on the subject of advanced CKD in older patients with diabetes.[7] In this article, the authors review some specific aspects of diabetic nephropathy in the elderly, including its impact on patients and national resources, pathology, natural history, and treatments.

IMPACT OF DIABETES ON OLDER PATIENTS AND NATIONAL RESOURCES

Persons with diabetes typically develop serious comorbidities, especially heart, eye, and peripheral vascular diseases. In its 2007 National Diabetes Fact Sheet, the Centers for Disease Control (CDC) reported that in 2004, heart disease and prior stroke were respectively noted on 68% and 14% of diabetes-related death certificates among people aged 65 years or older.[8] Moreover, the CDC indicated that, in 2005, 27% of adults with diabetes who were 75 years or older recounted some degree of visual impairment compared with 15% of diabetic patients who were between 18 and 44 years of age.[9] Individuals aged 65 years or older account for 55% of diabetic subjects who had nontraumatic lower extremity amputations.[10] Caring for elderly patients with diabetic renal disease imposes a huge financial burden on governments and family members. For example, the American Diabetes Association (ADA) indicated that the total estimated cost of diabetes in 2007 was $174 billion, including $58 billion to treat diabetes-related chronic complications.[11] Diabetic nephropathy in the elderly is mainly due T2-DM and its distribution is uneven among racial groups. American Indians, African Americans, and Mexican Americans have a greater incidence than Caucasians by as much as three to one depending on the minority cohort selected for comparison.[2] Genetic susceptibility, suboptimal care in minority groups, delayed diagnosis of T2-DM, and environmental factors are reasons proposed to explain such disparity.

PATHOLOGY

Renal biopsies obtained from individuals with T2-DM are similar to and may be indistinguishable from those seen in T1-DM.[12,13] In both types of diabetes, kidney injury is noted in glomeruli, arterioles, tubules, and the interstitium. Glomerular lesions consist of diffuse and nodular forms of intracapillary glomerulosclerosis. The diffuse type is characterized by mesangial widening and thickening of the capillary wall and glomerular basement membrane. With progression, capillary wall thickening and mesangial expansion lead to capillary narrowing and reduced glomerular circulation. Nodular lesions, termed intercapillary glomerulosclerosis by Kimmestiel and Wilson, occur at the periphery of the glomeruli and are well delineated by periodic acid–Schiff-positive staining that defines globular structures while exaggerating diffuse lesions. Albumin, demonstrable by immunofluorescence microscopy, is passively entrapped by the thickened basement membrane. In addition, hyaline deposits (so-called "exudative" or "insudative" lesions) are present in arterioles (hyaline arteriosclerosis), capillary walls (fibrin caps), and Bowman capsules (capsular drops).[14] Arteriolar hyalinosis, prominent in diabetic nephropathy, affects afferent as well as efferent arterioles.[14]

Mesangial expansion is the defining histologic feature of diabetic nephropathy.[15] Mesangial fractional volume (Vv [mes/glom]), an estimate of mesangial expansion, is the structural parameter that best correlates with GFR, and is closely related to the presence of proteinuria and hypertension.[15] Although diabetes is primarily a vascular disease, diabetic nephropathy is also associated with tubular basement membrane thickening and interstitial space expansion that are present early in diabetic nephropathy.[16] Decline in renal function in diabetic renal disease is a product of several interacting forces, including glomerular capillary narrowing, hyaline arteriosclerosis, glomerular sclerosis or occlusion, and interstitial fibrosis.[17]

The histologic diagnosis of diabetic nephropathy in older patients may be challenging because mesangial matrix expansion and thickening of the glomerular basement membrane have also been attributed to kidney senescence.[18] Likewise, tubular atrophy and interstitial fibrosis may be aging-related or due to chronic inflammation or vascular disease.[19]

In some reports, the pathology of renal disease in T2-DM is more complex than in T1-DM. Parving and colleagues[20] described a high prevalence of nondiabetic glomerular diseases in Danish patients with T2-DM undergoing renal biopsy for evaluation of proteinuria; 23% had a variety of nondiabetic glomerulopathies, such as "minimal lesion" and mesangioproliferative glomerulonephritis. Fioretto and Mauer performed renal function studies and renal biopsy examinations in a large cohort of T2-DM patients (age 58 ± 7 years) with microalbuminuria and proteinuria. These investigators described marked heterogeneity in renal structure among those patients. Only a minority had the typical lesions seen in individuals with T1-DM. The remaining subjects had mild or no diabetic glomerulopathy with or without tubulointerstitial, arteriolar, and global glomerulosclerosis changes. Fewer than 10% of their proteinuric patients had nondiabetic renal disease.[21] Elderly patients with T2-DM may have renal ischemia due to renal artery stenosis. Sawicki and colleagues[22] reported that the prevalence of renal artery stenosis in subjects with T2-DM and hypertension was greater than 10%. Bilateral artery stenosis was found in 43% of these cases.

NATURAL HISTORY

The natural history of diabetic nephropathy has been extensively studied in T1-DM because it is usually possible to specify the exact time of onset as that of the start of life-sustaining insulin administration. By contrast, establishing an onset date for T2-DM is often accidental because surveys indicate that as many as half of prevalent patients with diabetes are unaware of their disease. As initially described by Mogensen for T1-DM, there are 5 distinct stages of nephropathy. Two main variables, proteinuria and GFR, are employed to follow evolution of diabetic nephropathy.

Stage 1: Glomerular Hyperfiltration and Renal Hypertrophy

Glomerular hyperfiltration and renal hypertrophy typify the first stage.[23] At its onset, approximately one third of patients with T1-DM have an increased GFR that is 20% to 40% higher than that of age-matched normal individuals.[24] Intensive insulin therapy reduces hyperglycemia and may progressively reduce glomerular hyperfiltration over the next few months.[24] An increased GFR is predictive of clinical nephropathy in some subjects.[25] Neither short- nor long-term intensive insulin therapy has been shown to reduce glomerulomegaly in T1-DM patients.[26]

Stage 2: Early Glomerular Lesions or Silent Stage with Normal Albumin Excretion

Early glomerular lesions, such as glomerular basement membrane thickening and mesangial matrix widening, characterize the second stage of diabetic nephropathy.[27] These histologic changes emerge 18 to 36 months after the inception of T1-DM[28] and may be become prominent after 3.5 to 5 years.[29] Nephropathy usually is silent with a normal urinary albumin excretion rate (AER), but microalbuminuria (defined later) may be present after exercise or during episodes of poor control of hyperglycemia.

Stage 3: Microalbuminuria Stage or Incipient Diabetic Nephropathy

Microalbuminuria, defined as urinary AER greater than 30 mg/24 h or 20 μg/min and less than 300 mg/24 h or 200 μg/min, characterizes the third stage, which is also called incipient diabetic nephropathy.[1] Microalbuminuria is the first laboratory evidence of diabetic renal disease. Hypertension may also be a feature of the microalbuminuric stage. With great unpredictability in total daily excretion, microalbuminuria is an inconstant finding and is increased by hypertension, strenuous exercise, fever, poor glycemic control, congestive heart failure, and high salt intake.[30] Therefore, a diagnosis of incipient nephropathy in patients with T1-DM or T2-DM should only be made when microalbuminuria is detected in two or more urine specimens over the course of three or more months. Measurements of urinary albumin excretion can be performed by 24-hour, overnight, or short-term urine collections.[31] Determinations of the albumin to creatinine ratio (30–300 mg/g) or albumin concentration from an early-morning urine sample are acceptable for screening, but a timed urine collection is regarded as more accurate.[31] Approximately 25% to 40% of subjects with T1-DM express constant microalbuminuria after 5 to 10 years of diabetes.[32] Several studies suggest that a significant subset of microalbuminuria patients may convert to normoalbuminuria without obvious explanation.[33,34] In both types of diabetes, persistent microalbuminuria is a serious sign of renal damage that predicts a progressive downhill course toward clinical nephropathy and ultimately, ESRD.[1,35] In consequence, detection of microalbuminuria represents an essential step in the management strategy of diabetic renal disease.

Stage 4: Clinical or Overt Diabetic Nephropathy: Proteinuria and Decreasing Glomerular Filtration Rate

Conversion from the third to the fourth stage of diabetic nephropathy is silently characterized by an increase in proteinuria to greater than 300 mg/24 h, accompanied by progressive decline of glomerular filtration, often with worsening hypertension.[1,36] Urinary protein excretion is variable, ranging from as little as 500 mg/d to nephrotic amounts as high as 20 to 40 g/d. Persistent urinary protein loss, hypoproteinemia, reduced interstitial colloid pressure, and decreased ratio between interstitial and plasma albumin may lead to a nephrotic syndrome (proteinuria >3.5 g/d plus hyperlipidemia).[37] Diagnoses of other than diabetic renal disease should be pursued whenever a nephrotic syndrome occurs in an individual with T1-DM of less than 5 years, and in both types in the absence of retinopathy. In contrast, a diagnosis of nephropathy in T1-DM or T2-DM is less probable when progressive renal deterioration is not associated with macroalbuminuria.[38] Percutaneous renal biopsy to clarify the specific renal disorder is indicated in such instances. Systolic and diastolic hypertensions intensify the rate of renal function deterioration. Without aggressive blood pressure control, GFR typically declines in a linear fashion at a rate ranging from 7.5 to 28 mL/min/y.[36,39,40]

Stage 5: End-Stage Renal Disease

After 20 to 40 years of suboptimally managed T1-DM, historically approximately 30% to 40% of patients developed ESRD. In recent times, however, the interval between the onset of persistent proteinuria and the final stage of diabetic nephropathy has been extended significantly by early and intensive treatment of hypertension and enhanced control of hyperglycemia.

NEPHROPATHY IN TYPE 2 DIABETES

Delayed diagnosis and a muted presence complicate the construction of the natural history of T2-DM. Studies relating renal hemodynamics and hypertrophy in newly diagnosed patients with T2-DM have been inconsistent. Microalbuminuria is prevalent in older diabetic patients. A study comparing 187 diabetic subjects and 1073 nondiabetic individuals (mean age 74 years) revealed that 29.7% of the diabetics had microalbuminuria.[41] de Fine Olivarius and colleagues[42] reported in a study of 1267 newly diagnosed subjects with T2-DM (mean age 66 years) that the prevalence of microalbuminuria was 28.8% in women and 33.6% in men. Proteinuria was present in 6.6% of men and 4.6% of women.[42] A urinary AER of 15 mg/min or more is a short-term predictor of mortality in diabetics aged 69 to 74 years.[43] Fourteen percent to 24% of patients newly diagnosed with T2-DM have microalbuminuria, which is associated with hyperglycemia, elevated blood pressure, smoking, and hyperlipidemia.[44] Microalbuminuria in T2-DM is partially reversed by reduction of hyperglycemia and hypertension.[45] According to a 2004 position statement of the ADA, macroalbuminuria may be less specific for the presence of diabetic renal disease in T2-DM than in T1-DM.[46]

T2-DM individuals who develop nephropathy do so usually within 5 to 10 years of diagnosis though, as noted earlier, the diagnosis of T2-DM is often delayed until some other event stimulates medical attention. In an unpublished study correlating the interval between diagnosis and the time until onset of ESRD, the authors found that the older the diabetic person at the time diabetes was first diagnosed, the shorter the time until the need for dialysis. Why this is true provokes speculation. First, a delayed diagnosis and lack of treatment of diabetes may mask inception of complications. Second, older diabetic patients may have acceleration of diabetic nephropathy due to kidney senescence, atherosclerosis, hypertension, and ischemia created by renal artery stenosis.[17,18,22]

TREATMENT OF DIABETIC NEPHROPATHY

The experience of the past 2 decades convincingly demonstrates the effectiveness of renoprotection, which consists of lifestyle modification, intensive control of hyperglycemia, aggressive lipid reduction, and adequate lowering of hypertensive blood pressure with a drug regimen including an angiotensin-converting enzyme inhibitor (ACEI) or an angiotensin receptor blocker (ARB). Key components of renoprotection including intensive control of hyperglycemia and adequate lowering of hypertensive blood pressure to less than 130/80 mm Hg have modified the natural course of diabetic nephropathy by reversing functional changes and by stabilizing progression of structural abnormalities.

Nearly all studies demonstrating beneficial effects of metabolic and blood pressure controls on diabetic renal disease have been performed in young to middle-aged cohorts. In consequence, the management of diabetic renal disease in older people is frequently based on extrapolations of data gathered in selected and motivated younger people. Moreover, people older than 70 years have been virtually excluded in trials supporting major United States practice guidelines for the use of ACEIs and ARBs in CKD. In managing diabetes and diabetic nephropathy in the elderly, clinicians should keep in mind several key points. (1) Elderly diabetic patients constitute a diverse group expressing various clinical and functional situations. (2) The European Diabetes Working Party for Older People and The American Geriatric Society Panel on Improving Care for Elders with Diabetes recommend that treatment of elderly patients with diabetes focus on specific problems and priorities.[47,48] (3) The American Geriatric Society has also introduced the concept of time horizon for the benefits of certain treatments. Glycemic control may take as long as 8 years to have positive results on microvascular complications. Benefits of good blood pressure and lipid control may not be noticeable before 2 or 3 years.[48] (4) Many elderly patients with diabetes are frail and are also at greater risk for developing several common geriatric syndromes, such as depression, cognitive impairment, urinary incontinence, injurious falls, and persistent pain. The Assessing Care of Vulnerable Elders (ACOVE) project defines a frail elderly patient as a vulnerable person who is older than 65 years and is at increased risk of death or functional decline within 2 years.[49] (5) In consequence, renoprotection in a geriatric population should be tailored according to patients' autonomy, degree of frailty, life expectancy, comorbidity index, and the stage of diabetic nephropathy.

LIFESTYLE MODIFICATION

Although neglected at times by health care providers and patients, an important component of the management of diabetic nephropathy is lifestyle modification, including weight reduction, exercise, smoking cessation, and a decrease in alcohol consumption if excessive.[50] The Steno-2 study found that, in patients (mean age: 63 years) with T2-DM and microalbuminuria, intensive intervention with behavior modification and multiple drug combinations had sustained beneficial effects with respect to vascular complications and on rates of death from cardiovascular causes.[51] Apart from an increased risk of morbidity and premature death associated with the development of macrovascular complications, smoking is also linked to the premature development of microvascular complications of diabetes. Lifestyle modification can facilitate glycemia and blood pressure control as well as lipid reduction.

GLYCEMIC CONTROL

Two large-scale prospective trials, the Diabetes Control and Complication Trial (DCCT) conducted in T1-DM (age 27 ± 7 years) and the United Kingdom Prospective Diabetes Study (UKPDS) including patients with T2-DM (age 53.4 ± 8 years), decisively document that strict metabolic control of hyperglycemia prevents diabetic nephropathy.[52,53]

The ADVANCE (Action in Diabetes and Vascular Disease: Preterax and Diamicron) study showed recently that in T2-DM patients of an average age of 66 years, intensive glucose control (glycated hemoglobin 6.5 versus 7.3%) led to a 10% relative reduction in the combined outcome of major macrovascular events (death from cardiovascular causes, nonfatal myocardial infarction, or nonfatal stroke) and a 21% reduction in the incidence of diabetic nephropathy over a 5-year period.[54] Severe hypoglycemia, although occasional, was more common in the intensive-control group. Enthusiasm created by ADVANCE was tempered by another study published in the same 2008 issue of the New England Journal of Medicine. The ACCORD (Action to Control Cardiovascular Risk in Diabetes) study randomized 10,251 participants (mean age

62.2 years) with a median glycated hemoglobin of 8.1% to a strategy of intensive gly-cemic control (hemoglobin A1c [HbA1c] target <6.0%) or standard control (HbA1c target 7.0%–7.9%). Compared with standard therapy, the use of intense treatment to target normal HbA1c levels for 3.5 years increased mortality and did not significantly reduce major cardiovascular events.[55] The finding of higher mortality in the intensive-therapy group led to discontinuation of the intensive therapy after a mean of 3.5 years of follow-up. This study indicates that the potential risks of intensive glycemic control may outweigh its benefits in frail patients and those with long duration of diabetes, known history of hypoglycemia, and advanced age. The ADA suggest that clinicians should consider less stringent HbA1c goals than the usual target of less than 7.0% for individuals with any of the aforementioned characteristics.[50]

Prudence is recommended in treating hyperglycemia with advanced CKD. Degra-dation of endogenous and exogenous insulin is impaired in renal failure. As renal func-tion declines, progressive reductions in oral hypoglycemic agent and insulin doses are necessary to prevent hypoglycemia.[56] In consequence, oral agents with long half-lives should be avoided altogether because of the risk of persistent and severe episodic hypoglycemia. Metformin is contraindicated in renal insufficiency because of the risk of fatal lactic acidosis. Thiazolidinediones, agents that reduce insulin resistance, may induce fluid retention, edema, and congestive heart failure. Findings from a large population-based cohort of United States seniors (mean age 76.3 years) are compat-ible with an increased risk of all-cause mortality and congestive heart failure in patients initiating therapy with rosiglitazone compared with similar patients initiating therapy with pioglitazone.[57] In a Canadian population-based study of older patients (age ≥66 years), treatment with rosiglitazone was associated with an increased risk of congestive heart failure, acute myocardial infarction, and mortality when compared with combinations of other oral hypoglycemic agents.[58] Insulin therapy may represent a major psychological burden for some elderly subjects.

BLOOD PRESSURE CONTROL

The prevalence of hypertension in individuals with T2-DM is higher than that in the general population. At the age of 45 years, approximately 40% of patients with T2-DM are hypertensive; the proportion increases to 60% by the age of 75.[59–61] Systolic and diastolic hypertensions significantly escalate progression of diabetic nephrop-athy. Randomized clinical trials well document the benefits of lowering blood pressure to less than 140 mm Hg and less than 80 mm Hg in diabetic patients of all ages.[62–66] Aggressive and successful treatment of arterial hypertension prevents the transition from microalbuminuria to albuminuria, decreases albuminuria and nephrotic-range proteinuria, and slows the rate of deterioration of renal function. Moreover, the risk of fatal or nonfatal cardiovascular events is reduced in diabetic patients when systolic hypertension is reduced.

In general, ACEIs and ARBs are the drugs of choice for the treatment of arterial hypertension in patients with diabetic nephropathy.[63,67–71] Apart from reducing arterial blood pressure, both drug types are renoprotective owing to their ability to decrease intraglomerular pressure. The micro-HOPE study, a subgroup analysis of HOPE (Heart Outcomes Evaluation Prevention), revealed that 10 mg of ramipril compared with placebo in 1808 patients with T2-DM and a mean age of 65.3 years reduced the risk of overt nephropathy by 25% and that of cardiovascular death by 37%.[72] Winkelmayer and colleagues[73] assessed the nephroprotective efficacy and safety of ARB therapy in elderly patients by conducting age-specific subgroup analyses using data from the Reduction of End points in NIDDM with the Angiotensin II Antagonist

Losartan (RENAAL) study. Of 1513 participants, 421 (27.8%) were older than 65 years (maximum age 74 years). In those patients older than 65 years, losartan reduced the risk of ESRD by 50%. Of great import, the investigators did not find evidence that older patients were more likely to experience adverse events from losartan, such as increase in serum creatinine or hyperkalemia, than were younger patients.

The effects of an ACEI (enalapril or ramipril) and an ARB (telmisartan) on the progression of diabetic nephropathy have been compared. The DETAIL (Diabetics Exposed to Telmisartan and Enalapril) and ONTARGET (ONgoing Telmisartan Alone or in combination with Ramipril Global Endpoint Trial) studies included patients older than 65 years. In DETAIL, a long-term, head-to-head comparison of renal outcomes of Telmisartan and Enalapril in individuals with T2-DM and early nephropathy, telmisartan was not inferior to enalapril in preventing the progression of renal dysfunction measured as the decline of the GFR.[74] In the ONTARGET study, the number of events for the composite primary outcome, that is, dialysis, doubling of serum creatinine, and death, was similar for telmisartan and ramipril. Although combination therapy using those drugs reduced proteinuria to a greater extent than monotherapy, it worsened major renal outcomes.[75] ACEIs and ARBs initially can decrease GFR modestly. Potassium and serum creatinine should be checked 1 week after starting or changing these drugs to look for hyperkalemia and decreased GFR.

When diabetic patients with albuminuria and nephropathy are unable to tolerate ACEIs or ARBs, nondihydropyridine calcium channel blockers (DCCBs), such as diltiazem, verapamil, or β-blockers, should be used. Initial therapy with DCCBs should be avoided. For instance, in the Irbesartan Diabetic Nephropathy Trial, amlodipine was not more effective than placebo in slowing the progression of diabetic nephropathy.[69] The use of DCCBs should be restricted to situations in which ARBs and ACEIs cannot effectively lower arterial blood pressure.

β-Blockers are effective therapy for hypertension in diabetic subjects. In the UKPDS study of patients with T2-DM, atenolol was as useful as captopril in lowering blood pressure and protecting against cardiovascular disease.[76] β-Blockers, unfortunately, may induce worsening of insulin resistance, deterioration of glycemic control, possible exacerbation of peripheral vascular disease, and the masking of hypoglycemic symptoms.[76,77] Peripheral α-blockers, such as doxazosin, are as effective in decreasing blood pressure as ACEIs and calcium channel blockers, and have a beneficial metabolic profile,[78] but unfortunately they can induce orthostatic hypotension. Furthermore, in the Antihypertensive and Lipid Lowering Treatment to Prevent Heart Attack study, the doxazosin treatment arm was discontinued because of a significantly increased risk of heart failure compared with chlorthalidone.[79]

In general, hypoproteinemic diabetic patients with renal insufficiency are prone to stunning fluid retention of 25 kg or more making blood pressure control refractory to the usual antihypertensive therapy. Dietary salt restriction and a combination of loop diuretics plus metolazone, a quinazoline diuretic, are usually necessary.

DIETARY PROTEIN AND LIPID RESTRICTION

Studies in induced diabetic and subtotally nephrectomized rats noted that that a low-protein diet decreases intraglomerular pressure, and prevents progressive glomerular injury and albuminuria.[80] From a meta-analysis of five studies, Pedrini and colleagues[81] concluded that dietary protein restriction delayed progression of diabetic nephropathy in patients with T1-DM. By contrast, the Modified Diet in Renal Disease Study, in which only 3% of the subjects had T2-DM and none had T1-DM, failed to show a clear benefit of protein restriction.[82] Pijls and colleagues,[83] in a small-scale, randomized controlled study conducted in T2-DM patients younger than 79 years of age, concluded that in the longer term prevention or delay of renal damage in subjects with T2-DM, protein restriction was neither feasible nor efficacious. The current ADA recommendation suggests limiting protein intake to 0.8 to 1.0 g/kg/d in those with diabetes and CKD. Severe protein restriction may be dangerous in elderly individuals because they tend to decrease spontaneously their caloric and protein intakes. In patients with nephrotic-range proteinuria or nephrotic syndrome, protein restriction should be avoided because of the risk of malnutrition.

Abnormal lipid metabolism is highly prevalent in diabetics with renal disease, especially in those with a nephrotic syndrome. Several studies in humans link dyslipidemia with progression of CKD.[84] Hyperlipidemia may accelerate progression of CKD by promoting intrarenal atherosclerosis or through direct deleterious effects of lipids on renal cells. Reabsorption of fatty acids, phospholipids, and cholesterol contained in the filtered proteins (albumin and lipoproteins) by tubular epithelial cells can stimulate tubulointerstitial inflammation, foam cell formation, and tissue injury. In addition, accumulation of lipoproteins in the glomerular mesangium can also promote matrix proliferation and glomerulosclserosis.[85]

Several studies in patients with CKD have shown statins to be renoprotective. The pleiotropic effects of statins seem to extend beyond lipid-lowering and play a significant role in renoprotection. Statins seem to modulate glomerular mesangial and inflammatory processes independent of lipid reduction.[85] Statins may induce tubular proteinuria. Vidt and colleagues[86] reported that 0.2% of patients on 5 mg rosuvastatin and 1.2% of subjects on 40 mg rosvastatin developed proteinuria. A recent review by Kasiske and colleagues[87] did not find any evidence suggesting that statins caused kidney injury when used in doses currently approved by the US Food and Drug Administration. Treatment of dyslipidemia is paramount in the overall management of diabetes mellitus because it decreases the risk of cardiovascular diseases. In the Heart Protection Study, which included diabetic patients between 40 and 80 years old and treated with 40 mg of simvastatin daily, a reduction in the risk for myocardial infarction and stroke was observed within 12 months, irrespective of age or serum creatinine levels.[88] The Kidney Disease Outcomes Quality Initiative Clinical Practice Guidelines recommend that all patients with diabetes and stages 1 through 4 CKD be treated,[89] although there is no evidence to support treatment in individuals with stage 4 CKD. The ACOVE-3 strongly recommended dyslipidemia treatment in all frail diabetic patients.[49]

The effects of statins on hemodialysis patients with ESRD-DM have been disappointing up to now. In 2005, Wanner and colleagues[90] published the first prospective, randomized, placebo-controlled trial of a statin in T2-DM individuals on maintenance hemodialysis (MHD). A total of 1255 T2-DM patients (age 65.7 ± 8.3 years) on MHD for less than 2 years were assigned to receive atorvastatin (20 mg) or a matching placebo. Following 4 weeks of treatment, the median level of low-density lipoprotein (LDL) cholesterol was reduced by 42%, whereas among those receiving placebo it was reduced by 1.3%. After a medium follow-up of 4 years, such LDL reduction nevertheless did not significantly influence any primary end point, a composite of cardiovascular death, fatal stroke, nonfatal myocardial infarction, or stroke, which occurred in 37% of subjects in the atorvastatin group versus 38% in the placebo group. Similar results have been reported by another group of investigators employing rosuvastatin. Fellström and colleagues[91] conducted an international, multicenter, randomized, double-blind, prospective trial involving 2776 patients, 50 to 80 years of age, who were undergoing MHD. They randomly assigned patients to receive rosuvastatin, 10 mg daily, or placebo. Diabetes was the cause of ESRD in 20.6% of subjects on rosuvastatin and 18% of individuals receiving placebo. Although the initiation of treatment with rosuvastatin lowered the LDL cholesterol level, it did not have any significant effect on the composite primary end point of death from cardiovascular causes, nonfatal myocardial infarction, or nonfatal stroke.

PREVENTION OF NEPHROTOXICITY

Drug use increases with advancing age. Elderly diabetic patients are frequently exposed to nephrotoxic drugs such as nonsteroidal anti-inflammatory drugs (NSAIDs), cyclooxygenase-2 (COX-2) inhibitors, and radiocontrast agents. Senior citizens complaining of pain are prescribed NSAIDs by their physicians or buy them over the counter. NSAIDs and COX-2 inhibitors can cause hemodynamically mediated acute kidney injury by inhibiting the synthesis of prostaglandins that act to preserve renal blood flow and GFR in individuals with volume depletion, pre-existing CKD, congestive heart failure, and liver cirrhosis.[92,93] Other clinical syndromes associated with NSAIDs use include acute interstitial nephritis, sodium and potassium retention that can precipitate edema, poor blood pressure control, hyperkalemia, and heart failure. COX-2 inhibitors and NSAIDs should be used cautiously or not at all in elderly patients with diabetic renal disease, particular in those receiving diuretics, ACEIs, or ARBs.

The incidence of radiocontrast-induced renal failure is higher in diabetic patients than in nondiabetic subjects.[94] Recognition of the risk of radiocontrast medium should limit use whenever possible. Besides diabetes, other risk factors include age older than 75 years, hypovolemia, intra-arterial infusion of radiocontrast, CKD, and contrast load. Volume expansion with isotonic sodium chloride and bicarbonate, before and after contrast material administration, may reduce the risk of acute kidney injury.[95] A systematic review of several studies of acetylcysteine for the prevention of contrast-induced nephropathy yields inconsistent results.[96]

UREMIA THERAPY

Internists, family practitioners, and health care extenders should refer their patients with diabetic nephropathy to nephrologists for management of CKD and pre-ESRD education whenever creatinine clearance drops to less than 60 mL/min. Delayed referral to renal specialists negates early arteriovenous fistula construction for hemodialysis and increases morbidity, mortality, and health care resources.[97,98]

When creatinine clearance falls to 30 mL/min, anemia, if present, will improve with an erythropoiesis stimulating agent. At this time, subjects with diabetic nephropathy can learn about available options in renal replacement (RRT), including home or center hemodialysis, continuous ambulatory peritoneal dialysis (CAPD), continuous cyclic peritoneal dialysis (CCPD), and living related or deceased donor kidney transplantation. The modality of RRT must be individualized according to patient's age, preference, education, geographic location, family and social support, and extent of comorbid conditions, particularly cardiovascular disease.

An imperfectly defined number of elderly patients, severely incapacitated by other serious diabetic complications, may refuse or discontinue renal RRT and choose death. Nephrologists and health care providers working in dialysis units should learn how to counsel and help patients refusing dialytic therapy. They should adopt end-of-life care from other disciplines and work with local palliative care and hospice services. It is extremely useful to follow the consensus guidelines published by the Renal Physicians Association/American Society of Nephrology Working Group.[99]

MHD, frequently assigned but not selected by patients, is the most used modality. In its 2008 annual report the USRDS indicated that of 184,258 diabetic ESRD patients receiving uremia therapy in 2006, 76.3% were treated with MHD but only 4.6% were on peritoneal dialysis (PD).[2] About 18.6% of individuals with ESRD-DM had a functioning kidney transplant in the United States in 2006.[2] Although home hemodialysis is, by consensus, superior to dialysis facility, only 737 diabetic subjects chose this modality.[2] Controversy exists as to which dialysis modality, PD or MHD, offers the best survival to subjects with ESRD-DM. Analysis of prevalent patients from 1987 to 1989 indicated that CAPD was associated with a 19% higher all-cause mortality than hemodialysis.[100] This increased risk was greatest in diabetic patients of any age and in those without diabetes older than 55 years.[100] Suboptimal delivery of dialysis and poor management of comorbidities are explanations proposed for these differences. Analyzing data from 6 large-scale registry studies and 3 prospective cohort studies conducted in the United States, Canada, Denmark, and the Netherlands, Vonesh and colleagues[101] reported in 2006 that PD was generally found to be associated with equal or better survival among nondiabetic patients and younger diabetic individuals in all four countries. However, among older diabetic subjects, results varied by country. Whereas in the United States MHD was associated with better survival for diabetics aged 45 years or older, the Canadian and Danish registries showed no difference in survival between PD and MHD among older diabetic patients.

Kidney transplantation is generally accepted as the best option in RRT for all patients, affording greater survival than the best dialytic therapy. In 2007 Rao and colleagues,[102] using the Scientific Registry of Transplant Recipients database, reported a retrospective analysis of 5567 kidney transplant candidates aged 70 years or older. During 1990 to 2004, 2078 candidates received a deceased donor kidney and 360 a living donor transplant. Of the 2078 deceased donor transplant recipients, 688 (33%) received expanded criteria donor kidneys. Mortality risk was compared for those transplanted with that of candidates remaining on the transplant list. Elderly transplant recipients enjoyed a 41% lower overall risk of death than age-matched patients on the transplant waiting list. The relative mortality risk for recipients 70 years or older with ESRD-DM was 47% lower compared with corresponding wait-listed candidates. Although kidney transplant outcomes in the geriatric population have improved, their transplantation rate remains limited. Concerns about limited life expectancy, high comorbidity rates, and relative organ shortage are suggested reasons. Furthermore, in April 2009 McCullough and colleagues[103] recounted that between 1998 and 2006, 23% of patients with ESRD-DM under the age of 50 years received a kidney alone or simultaneous pancreas-kidney transplant (SPK) whereas only 6% of diabetic patients aged 50 to 75 years with ESRD were transplanted. Although a successful combined pancreas and kidney transplant offers excellent glycemic control and better quality of life, only 606 diabetic patients aged 50 to 75 years received an SPK between 1998 and 2006.[103]

Caring for geriatric patients afflicted by diabetic nephropathy is demanding and requires a long-term commitment by patients and health care professionals. This care is better accomplished by a team consisting of a primary care physician or geriatrician, an endocrinologist, a nephrologist, a cardiologist, an ophthalmologist, a podiatrist, a nutritionist, and a nurse-educator. Evidence-based data suggest that the care of elderly patients afflicted by diabetic nephropathy has been suboptimal in the United States.[5] Much effort should be made to diagnose T2-DM early, and educate diabetic subjects and primary care providers about the effectiveness of glycemic control and blood pressure lowering to prevent or delay diabetic nephropathy and ESRD.

REFERENCES

1. Mogensen CE. Definition of diabetic renal disease in insulin-dependent diabetes mellitus based on renal function tests. In: Mogensen CE, editor. The kidney and hypertension in diabetes mellitus. 5th edition. Boston (MA): Kluwer; 2000. p. 13–28.
2. United States Renal Data System. USRDS 2008 annual data report. Bethesda (MD): National Institutes of Health, National Institute of Diabetes and Digestive and Kidney Diseases; 2008.
3. McDonald M, Hertz RP, Unger AN, et al. Prevalence, awareness, and management of hypertension, dyslipidemia, and diabetes among United States adults aged 65 and older. J Gerontol A Biol Sci Med Sci 2009;64(2):256–63.
4. Coresh J, Selvin E, Stevens LA, et al. Prevalence of chronic kidney disease in the United States. JAMA 2007;298(17):2038–47.
5. Patel UD, Young EW, Ojo AO, et al. CKD progression and mortality among older patients with diabetes. Am J Kidney Dis 2005;46(3):406–14.
6. Corsonello A, Pedone C, Corica F, et al. Gruppo Italiano di Farmcovigilanza nel-l'Anziano (GIFA): concealed renal failure and adverse drug reactions in older patients with type 2 diabetes mellitus. J Gerontol A Biol Sci Med Sci 2005;60:1147–51.
7. Abaterusso C, Lupo A, Ortalda V, et al. Treating elderly people with diabetes and stages 3 and 4 chronic kidney disease. Clin J Am Soc Nephrol 2008;3:1185–94.
8. Centers for Disease Control and Prevention. National diabetes fact sheet: general information and national estimates on diabetes in the United States. Atlanta, GA: U.S. Department of Health and Human Services, Centers for Disease Control and Prevention; 2007.
9. Centers for Disease Control and Prevention. Diabetes data and trends. Available at: http://www.cdc.gov/diabetes/statistics/newTrends.htm. Accessed April 18, 2008.
10. Sugarman JR, Reiber GE, Baumgardner G, et al. Use of therapeutic footwear benefit among diabetic medicare beneficiaries in three states, 1995. Diabetes Care 1998;21:777–81.
11. American Diabetes Association. Economic costs of diabetes in the U.S. in 2007. Diabetes Care 2008;31(3):596–615.
12. White KE, Bilous RW. Type 2 diabetic patients with nephropathy show structural-functional relationships that are similar to type 1 disease. J Am Soc Nephrol 2000;11:1667–73.
13. Østerby R, Gall M-A, Schmitz A, et al. Glomerular structure and function in proteinuric type 2 (non-insulin-dependent) diabetic patients. Diabetologia 1993;36:1064–70.
14. Olsen S. Light microscopy of diabetic glomerulopathy: the classic lesions. In: Mogensen CE, editor. The kidney and hypertension in diabetes mellitus. 2nd edition. Boston (MA): Kluwer Academic; 2000. p. 201–10.
15. Mauer SM, Steffes MW, Ellis EN, et al. Structural functional relationships in diabetic nephropathy. J Clin Invest 1984;74:1143–55.
16. Brito PL, Fioretto P, Drummond K, et al. Proximal tubular basement width in insulin-dependent diabetes mellitus. Kidney Int 1998;53:754–61.
17. Lane PH, Steffes MW, Fioretto P, et al. Renal expansion in insulin-dependent diabetes mellitus. Kidney Int 1998;53:754–61.
18. Zhou XJ, Laszik ZG, Silva FG. Anatomical changes in the aging kidney. In: Macias-Nunez JF, Cameron JS, Oreopoulos DG, editors. The aging kidney in health and disease. New York: Springer; 2007. p. 39–54.

19. Nadasdy T, Laszik ZG, Blick KE. Tubular atrophy in the end-stage kidney: a lectin and immunohistochemical study. Hum Pathol 1994;25:22–8.
20. Parving H-H, Gall MA, Skøtt P, et al. Prevalence and causes of albuminuria in non-insulin-dependent diabetic patients. Kidney Int 1992;41(4):758–62.
21. Fioretto P, Mauer M. Histology of diabetic nephropathy. Semin Nephrol 2007; 27(2):195–207.
22. Sawicki P, Kaiser S, Heinemann L, et al. Prevalence of renal artery stenosis in diabetes mellitus: an autopsy study. J Intern Med 1991;229:489–92.
23. Cambier P. Application de la théorie of Rehberg a l'étude clinique des affections rénales du diabète. Ann Med 1943;35:273–99 [French].
24. Christiansen JS, Frandsen M, Parving HH. The effect of intravenous insulin infusion on kidney function on insulin-dependent diabetes mellitus. Diabetologia 1981;20:199–204.
25. Rudberg S, Persson B, Dahlquist G. Increased glomerular filtration rate as a predictor of diabetic nephropathy: an-8 year prospective study. Kidney Int 1992;41:822–8.
26. Christensen CK, Christiansen JS, Schmitz A, et al. Effect of continuous subcutaneous insulin infusion on kidney function and size in IDDM patients: a 2-year controlled study. HNO 1987;1:91–5.
27. Fioretto P, Steffes MW, Sutherland DE, et al. Sequential renal biopsies in insulin-dependent patients: structural factors associated with clinical progression. Kidney Int 1995;48:1929–35.
28. Østerby R. Early phases in the development of diabetic glomerulopathy: quantitative electron microscopic study. Acta Med Scand 1974;S574(Suppl): 3–82.
29. Østerby R, Gunderson HJG. Glomerular size and structure in diabetes mellitus: 1. Early abnormalities. Diabetologia 1975;11:225–9.
30. Mogensen CE, Vestbo E, Poulsen PL, et al. Microalbuminuria and potential confounders. A review and some observations on variability of urinary albumin excretion. Diabetes Care 1995;15:572–81.
31. Eshøj O, Feldt-Rasmussen B, Larsen ML, et al. Comparison of overnight, morning and 24-hour urine collection in the assessment of diabetic microalbuminuria. Diabet Med 1987;4:531–3.
32. Mogensen CE. Microalbuminuria as a predictor of diabetic nephropathy. Kidney Int 1987;31:673–89.
33. Tabei BP, Al-Kassab AS, Ilag LL, et al. Does microalbuminuria predict diabetic nephropathy? Diabetes Care 2001;24:1560–6.
34. Arun CS, Stoddart J, Mackin P, et al. Significance on microalbuminuria in long-duration type 1 diabetes. Diabetes Care 2003;26:2144–9.
35. Messent JW, Elliott TG, Hill RD, et al. Prognostic significance of microalbuminuria in insulin-dependent diabetes mellitus: a twenty-three year follow-up study. Kidney Int 1992;41:836–9.
36. Parving HH, Smidt UM, Friisberg B, et al. A prospective study of glomerular filtration rate and arterial blood pressure in insulin-dependent diabetes with diabetic nephropathy. Diabetologia 1981;20:457–61.
37. Hommel E, Mathiesen ER, Aukland K, et al. Pathophysiological aspects of edema formation in diabetic nephropathy. Kidney Int 1990;38:1187–92.
38. Viberti GC, Wiseman MJ, Pinto JR, et al. Diabetic Nephropathy. In: Kahn CR, Weir GC, editors. Joslin's diabetes mellitus. 13th edition. Philadelphia: Lea & Febiger; 1994. p. 691–737.

39. Mogensen CE. Progression of nephropathy in long-term diabetics with proteinuria and effect of initial antihypertensive treatment. Scan J Lab Invest 1976;36:383–8.

40. Viberti GC, Bilous RW, Mackintosh C, et al. Monitoring glomerular function in diabetic nephropathy: a prospective study. Am J Med 1983;74:256–64.

41. Wasén E, Isoaho R, Mattila K, et al. Renal impairment associated with diabetes in the elderly. Diabetes Care 2004;27:2648–53.

42. de Fine Olivarius N, Andreasen AH, Keiding N, et al. Epidemiology of renal involvement in newly-diagnosed middle-aged and elderly diabetic patients. Cross-sectional data from the population-based study "Diabetes Care in General Practice". Diabetologia 1993;36:1007–16.

43. Damsgaard EM, Frøland A, Jørgensen OD, et al. Prognostic value of urinary albumin excretion rate and other risk factors in elderly diabetic patients and non-diabetic control subjects surviving the first 5 years after assessment. Diabetologia 1994;37(12):1030–6.

44. Standl E, Stiegler H. Microalbuminuria in a random cohort of newly diagnosed type 2 (non-insulin-dependent) diabetic patients living in the greater Munich area. Diabetologia 1993;36:1017–23.

45. UK Prospective Diabetes Study (UKPDS): X. Urinary albumin excretion over 3 years in diet-treated type 2, (non-insulin-dependent) diabetic patients, and association with hypertension, hyperglycemia, and hypertriglyceridaemia. Diabetologia 1993;36:1021–9.

46. American Diabetes Association. Nephropathy in diabetes (position statement). Diabetes Care 2004;27(1):S79–83.

47. European Diabetes Working for Older People. Clinical guidelines for type 2 diabetes mellitus. Available at: http://www.eugms.org/index.php?pid=30; 2004. Accessed January 8, 2008.

48. Brown SF, Mangione CM, Saliba D, et al. California Healthcare Foundation/American Geriatrics Society Panel Improving Care for Elders with Diabetes. Guidelines for improving the care of older persons with diabetes mellitus. J Am Geriatr Soc 2003;51(Suppl 5):S265–80.

49. Wenger NS, Shekelle PG, Roth CP, The ACOVE investigators: introduction to the assessing care of vulnerable elders-3 quality indicator measurement set. J Am Geriatr Soc 2007;55(Suppl 2):S247–52.

50. American Diabetes Association. Standards of medical care in diabetes. Diabetes Care 2009;32(Suppl 1):S13–61.

51. Gaede P, Lund-Andersen H, Parving HH, et al. Effect of multifactorial intervention on mortality in type 2 diabetes. N Engl J Med 2008;358:580–91.

52. Diabetes Control and Complications Trial Research Group. The effect of intensive treatment of diabetes on the development and progression of long-term complications in insulin-dependent diabetes mellitus. N Engl J Med 1993;329:977–86.

53. Intensive blood-glucose control with sulphonylureas or insulin compared with conventional treatment and risk of complications in patients with type 2 diabetes (UKPDS 33) UK Prospective Diabetes Study Group. Lancet 1998;352:837–53.

54. The ADVANCE Collaborative Group. Intensive blood glucose control and vascular outcomes in patients with type 2 diabetes. N Engl J Med 2008;358:2560–72.

55. Action to Control Cardiovascular Risk in Diabetes Study Group. Effects of intensive glucose lowering in type 2 diabetes. N Engl J Med 2008;358:2545–59.

56. Biensenbach G, Raml A, Schmekal B, et al. Decreased insulin requirement in relation to GFR in nephropathic type 1 and insulin treated type 2 diabetic patients. Diabet Med 2003;20:642–5.

57. Winkelmayer WC, Setoguchi S, Levin R, et al. Comparison of cardiovascular outcomes in elderly patients with diabetes who initiated roziglitazone vs. pioglitazone therapy. Arch Intern Med 2008;168(21):2368–75.

58. Lipscombe LL, Gomes T, Lévesque LE, Hux JE, et al. Thiazolidinediones and cardiovascular outcomes in older patients with diabetes. JAMA 2007;298(22):2634–43.

59. Hypertension in Diabetes Study Group. HDS 1. Prevalence of hypertension in newly presenting type 2 diabetic patients and the association with risk factors for cardio-vascular and diabetic complications. J Hypertens 1993;11:309–17.

60. Sproston K, Primatesta P, editors. Health survey for England 2003. Summary of key findings. p. 8–10.

61. Harris MI, Cowie CC, Stern MP, editors. Diabetes in America. 2nd edition. Washington, (DC): National Institutes of Health, National Institute of Diabetes, and Digestive and Kidney Diseases; 1995. p. 117–64.

62. Chobanian AV, Bakris GL, Black HR, et al. Report of the Joint National Committee on prevention, detection, evaluation, and treatment of high blood pressure: the JNC 7 report. JAMA 2003;289:2560–72.

63. Tight blood pressure control and risk of macrovascular and microvascular complications in type 2 diabetes (UKPDS 38) UK Prospective Diabetes Study Group. BMJ 1998;317:703–13.

64. Hansson L, Zanchetti A, Caruthers SG, et al. Effects of intensive blood-pressure lowering and low-dose aspirin in patients with hypertension: principal results of the Hypertension Optimal Treatment (HOT) randomized trial: HOT Study Group. Lancet 1998;351:1755–62.

65. Adler AI, Stratton IM, Neil HA, et al. Association of systolic blood pressure with macrovascular and microvascular complications of type 2 diabetes (UKPDS 36): prospective observational study. BMJ 2000;321:412–9.

66. Young JH, Klag MJ, Muntner P, et al. Blood pressure and decline in kidney function: findings from the Systolic Hypertension in the Elderly Program (SHEP). J Am Soc Nephrol 2002;13:2776–82.

67. Lewis EJ, Hunsicker LG, Bain RP, et al. The effect of angiotensin-converting enzyme inhibition on diabetic nephropathy. N Engl J Med 1993;329:1456–62.

68. Laffel LM, McGill JB, Gans DJ. The beneficial effect of angiotensin-converting enzyme inhibition in normotensive IDDM patients with microalbuminuria. North American Microalbuminuria Study Group. Am J Med 1995;99:497–504.

69. Lewis EJ, Hunsicker LG, Clarke WR, et al. Renoprotective effect of the angiotensin-receptor antagonist irbesartan in patients with nephropathy due to type 2 diabetes. N Engl J Med 2001;345:851–60.

70. Brenner BM, Cooper ME, de Zeeuw D, et al. Effects of Losartan on renal and cardiovascular outcomes in patients with type 2 diabetes and nephropathy. N Engl J Med 2001;345:861–9.

71. Parving HH, Lehnert H, Brochner-Mortensen J, et al. The effect of irbesartan on the development of diabetic nephropathy in patients with type 2 diabetes. N Engl J Med 2001;345:870–8.

72. Heart Outcomes Prevention Evaluation Study Investigators. Effects of ramipiril on cardiovascular and microvascular outcomes in people with diabetes mellitus: results of the HOPE study and MICRO-HOPE substudy. Lancet 2000;355:253–9.

73. Winkelmayer WC, Zhang Z, Shahinfar S, et al. Efficacy and safety on angiotensin II receptor blockade in elderly patients with diabetes. Diabetes Care 2006;29(10):2210–7.

74. Barnett AH, Bain SC, Bouter P, et al. Diabetics Exposed to Telmisartan and Enalapril Study Group. Angiotensin-receptor blockade versus converting-enzyme inhibition in type 2 diabetes and nephropathy. N Engl J Med 2004;351(19): 1952–61.

75. Mann JF, Schmieder RE, McQueen M, et al. Renal outcomes with telmisartan, ramipiril, or both, in people at high vascular risk (the ONTARGET study): a multicentre, randomised, double-blind, controlled trial. Lancet 2008;372(9638): 547–53.

76. UK Prospective Diabetes Study Group. Efficacy of atenolol and captopril in reducing risk of macrovascular and microvascular complications in type 2 diabetes: UKPDS 39. BMJ 1998;317:713–20.

77. Holzgreve H, Nakov R, Beck K, et al. Antihypertensive therapy with verapamil SR plus trandolapril versus atenolol plus chlorthalidone on glycemic control. Am J Hypertens 2003;16:381–6.

78. Giordano M, Matsuda M, Sanders L, et al. Effects of angiotensin-converting enzyme inhibitors, Ca+ channel antagonists, and alpha-adrenergic blockers on glucose and lipid metabolism in NIDDM patients with hypertension. Diabetes 1995;44:665–71.

79. Major cardiovascular in hypertensive patients randomized to doxazosin vs. chlorthalidone: the antihypertensive and lipid-lowering treatment to prevent heart attack trial (ALLHAT) ALLHAT Collaborative Research Group. JAMA 2000;283:1967–75.

80. Hostetter TH, Meyer TW, Rennke HG, et al. Chronic effects of dietary in the rat with intact and reduced renal mass. Kidney Int 1986;30:509–17.

81. Pedrini MT, Levey AS, Lau J, et al. The effect of dietary protein restriction on the progression of diabetic and nondiabetic renal diseases: meta-analysis. Ann Intern Med 1996;124:627–32.

82. Klahr S, Levey AS, Beck GJ, et al. The effects of dietary protein and blood-pressure control on the progression of chronic renal disease. Modification of Diet in Renal Study Group. N Engl J Med 1994;330:877–84.

83. Pijls LT, de Vries H, van Eijk JT, et al. Protein restriction, glomerular filtration rate and albuminuria in patients with type diabetes mellitus: a randomized trial. Eur J Clin Nutr 2002;56(12):1200–7.

84. Kurukulasuriya LR, Athappan G, Saab G, et al. HMG CoA reductase inhibitors and renoprotection: the weight of the evidence. Ther Adv Cardiovasc Dis 2007;1(1):49–59.

85. Vaziri ND. Dyslipidemia of chronic renal failure: the nature, mechanism, and potential consequences. Am J Physiol Renal Physiol 2006;290:F262–72.

86. Vidt DG, Cressman MD, Harris S, et al. Rosuvastatin-induced arrest in progression of renal disease. Cardiology 2004;102:52–60.

87. Kasiske BL, Wanner C, O'Neill WC, National Lipid Association Statin Safety Task Force Kidney Expert Panel. An assessment of statin safety by nephrologists. Am J Cardiol 2006;97:S82–5.

88. Collins R, Armitage J, Parish S, et al. Heart Protection Study Group Collaborative Group. MRC/BHF Heart Protection Study of cholesterol-lowering with simvastatin in 5963 people with diabetes: a randomized placebo-controlled trial. Lancet 2003;361:2005–16.

89. KDOQI clinical practice guidelines and clinical practice recommendations for diabetes and chronic kidney disease. Am J Kidney Dis 2007;49:S1–179.

90. Wanner C, Krane V, März W, et al. German Diabetes and Dialysis Study Investigators. Atorvastatin in patients with type 2 diabetes mellitus undergoing hemodialysis. N Engl J Med 2005;353:238–48.

91. Fellström BC, Jardine AG, Schmieder RE, et al. Aurora Study Group. Rosuvastatin and cardiovascular events in patients undergoing hemodialysis. N Engl J Med 2009;360:1395–407.

92. Oates JA, Fitzgerald GA, Branch RA, et al. Clinical implications of prostaglandin and thromboxane A2 formation. N Engl J Med 1988;319(12):761–7.

93. Perazella MA, Eras J. Are selective COX-2 inhibitors nephrotoxic. Am J Kidney Dis 2000;35(5):937–40.

94. Parfrey PS, Griffiths SM, Barrett BJ, et al. Contrast material-induced renal failure in patients with diabetes mellitus, renal insufficiency and both. A prospective controlled study. N Engl J Med 1989;321:395–7.

95. Weisbord SD, Palevsky PM. Prevention of contrast-induced nephropathy with volume expansion. Clin J Am Soc Nephrol 2008;3(1):273–80.

96. Bagshaw SM, Ghali WA. Acetylcysteine for prevention of contrast-induced nephropathy after intravascular angiography: a systemic review and meta-analysis. BMC Med 2004;2:38.

97. Jungers P, Zingraff J, Albouze P. Late referral to maintenance hemodialysis: detrimental consequences. Nephrol Dial Transplant 1993;8:1089–93.

98. Woods JD, Port FK. The impact of vascular access for hemodialysis on patient survival. Nephrol Dial Transplant 1997;12:657–9.

99. Shared decision-making in the appropriate initiation of and withdrawal from dialysis. Renal Physicians Association and American Society of Nephrology, Washington, DC, 2000.

100. Bloemberg WE, Port FK, Mauger EA, et al. A comparison of mortality between patients treated with hemodialysis and peritoneal dialysis. J Am Soc Nephrol 1995;6:177–83.

101. Vonesh EF, Snyder JJ, Foley RN, et al. Mortality studies comparing peritoneal dialysis and hemodialysis: what do they tell us. Kidney Int Suppl 2006;103: S3–11.

102. Rao PS, Merion RM, Ashby VB, et al. Renal transplantation in elderly patients older than 70 years of age: results from the Scientific Registry of Transplants Recipients. Transplantation 2007;83(8):1069–74.

103. McCullough KP, Keith DS, Meyer KH, et al. Kidney and pancreas transplantation in the United States, 1998-2007: access for patients with diabetes and end-stage renal disease. Am J Transplant 2009;9:894–906.

Hypertension in the Elderly

Maria Czarina Acelajado, MD[a,c,*], Suzanne Oparil, MD[b]

KEYWORDS

- Elderly • Hypertension • Pathophysiology
- Diagnosis • Management

Hypertension is an important modifiable risk factor for cardiovascular morbidity and mortality and for chronic occlusive peripheral arterial disease, congestive heart failure, aortic aneurysm, and chronic kidney disease. The risk of death from ischemic heart disease (IHD) or stroke increases dramatically in a log-linear fashion for blood pressure (BP) levels higher than 115/75 mm Hg, even in individuals without known vascular disease at baseline.[1] The probability of dying from IHD or stroke is doubled for every 20 mm Hg increase in systolic BP (SBP) or 10 mm Hg elevation in diastolic BP (DBP) in middle-aged and elderly persons. An SBP reduction of 5 mm Hg in the population can decrease stroke mortality by 14% and CVD mortality by 9%.[2]

The elderly comprise a significant subset of the population with hypertension, because the prevalence of hypertension increases with advancing age. Data from the National Health and Nutrition Examination Survey from 1999 to 2004 show that 60% of all adults aged 60 to 69 years and up to 77% of those older than 80 years have hypertension.[3] The lifetime risk for developing hypertension in persons who are normotensive at age 55 to 65 years is very high, exceeding 90%,[4] and is mainly accounted for by an age-related increase in SBP. Although the DBP in the population plateaus in the fifth and sixth decades of life and then slowly declines thereafter, SBP levels continue to climb, leading to an increase in pulse pressure (PP) and the predominance of isolated systolic hypertension (ISH) in the elderly (**Fig. 1**).[5] In persons older than 50 years, the risk for death from IHD and stroke is positively related to SBP and inversely related to DBP,[6–8] underscoring the importance of increased PP as a predictor of mortality in older patients.[9,10] Furthermore, combining SBP with DBP and PP with mean arterial pressure predicts cardiovascular disease (CVD) risk better than each component taken singly, which, in elderly subjects with hypertension, emphasizes the importance of increased arterial stiffness in stratifying CVD risk.[11]

[a] Vascular Biology and Hypertension Program of the Division of Cardiovascular Disease, Department of Medicine, School of Medicine, University of Alabama at Birmingham, USA
[b] Vascular Biology and Hypertension Program of the Division of Cardiovascular Disease, Department of Medicine, School of Medicine, University of Alabama at Birmingham, USA
[c] Vascular Biology and Hypertension Program, 1530 3rd Avenue South, CH19 Room 115, Birmingham, Alabama 35294-2041, USA
* Corresponding author. Vascular Biology and Hypertension Program, 1530 3rd Avenue South, CH19 Room 115, Birmingham, Alabama 35294-2041.
E-mail address: czarina.acelajado@ccc.uab.edu (M.C. Acelajado).

Clin Geriatr Med 25 (2009) 391–412
doi:10.1016/j.cger.2009.06.001
0749-0690/09/$ – see front matter © 2009 Elsevier Inc. All rights reserved.

geriatric.theclinics.com

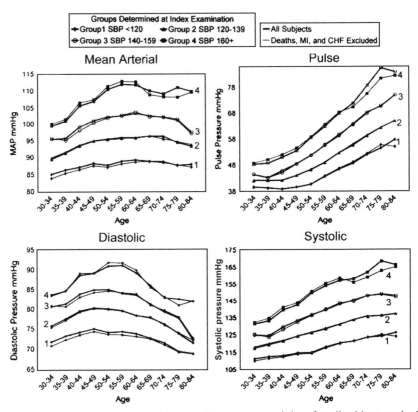

Fig. 1. Arterial pressure components by age: Group-averaged data for all subjects and with deaths, MI, and CHF excluded. Averaged blood pressure levels from all available data from each subject within 5-year age intervals (30–34 through 80–84) by SBP groupings 1 through 4. Thick line represents entire study cohort (2036 subjects); thin line represents study cohort with deaths and nonfatal MI or CHF excluded (1353 subjects). (*From* Franklin SS, Gustin W, Wong ND, et al. Hemodynamic patterns of age-related changes in blood pressure. The Framingham Heart Study. Circulation 1997;96:310; with permission.)

PATHOPHYSIOLOGY
Arterial Stiffness

The phenomenon of increased SBP and PP in old age is partially explained by structural changes in the arterial media that occur with aging. These include loss of vascular smooth muscle cells, increase in vessel wall collagen content and collagen fiber cross-linking, calcium deposition, and disruption and thinning of the elastic fibers.[12] These changes are most marked at the level of the large elastic arteries, such as the aorta,[13] and bring about increased arterial thickness resulting from remodeling and a loss of elastic properties, leading to abnormal dilation of the vessel. The result is a stiff artery that has decreased capacitance and limited recoil and is thus unable to accommodate the changes that occur during the cardiac cycle. As a result, the artery becomes ineffective in converting the intermittent nature of blood flow generated by the pumping heart into more continuous flow. During systole, the aged arterial tree exhibits limited expansion and fails to effectively buffer the pressures generated by the heart, causing an increase in peak BP. Further, the loss of recoil during diastole results in a reduction in DBP. The elevated pulsatile load resulting from these changes, that is, the increased PP, damages the heart and the vasculature, increasing cardiovascular risk.

The velocity of the pressure waves generated by cardiac contractions as they travel along the arterial tree, the pulse wave velocity (PWV), rises with increased vascular stiffness. In the normal subject, pressure waves travel distally from the heart along the arterial tree during systole and are reflected back to the heart from points of branching, areas of increased arterial stiffness, and high-resistance arterioles in the periphery during diastole.[14] In contrast, the increased vascular stiffness that occurs with aging causes an increase in PWV such that the reflected waves reach the heart earlier, in late systole. By this process, increased vascular stiffness augments systolic pressure, increases cardiac afterload, and amplifies the pulsatile nature of blood flow (**Fig. 2**).[15,16] PWV is assessed noninvasively by measuring the time delay in the arrival of a predefined part of the arterial pulse wave from a proximal to a distal vessel (**Fig. 3**). These measurements can be done simultaneously in both vessels or sequentially, using the R wave of the electrocardiogram as reference. The carotid-femoral PWV is most commonly measured, but brachial-ankle, aorta-femoral, and femoral-tibial PWV measurements are also used.[15] An elevation in PWV, particularly the carotid-femoral PWV, has been shown to be an independent predictor of cardiovascular mortality and morbidity in elderly patients with hypertension.[17,18]

Functional mechanisms also contribute to the age-related increases in arterial stiffness and SBP. Endothelial dysfunction is more common in the elderly, especially elderly persons with hypertension, and is due mainly to decreased bioavailability of nitric oxide (NO).[19] NO plays a key role in regulation of vasomotor tone and thrombosis by promoting vasodilation and inhibiting platelet aggregation.[20] Endothelial dysfunction is most commonly assessed sonographically by measuring the degree of arterial dilation after hyperemia, flow-mediated dilation (FMD). A peripheral artery, such as the brachial, is typically used. In elderly persons with ISH, the FMD is less

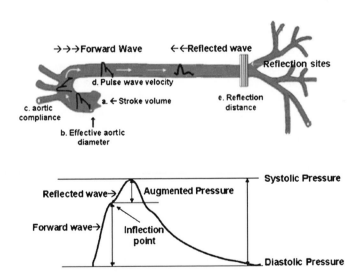

Fig. 2. Pulse wave and the nature of reflected waves. Pulse pressure is a function of the stroke volume, compliance and diameter of the aorta, PWV, and the distance from the reflection points to the heart. With the stiffened aorta with aging, the reflected waves reach the heart earlier, causing an augmentation of SBP and PP. (*From* Vasan RS. Pathogenesis of elevated peripheral pulse pressure. Hypertension 2008;51:34; with permission.)

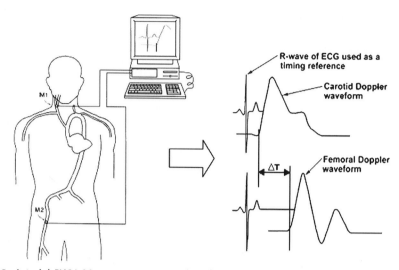

Fig. 3. Arterial PWV. Measurements are taken from 2 points, usually a proximal (M1) and a distal (M2) artery. PWV is measured as D/δT (m/s), where D is the distance between the 2 points and δT is the time delay between the arrival of the pulse wave at these 2 points. In machines that measure the PWV from M1 and M2 sequentially, the R wave of the electrocardiogram is used as reference. (*From* Wang X, Keith JC, Struthers AD, et al. Assessment of arterial stiffness, a translational medicine biomarker system for evaluation of vascular risk. Cardiovasc Ther 2008;26:216; with permission.)

than in age-matched normotensive and younger (mean age, 37 years) normotensive controls, signifying that endothelial dysfunction is present.[21] Because of impaired vasodilation, endothelial dysfunction contributes to the arterial stiffness found in elderly patients with hypertension.

Salt-sensitivity

Increased salt sensitivity, characterized by increases in BP in response to a sodium load, occurs in older individuals, particularly in those with hypertension, as a result of an aging-related decrease in renal function that limits the ability of the kidney to excrete a sodium load.[22] Other mechanisms that contribute to salt sensitivity and hypertension in the elderly include a decline in activity of membrane sodium-potassium and calcium adenosine triphosphate pumps, leading to an excess of intracellular calcium and sustained vasoconstriction, thereby increasing vascular resistance.[23] Decreased activity of the sodium pump and age-associated increases in salt sensitivity of BP can also result from an age-related increase in endogenous sodium pump inhibitors, such as marinobufagenin.[24] Genetic factors, such as polymorphisms of the angiotensin converting enzyme (ACE) gene, may also play a role in the pathogenesis of salt sensitivity in the elderly.[25,26] Lastly, the decline in estrogen production following menopause enhances salt sensitivity in elderly women, likely resulting from cessation of estrogen-related natriuretic effects, including NO synthesis and inhibition of angiotensin II receptor activation in the kidney.[27]

Neurohormonal Mechanisms

Neurohormonal mechanisms that play a major role in BP regulation in younger subjects, that is, the renin-angiotensin-aldosterone system and the sympathetic nervous system (SNS), are altered with aging. There is a progressive decline in baseline plasma renin activity and renin secretion after stimuli such as standing, salt-depletion, or furosemide administration.[28,29] Plasma renin activity at age 60 years is ~40% to 60% of the levels found in younger subjects under similar conditions.[30] Moreover, in the elderly, there is a sluggish aldosterone response to acute stimuli such as sodium deprivation or increased potassium intake. In contrast, net basal SNS activity increases with advancing age. Peripheral plasma norepinephrine concentration in individuals aged 65 years and older is double the level found in younger subjects.[31] This is attributed to increased catecholamine spillover into the plasma, coupled with reduced clearance of norepinephrine resulting from a combination of reduced renal function and decreased neuronal reuptake, particularly in the heart.

DIAGNOSIS

The Seventh Joint National Committee on Prevention, Detection, Evaluation, and Treatment of High Blood Pressure (JNC 7) has defined criteria for normal BP, prehypertension, and stage 1 and 2 hypertension (**Table 1**).[32] The diagnosis requires that the BP readings be taken after the patient has been seated quietly for 5 minutes, using an appropriately sized cuff, with the arm supported and at the level of the heart. The patient should have abstained from caffeine, smoking, and exercise half an hour before taking the BP. An elevated BP found as an average of two readings per visit on two or more clinic visits is recommended to establish a diagnosis of hypertension.

Once the diagnosis of hypertension is confirmed, the evaluation is now directed at assessing lifestyle, searching for other cardiovascular risk factors that may affect prognosis and treatment, identifying secondary causes of hypertension (**Box 1**), and looking for evidence of target-organ damage. This is especially true in the elderly, who typically present with multiple risk factors and comorbidities.

Routine laboratory examinations before initiating therapy include a 12-lead electrocardiogram, urinalysis, determination of blood glucose, hematocrit, creatinine, serum potassium, and calcium levels, and a lipoprotein profile.[32] If the patient presents with a clinical picture consistent with an identifiable cause of hypertension, ancillary diagnostic procedures may be done if clinically warranted. This is particularly true in patients whose BP is difficult to control.

Hypertension and Kidney Disease in the Elderly

Chronic kidney disease (CKD) is a major comorbidity among elderly patients with hypertension, with 77% of patients older than 60 years having both conditions.[3] Elevated BP is a strong and independent risk factor for the development of end-stage renal disease, with a greater risk associated with increased SBP versus an increased DBP.[33,34]

Table 1
Classification of blood pressure for adults

Blood Pressure Classification	SBP (mm Hg)	DBP (mm Hg)
Normal	<120	and <80
Prehypertension	120–139	or 80–89
Stage 1 hypertension	140–159	or 90–99
Stage 2 hypertension	>160	or >100

Data from Chobanian AV, Bakris GL, Black HR, et al. Seventh Report of the Joint National Committee on Prevention, Detection, Evaluation, and Treatment of High Blood Pressure. Hypertension 2003;42:1206–52.

> **Box 1**
> **Identifiable causes of hypertension**
>
> Chronic kidney disease
>
> Hyperaldosteronism
>
> Renovascular hypertension
>
> Cushing syndrome
>
> Obstructive sleep apnea
>
> Pheochromocytoma
>
> Coarctation of the aorta
>
> Increased intracranial pressure
>
> Thyroid/parathyroid disease
>
> *Data from* Chobanian AV, Bakris GL, Black HR, et al. Seventh Report of the Joint National Committee on Prevention, Detection, Evaluation, and Treatment of High Blood Pressure. Hypertension 2003;42:1206–52.

Furthermore, among patients with ISH, baseline serum creatinine and the presence of subclinical or overt proteinuria predict a higher mortality rate.[35] An increased PP in elderly patients has been found to be inversely related to the glomerular filtration rate [36] Further, a stepwise increase in the prevalence of ISH has been found with increasing stages of CKD, even in those who did not have hypertension before the onset of CKD.[37] These findings emphasize the important relationship of BP, particularly SBP and PP, with kidney function, particularly in the elderly.

TREATMENT
Goal of Antihypertensive Treatment

The goal of antihypertensive treatment is to lower the BP to reduce cardiovascular and renal morbidity and mortality. Lowering the BP produces benefit in both older and younger persons, with no difference between the age groups in the risk reduction achieved per unit of BP reduction.[38] JNC 7 recommends a BP goal of less than 140/90 in individuals with uncomplicated hypertension, regardless of age. In patients with hypertension and CKD or diabetes mellitus (DM), the goal BP is less than 130/80, irrespective of age. Further, JNC 7 advocates that attaining an SBP of less than 140 mm Hg should be the primary objective of antihypertensive treatment, because in most patients with hypertension, the DBP goal will be achieved once the SBP goal is reached.[32] This goal structure has been questioned for the elderly subgroup, because outcome trials that have shown treatment benefit in the elderly have generally used a threshold SBP greater than 160 mm Hg and a goal SBP of ~150 mm Hg **(Fig. 4)**.[6,39–42] Data on the benefit of reducing the SBP further are lacking. Further, in elderly patients with hypertension, reducing the SBP to less than 140 mm Hg may be achieved at the expense of an excessively low DBP, associated with an increased risk for death.[43] Randomized controlled trials with different treatment thresholds and goals are needed to address this important issue.

Lifestyle Modification

Lifestyle modification is an integral part of treatment of the elderly patient with hypertension. There is strong evidence that maintaining an ideal body weight, engaging in regular aerobic activity for a minimum of 30 minutes per session on most days of the

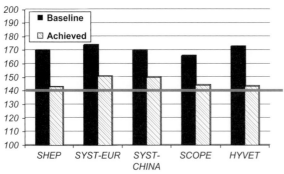

Fig. 4. Baseline- and achieved-SBP levels in clinical trials on hypertension involving elderly patients. SBPs achieved by active treatment in placebo-controlled trials (except Study on Cognition and Prognosis in the Elderly [SCOPE]) in elderly patients with hypertension. Gray line denotes goal BP set by JNC 7.

week, restricting sodium intake to 2.4 g (or 6 g of sodium chloride) per day, and limiting alcohol intake to two drinks per day will reduce BP (**Table 2**).[44–47] Evidence that lifestyle modification reduces CVD outcomes in patients with hypertension is less strong. Most trials of lifestyle modification have not lasted long enough or did not enroll a sufficient number of subjects to provide adequate data on clinical outcomes in patients with hypertension. In 10- to 15-year follow-up studies of the Trials of Hypertension Prevention I and II (TOHP I and TOHP II), which tested nonpharmacologic interventions in reducing BP in middle-aged subjects with prehypertension, it was shown that there was a 25% reduction in risk for CVD in the groups randomized to sodium reduction.[48] Further, combining a high potassium diet with sodium reduction was associated with lower cardiovascular risk on follow-up than either intervention alone.[49]

A landmark study of lifestyle modification in the elderly is the Trial of Nonpharmacologic Interventions in the Elderly (TONE),[45] in which 975 subjects with hypertension aged 60 to 80 years were randomized to one of four groups, that is, sodium reduction, weight loss, a combination of both, or usual care. Study participants were taking a single antihypertensive agent at the time of randomization, and 90 days after the first group-intervention session, weaning from the antihypertensive medication was initiated, with a goal of discontinuing the drug altogether. TONE tested the hypotheses that sodium reduction and/or weight loss would result in reductions in BP and

Table 2
Degree of BP reduction achieved with lifestyle modifications in elderly patients with hypertension

Intervention	Definition	Degree of SBP/DBP (mm Hg) Reduction
Dietary sodium restriction	Limit sodium intake to <80 mmol/d	3.4 to 7.2/1.9 to 3.2[45,46]
Increased physical activity	Aerobic activity lasting 30 min done thrice weekly	8.5/5.1[47]
Weight reduction	Weight loss of 4.5 kg	4/1.1[45]
Limiting alcohol intake	Limit alcohol intake to <2 drinks per day	1.2/0.7[44,a]

[a] Subjects involved were of mean age 58 ± 10.9 years.

therefore the need for reinstituting antihypertensive therapy and cardiovascular events and death. Specifically, the primary end points for the study were the occurrence of any of the following after attempted withdrawal of the antihypertensive medication: high BP reading (SBP > 190 mm Hg or DBP > 110 mm Hg at one study visit; or mean SBP > 170 mm Hg or mean DBP > 100 mm Hg at two sequential visits; or mean SBP > 150 mm Hg or mean DBP > 90 mm Hg at three sequential visits), resumption of antihypertensive drug, myocardial infarction (MI), stroke, congestive heart failure (CHF), angioplasty, or coronary bypass surgery.

In TONE, a goal of −4.5 kg was set for the participants in the weight-loss and combination arms, using a combination of diet and increased physical activity. Average weight loss among participants in the weight-loss arm was 3.5 kg and 47% achieved the goal of −4.5 kg after 9 months; 39% of subjects in the weight-loss arm did not experience an increase in BP or a need to reinstitute BP-lowering medications for 30 months after discontinuing antihypertensive drugs. Weight loss, best achieved by regular physical activity and avoidance of excessive caloric intake, was well tolerated and was not associated with adverse events. Weight loss is thus encouraged among obese or overweight elderly patients, and achievement and maintenance of the ideal body weight should be targeted.

Owing to greater salt sensitivity in the elderly, older age predicts treatment success in sodium intervention trials for the treatment of hypertension.[50] In TONE, the goal of sodium reduction to less than 80 mmol/d (1.8 g/d) was achieved by only 36% of the study participants in the sodium-reduction arm. Despite this, 72% of those assigned to a low-sodium diet had their BP controlled to less than 140/90 mm Hg, and 38% of these patients remained off antihypertensive medications for 30 months.[45] In another study performed in the United Kingdom, lowering dietary salt from 10 g/d to less than 5 g/d for 1 month reduced urinary sodium excretion by 83 mmol/d and lowered supine BP by 7.2/3.2 mm Hg in a population of elderly normotensive (n = 18) and hypertensive (n = 29) subjects.[46] Dietary sodium restriction has been shown to decrease BP and improve large elastic-artery compliance in elderly persons with hypertension,[51] consistent with the concept that dietary sodium may contribute to large-artery stiffness in these patients. In addition to reduction of sodium, a diet rich in fruits, vegetables, and low-fat dairy products, with limited cholesterol and saturated fat is advocated for patients with hypertension (the Dietary Approaches to Stop Hypertension, or the DASH diet),[52] except for those with CKD, for whom the increased potassium and protein may be harmful. Dietary modification, although difficult for most persons, is an important adjunct to medical hypertension treatment.

Regular aerobic exercise, consisting of a minimum of 30 minutes of interval training on a treadmill done thrice weekly, has been shown to be a useful adjunct to the treatment of hypertension in the elderly.[47] Adherence to the 12-week exercise program in this study lowered SBP by 8.5 mm Hg, DBP by 5.1 mm Hg, and PP by 3.2 mm Hg on 24-hour ambulatory BP monitoring among elderly patients with hypertension, and this was well tolerated by the study participants.

A position paper from the American Society of Hypertension advocates a comprehensive lifestyle intervention, that is, a combination of diet (reduced salt intake, high potassium intake, and moderate alcohol consumption, with limited cholesterol and saturated fat) and physical activity and weight loss to substantially lower BP and improve BP control, particularly among elderly patients with hypertension.[53] A 6-month lifestyle intervention has been shown to decrease BP by 4.2/4.9 mm Hg among elderly subjects with borderline elevations of DBP.[54] This beneficial effect on BP was achieved in the context of significant (−2.1 kg) weight loss but without significant reduction in urinary sodium excretion. Lifestyle interventions have been found to be safe and well tolerated among the elderly. Furthermore, the adoption of healthy life-style changes and weight reduction has been associated with other benefits, namely, improvement of lipid profile, glucose tolerance, cardiovascular risk, and well being of patients.

Pharmacologic Treatment

Randomized controlled trials have consistently demonstrated that antihypertensive therapy in the elderly is effective in preventing total mortality, stroke, and coronary events.[6] The Systolic Hypertension in the Elderly Program (SHEP) study examined the benefit of BP lowering using chlorthalidone with or without atenolol versus placebo in 4736 elderly subjects with ISH.[39] Subjects had to be older than 60 years, with baseline SBP > 160 mm Hg and DBP < 90 mm Hg. SHEP showed that chlorthalidone-based therapy lowered the incidence of cardiovascular death by 32%, stroke by 36%, heart failure by 54%, and myocardial infarction by 27%, after a mean follow-up of 4.5 years. In the European Trial on Systolic Hypertension in the Elderly (SYST-EUR), 4695 patients aged 60 years and older with ISH were randomized to the calcium-channel blocker (CCB) nitrendipine versus placebo, with the possible addition of hydrochlorothiazide and enalapril or matching placebo.[40] After a mean follow-up of 2 years, nitrendipine-based treatment reduced the SBP by 23 mm Hg and the DBP by 7 mm Hg. Active treatment significantly decreased the incidence of stroke by 42% and all fatal and nonfatal cardiac end points by 26%. A similar trial in China, Systolic Hypertension in China (SYST-CHINA), also using nitrendipine versus placebo, showed a reduction in SBP by 20 mm Hg and DBP by 5 mm Hg in the active treatment group, associated with a reduction in total strokes of 38% and in all fatal and nonfatal cardiovascular end points by 37%.[41] All-cause mortality was decreased by 39%.

At the time the results of these trials were combined with older studies involving elderly subjects with hypertension in a meta-analysis, active treatment produced significant reductions in total mortality (13%), stroke (30%), and coronary events (23%) compared with the control group, which was a placebo in seven of the eight studies included.[6] The number needed to treat for 5 years to prevent one major fatal or nonfatal cardiovascular event was fewer in men than in women (18 vs 38), in subjects older than 70 years than in those aged 60 to 69 years (19 vs 39), in those with preexisting CVD (16 vs 37), and in those with a PP higher than 90 mm Hg (63 vs 119). Thus, older persons and those with stiff vessels or preexisting CVD derived particular benefit from antihypertensive treatment.

The benefits of hypertension treatment persisted long after termination of the studies. For example, in a 14-year follow-up of the SHEP trial, subjects who had been randomized to chlorthalidone had a lower incidence of cardiovascular death compared with placebo, similar to the findings during the double-blind phase of the trial.[55] There was no significant difference in stroke or all-cause mortality between the treatment arms in the 14-year follow-up. Data from SYST-EUR demonstrated greater benefit of early initiation of antihypertensive treatment in ISH. After a mean follow-up of 2 years in the double-blind phase, 3517 of the 4409 subjects who were still alive entered a 4-year open-label phase, whereby they were given nitrendipine with the possible addition of enalapril or hydrochlorothiazide. The subjects who were initially randomized to active treatment and to placebo in the double-blind phase of the trial comprised the immediate and delayed treatment arms of the extended follow-up study, respectively. Immediate versus delayed treatment decreased the incidence of stroke by 28% and cardiovascular complications by 15%, with early initiation of treatment preventing 17 strokes or 25 cardiovascular events per 1000 patients treated.[56] This highlights the need for immediate recognition and prompt initiation of treatment of ISH once the diagnosis is confirmed, to provide the greatest impact on reducing cardiovascular risk.

Selection of Pharmacologic Agents

Thiazide-type diuretics, either alone or in combination with other agents, are recommended by JNC 7 as initial agents in the treatment of hypertension.[32] These agents are preferred because of an extensive volume of data showing that they decrease stroke and cardiovascular mortality in elderly patients with hypertension and because of their wide availability and low cost. In the Antihypertensive and Lipid-Lowering Treatment to Prevent Heart Attack Trial (ALLHAT), a total of 42,418 participants whose average age at enrollment was 67 years were randomized to chlorthalidone, lisinopril, amlodipine, or doxazosin. The doxazosin arm was terminated early because of an excess of combined cardiovascular events and heart failure compared with the chlorthalidone arm. Chlorthalidone was comparable to amlodipine and lisinopril in preventing major coronary events and in increasing survival and was superior to the other agents in preventing some secondary outcomes, for example, heart failure.[57] These effects were the same in the subgroup of participants older than 65 years as in younger participants.

Thiazide diuretics have benefits that are distinct from their effects on BP and CVD outcomes. They act on the distal nephron to increase calcium reabsorption and reduce calcium excretion in a manner that is related reciprocally to their effects on sodium reabsorption or natriuresis.[58] The effect of thiazides on calcium reabsorption constitutes the basis for their usefulness in preventing the formation of calcium-containing renal stones and may also explain their protective effects on rates of bone mineral loss and prevention of hip fracture.[59–61]

A downside of thiazide diuretic-based treatment in elderly patients with hypertension, who may have contracted intravascular volumes and impaired baroreflexes, is an increased incidence of orthostatic hypotension.[62] Also, thiazide diuretics are associated with various metabolic side effects, including electrolyte abnormalities (hypokalemia and hyponatremia being most common), dyslipidemia, insulin resistance, and new-onset DM.[63] In ALLHAT, chlorthalidone treatment was associated with a higher incidence of new-onset diabetes in patients with or without preexisting metabolic syndrome or dysglycemia compared with lisinopril or amlodipine.[57,64,65] Mean fasting blood glucose in the chlorthalidone arm was 3 to 7 mg/dL higher than that in the amlodipine and lisinopril arms after 2 years of follow-up. The odds ratios for developing new-onset DM (defined as plasma glucose levels >6.9 mmol/L) were lower for amlodipine and lisinopril than chlorthalidone treatment. However, after 4 to 6 years of follow-up, although subjects randomized to chlorthalidone still had increased odds of developing new-onset diabetes compared with those randomized to amlodipine or lisinopril, the odds ratios were no longer significantly different.[65]

Whether the metabolic effects of diuretics have adverse consequences for CVD outcomes has been questioned. For example, in ALLHAT, there was no significant increase in any outcome (stroke, total mortality, coronary heart disease, heart failure, and end-stage renal disease) in subjects who developed incident DM while on chlorthalidone compared with those who did not develop DM while on the same regimen.[65] Incident DM in patients who were randomized to chlorthalidone was associated with a lower relative risk of all-cause mortality, combined CVD, heart failure, and end-stage renal disease than was incident DM in the other two treatment arms (lisinopril and amlodipine). Likewise, in a 14-year follow-up study of SHEP, subjects who were randomized to chlorthalidone and who developed elevated glucose levels during the trial had no increased risk for cardiovascular mortality compared with subjects who did not develop incident DM on chlorthalidone treatment. In contrast, subjects with preexisting DM or those who developed DM while on placebo had an increased incidence of death from cardiovascular causes compared with subjects without DM.[66] These findings suggest that thiazide diuretics lead to elevated glucose levels and chemical DM by way of mechanisms distinct from those associated with the development of naturally occurring DM, and that the occurrence of new-onset DM in the context of thiazide diuretic treatment does not seem to increase the risk of clinically significant events, such as cardiovascular mortality.

Other classes of antihypertensive drugs, including ACE inhibitors and CCBs, have outcome benefit compared with placebo in elderly patients with hypertension.[40,41,67] A meta-analysis done by the Blood Pressure Lowering Treatment Trialists' Collaboration analyzed results of 31 trials that compared an ACE inhibitor or a CCB versus placebo or compared different antihypertensive drug regimens (ACE inhibitor versus diuretic or β-blocker, CCB versus diuretic or β-blocker, and ACE inhibitor versus CCB).[38] The Trialists examined the outcome benefit of various antihypertensive drugs on total major cardiovascular events (fatal and nonfatal stroke, nonfatal myocardial infarction or death from coronary heart disease, or heart failure) and compared the effects on the primary outcome between two age groups (<65 years and >65 years). The analysis showed treatment benefit in younger (<65 years) and older (>65 years) subjects with hypertension, with no strong evidence that the outcome benefit in the elderly differed greatly between antihypertensive drug classes, which included diuretics or β-blockers (the conventional antihypertensive agents), CCBs, and ACE inhibitors. The degree of BP lowering provided the same incremental reduction in risk for cardiovascular events in elderly subjects with hypertension as in younger subjects; hence the beneficial effects were attributed primarily to BP reduction achieved rather than the choice of drug. Thus, no strong evidence was found in this study to support the use of one antihypertensive class over another in treating elderly patients with hypertension, so long as a similar degree of BP lowering is achieved.

In contrast, several large outcome trials provide evidence for benefits of antihypertensive treatment that are unrelated to BP reduction. The Losartan Intervention For Endpoint reduction in hypertension study (LIFE) compared the effects of losartan-based treatment to atenolol-based treatment on CVD outcomes in 9193 participants (mean age, 70 years) with essential hypertension and left ventricular hypertrophy by electrocardiogram.[68] Losartan-based treatment produced significantly greater reductions in CVD outcomes (driven by stroke) than atenolol-based treatment despite an average difference of only 1 mm Hg between the treatment groups, suggesting that losartan exerts benefits beyond BP lowering. The lack of BP difference between treatment groups was substantiated by 24-hour ambulatory BP monitoring (ABPM) in a substudy of 110 LIFE participants in a single site in Denmark.[69] Similarly, in the Anglo-Scandinavian Cardiac Outcomes Trial–Blood Pressure Lowering Arm (ASCOT-BPLA), which compared amlodipine with or without perindopril versus atenolol with or without bendroflumethiazide in 19,257 high-risk subjects with hypertension, found that treatment based on amlodipine was superior in preventing a composite of cardiovascular mortality, myocardial infarction, and stroke with a similar degree of BP reduction.[70] Further, the Avoiding Cardiovascular Events through Combination Therapy in Patients Living with Systolic Hypertension (ACCOMPLISH) Trial demonstrated that an ACE inhibitor-CCB combination (benazepril and amlodipine) was superior to a combination of an ACE inhibitor and a diuretic (benazepril and hydrochlorothiazide) in preventing a composite of fatal and nonfatal cardiovascular end points in the absence of a BP difference between groups.[71] A 24-hour ABPM analysis of a large subset of ACCOMPLISH participants showed that the BP differences between the treatment arms was small and favored the ACE inhibitor-diuretic combination, an effect that was not concordant with the CVD outcomes.[72] These findings demonstrate that differences in CVD outcomes are not entirely explained by better BP control in many antihypertensive treatment trials.

The usefulness of β-blockers as first-line treatment of hypertension in older persons has been questioned. A meta-analysis of trials that involved older subjects with hypertension demonstrated that β-blocker–based treatment, particularly with atenolol, was associated with a 16% higher risk of stroke compared with other anti-hypertensive drug classes.[73] Further, when compared with placebo, β-blockers reduced mortality risk in subjects with hypertension by only 19%, only half the risk reduction achieved with other antihypertensive drug classes. In an older meta-analysis of 10 trials involving a total of 16,154 elderly patients with hypertension who were treated with a diuretic versus a β-blocker, diuretic-based treatment was found to be more effective in reducing fatal and nonfatal stroke, cardiovascular mortality, and all-cause mortality.[74] Thus, there is no convincing evidence that traditional β-blockers, particularly atenolol, given as initial treatment of hypertension, are more effective than placebo in reducing outcomes in the elderly. Studies involving newer β-blockers, such as carvedilol and nebivolol, have shown some advantage over atenolol or metoprolol in elderly patients with ISH in reducing PP[75] and improving endothelial function assessed by FMD,[76] but whether this translates into clinically relevant outcomes remains to be determined. Moreover, β-blocker use has been associated with increased insulin resistance and worsening glycemic control in diabetic patients, and again these effects are less pronounced with newer agents (eg, carvedilol) versus older ones (eg, metoprolol).[77] Despite these caveats, β-blockers are important agents for use in the treatment of elderly patients with hypertension with comorbidities such as coronary artery disease and CHF and as second- or third-line agents in others.

The debate about which antihypertensive drug class should be used first in elderly patients with hypertension has been rendered moot by the repeated demonstration that most elderly patients with hypertension need more than one drug for BP control. The JNC 7 guidelines recommend initiating treatment with combination therapy if the baseline SBP is more than 20 mm Hg or DBP is more than 10 mm Hg higher than the goal.[32] Combining antihypertensive drugs with complementary mechanisms of action has many benefits, including greater antihypertensive efficacy and lower rates of dose-related adverse events, because lower doses of the individual components than would be used in monotherapy can be administered.[78] The use of fixed-dose combination pills may also lower overall cost (because of reduction in number of copays required) and improve medication adherence in elderly individuals with hypertension.[79] JNC 7 encourages the use of diuretics, both as first-line treatment and in combination with other drugs. The choice of a second agent or a first-line drug, if a patient cannot take thiazide-type diuretics, may be dependent on the presence of compelling indications that require the use of a certain drug class for treatment of a concomitant condition (Table 3). Most common antihypertensive regimens involve an ACE inhibitor or an angiotensinogen II receptor blocker combined with a diuretic or a CCB. Triple combinations that include a diuretic, rennin-angio-tensin-aldosterone-system blocker, and a CCB are currently under development.

ACCOMPLISH, performed in high-risk elderly patients (average age on entry was 68 years), has challenged the "diuretics first" concept by demonstrating that the ACE-CCB combination lowered the primary end point by 19.6% compared with the control

Table 3
Compelling Indications for antihypertensive drugs

Compelling Indications	Diuretic	β-Blocker	ACE Inhibitor	ARB	CCB	Aldosterone Antagonist
Heart failure	✔	✔	✔	✔	—	✔
Postmyocardial infarction	—	✔	✔	—	—	✔
High coronary disease risk	✔	✔	✔	—	✔	—
Diabetes	✔	✔	✔	✔	✔	—
Chornic kidney disease	—	—	✔	✔	—	—
Recurrent stroke prevention	✔	—	✔	—	—	—

Abbreviation: ARB, Angiotensinogen II receptor blocker.
Data from Chobanian AV, Bakris GL, Black HR, et al. Seventh Report of the Joint National Committee on Prevention, Detection, Evaluation, and Treatment of High Blood Pressure. Hypertension 2003;42:1206–52.

group. ACCOMPLISH has been criticized on the basis of its use of low-dose hydrochlorothiazide. Chlorthalidone, used in ALLHAT and other National Heart, Lung, and Blood Institute–sponsored trials, has a longer duration of action than hydrochlorothiazide, and it is more effective in lowering BP.[80] In the Multiple Risk Factor Intervention Trial (MRFIT), hydrochlorothiazide was associated with an unfavorable trend in mortality, and hence the protocol was amended after about 5 years of randomization, and chlorthalidone was used in place of hydrochlorothiazide.[81] Consequently, this change was associated with a more favorable mortality trend.[82] The 24-hour ABPM results of ACCOMPLISH suggest that the putative inferior pharmokinetic properties of hydrochlorothiazide could not be responsible for the inferior outcome of that arm of the study because BP tended to be lower in the diuretic arm.[72] Further, CCBs are considered metabolically neutral because they do not induce the metabolic side effects of thiazide diuretics; hence their use in patients with hypertension, particularly those with metabolic syndrome, may be advantageous. Lastly, in a meta-analysis of 13 trials, nine of which involved subjects who had hypertension and were older than 60 years, CCBs have been found to decrease the risk of stroke more effectively than other antihypertensive agents.[83]

Health care providers have a variety of effective drug combinations with which to treat hypertension in the elderly, with even more to come. The polypill concept, which advocates combining agents to treat multiple cardiovascular conditions, for example, hypertension, dyslipidemia, and coagulation, in a single preparation, has been widely espoused for the elderly because of their heavy burden of risk factors and their need for more convenient dosing regimens.[84] A phase II trial, The Indian Polycap Study (TIPS), has been completed with a form of polypill, the Polycap, which incorporates a low-dose thiazide (12.5 mg), atenolol (50 mg), ramipril (5 mg), simvastatin (20 mg), and aspirin (100 mg) in a single pill taken once daily.[85] The trial enrolled subjects aged 45 to 80 years without CVD and with at least one risk factor and has shown effective reduction of multiple risk factors, which is comparable to the individual drugs taken separately. Further, the Polycap had excellent tolerability. This approach may supercede individualized antihypertensive therapy for many elderly patients in a variety of health care settings, but further studies are needed to evaluate its effects on hard outcomes, such as reduction of mortality. Expert panels that are currently developing guidelines for antihypertensive treatment are weighing the totality of evidence supporting different approaches to initiating treatment in the elderly. Revised guidelines from JNC 8 are expected in the year 2010.

Treating Hypertension in the Oldest Old

Evidence concerning the risks and benefits of treating hypertension in the oldest old, that is, older than 80 years, has been limited, because this age group has usually been excluded from participating in clinical trials. The Swedish Trial in Old Patients with Hypertension (STOP-Hypertension) study, which randomized elderly subjects with hypertension, up to age 84 years, to any of 3 β-blockers, a diuretic combination, or placebo, showed that those on active treatment had lower BP levels and fewer primary end points (stroke, myocardial infarction, or any other cardiovascular cause of death).[86] Data from STOP-Hypertension and from other randomized controlled trials that included participants older than 80 years showed that in this age group, antihypertensive treatment decreased the risk of stroke by 36%, but was associated with a nonsignificant 6% excess risk for death from any cause.[87] However, the Hypertension in the Very Elderly Trial (HYVET), which enrolled 3845 patients aged 80 years and older with a baseline SBP more than 160 mm Hg, demonstrated that, compared with placebo, thiazide-based antihypertensive treatment (indapamide with or without perindopril) significantly reduces the risk for death from stroke (by 39%) and death from any cause (by 21%) and incidence of heart failure (by 64%).[88] Treatment goal was 150/80, and this was achieved in nearly 50% of subjects after 2 years of the trial. The subjects tolerated treatment well, with comparable rates of adverse events in both arms of the study. Because of the large sample size, this study provided conclusive proof of the benefit of treating hypertension in the very old.

Some features of the HYVET design merit comment. The study excluded subjects with clinical dementia and those who required nursing care, which make up a significant proportion of persons in this age group. Because of this, the results may not be universally applicable to patients with hypertension who are older than 80 years. Health care providers will need to use clinical judgment in deciding whom to treat and how aggressively to treat BP in elderly persons with hypertension with important physical or cognitive impairment.

COMPLEXITIES OF BLOOD PRESSURE TREATMENT IN THE ELDERLY

The treatment of hypertension in the elderly presents many challenges. Elderly persons with hypertension usually take several medications for a variety of concomitant conditions, mostly chronic, and this makes them more likely to mismanage their antihypertensive medications. Many medications frequently taken by elderly patients, such as nonsteroidal antiinflammatory drugs (NSAIDs), interfere with the actions of antihypertensive medications. Orthostatic hypotension occurs commonly in the elderly and may be exacerbated by antihypertensive treatment, creating a barrier against achieving adequate BP control. High BP also exacerbates aging-related cognitive decline and may predispose to the development of dementia in the elderly. The higher incidence of cognitive and memory impairment in the elderly necessitates the use of simple antihypertensive regimens to improve medication adherence and BP control.

Medication Nonadherence

Nonadherence to medications may partially explain the poor BP control rates seen in the elderly. It is estimated that as many as 24% of patients with chronic cardiovascular conditions, including hypertension, do not take their medications as prescribed.[89] Polypharmacy, which is common in the elderly, compounds the problem, and typically, rates of adherence drop as the number of pills taken per day increases.

Simplification of treatment regimens by using combination pills has been shown to improve adherence.[90–92] Patients who have been seen by their physician in the previous year have also been shown to be more adherent to treatment, highlighting the important role of physicians in promoting adherence. Lastly, behavioral techniques, such as getting feedback from patients regarding their medication use and the adoption of shared decision-making between the patient and the health care provider in the formulation of treatment regimens,[93] may help improve adherence rates, particularly in the elderly population.

Effect of Concomitant Medications on BP Control

Classes of drugs that commonly interfere with the efficacy of antihypertensive medications include, but are not limited to, NSAIDs, certain cold formulations, steroids, estrogen-containing drugs, alcohol, erythropoeitin, and certain herbal preparations.[32]

Osteoarthritis is common in the elderly population. Usual treatment of this condition includes NSAIDs and selective cyclooxygenase-2 inhibitors (COX-2), which provide pain control and antiinflammatory action. These drugs are notorious for worsening BP control in patients with hypertension by inhibiting prostaglandin E_2 and prostacyclin production by the kidney, resulting in sodium retention and vasoconstriction.[94] NSAIDs also interfere with the actions of many antihypertensive drug classes, causing SBP elevations as great as 6 mm Hg.[95] The BP-lowering effects of ACE inhibitors are blunted to a greater degree by concomitant NSAID intake compared with other antihypertensive drug classes.[96,97] Nonselective NSAIDs and COX-2 inhibitors produce these effects.[98] The degree of BP elevation is related to the type of NSAID and seems to be greatest for piroxicam and indomethacin.[96,99]

Aspirin, which is also commonly prescribed in the elderly population, can produce the same BP elevations as NSAIDs by virtue of its similar inhibitory effects on vasodilator prostaglandins. However, low-dose aspirin, the dose most commonly used in primary and secondary prevention of cardiovascular outcomes, has not been shown to have a significant influence on BP control in elderly persons with hypertension undergoing treatment to lower BP.[100]

Orthostatic Hypotension

In healthy elderly subjects, there is a tendency for the SBP to decrease by up to 5 mm Hg on standing, whereas DBP is maintained.[101] The prevalence of orthostatic hypotension, defined as a supine-to-standing SBP decrease greater than 20 mm Hg or DBP decrease greater than 10 mm Hg,[32] among elderly subjects with hypertension, has been reported to range from 12% to 55%. Orthostatic hypotension increases in prevalence with advancing age and with increasing numbers of medications taken.[102–104]

Orthostatic hypotension in the elderly has been attributed to an age-related diminution of baroreflex activation that occurs with standing.[105,106] Orthostatic hypotension is associated with dizziness, difficulty walking, frequent falls, history of myocardial infarction or transient ischemic attack, syncope, and the presence of carotid artery stenosis on ultrasonography.[104]

The risk for developing orthostatic hypotension requires that medications for hypertension be started at low doses and titrated slowly to achieve the goal BP. Alpha-blockers, combination α-β-blockers, diuretics, and nitrates are known to cause or aggravate orthostatic hypotension. In addition, certain antidepressants (trazodone, paroxetine, sertraline, venlafaxine) and antipsychotics (risperidone, olanzapine, quetiapine) have been found to cause a drop in BP on standing.[62] The presence of orthostatic hypotension in an elderly person with hypertension clearly puts the patient at an increased risk, warrants a review of his/her drug regimen, and clearly poses a challenge to achieving optimum BP control. Elderly patients with hypertension should be evaluated for postural hypotension periodically by checking standing BPs.

Dementia

Cognitive impairment is associated with aging, and dementia occurs commonly among elderly adults, with an estimated overall prevalence of ~8%.[107] Hypertension plays a role in the pathogenesis of cognitive impairment in the elderly. An elevated BP in midlife is predictive of dementia in the later years.[108] In elderly adults, a high SBP (>180 mm Hg) and a low DBP (<70 mm Hg) are risk factors for dementia.[109] Antihypertensive treatment is associated with a reduction in risk for cognitive impairment. In the SYST-EUR trial, treatment of hypertension reduced the incidence of dementia by 65% compared with the placebo control group.[110] However, in the much older patients enrolled in HYVET, the reduction of dementia with antihypertensive treatment was not statistically significant.[111] This was attributed to the trial's early termination, which may not have allowed sufficient time for the benefits of antihypertensive treatment on the rate of cognitive decline to become fully manifest.

The higher incidence of cognitive impairment in the elderly warrants that BP treatment regimens be simplified to improve adherence and therefore BP control. This may be accomplished by the use of combination pills, where applicable, and once-daily dosing. It is the physician's responsibility to ensure that the patient and/or his caregiver comprehend the treatment plan, including the dosing of medications, during the office visit.

SUMMARY

Hypertension is an important risk factor for cardiovascular morbidity and mortality, particularly in the elderly, in whom it is highly prevalent. BP elevation in the elderly is a result of structural and functional changes in the arterial tree and alterations in salt-sensitivity and neurohormonal mechanisms that occur with aging. Treatment of hypertension has been shown to significantly affect the elderly population, as shown by dramatic reductions in stroke, heart failure, myocardial infarction, and all-cause mortality. Hypertension treatment also decreases the incidence of cognitive impairment and dementia in the elderly. The adoption of a healthy lifestyle, which includes diet, physical activity, and maintenance of ideal body weight, is a cornerstone of hypertension management, with benefits extending beyond BP lowering. A comprehensive lifestyle intervention may reduce the need for antihypertensive medications in the elderly. Evidence indicates that several classes of antihypertensive drugs are effective in preventing cardiovascular events, but that no single drug is adequate to control BP in most elderly patients with hypertension. Accordingly, treatment decisions should be guided by the presence of compelling indications such as diabetes or heart failure and by the tolerability of individual drugs or drug combinations in individual patients. The concomitant intake of certain medications, especially NSAIDs, that counter the effects of antihypertensive drugs and the frequent occurrence of orthostatic hypotension complicate treatment in older patients and drive down BP control rates. The rapid growth of the elderly population mandates that clinicians should be prepared to handle the increase in disease burden from hypertension in the years to come.

REFERENCES

1. Lewington S, Clarke R, Qizilbash N, et al, for the Prospective Studies Collaboration. Age-specific relevance of usual blood pressure to vascular mortality: a meta-analysis of individual data for 1 million adults in 61 prospective studies. Lancet 2002;360:1903–13.
2. Whelton PK, He J, Appel LJ, et al. Primary prevention of hypertension: clinical and public health advisory from the National High Blood Pressure Education Program. JAMA 2002;288:1882–8.
3. Ostchega Y, Dillon CF, Hughes JP, et al. Trends in hypertension prevalence, awareness, treatment, and control in older U.S. adults: data from the National Health and Nutrition Examination Survey 1988 to 2004. J Am Geriatr Soc 2007;55:1056–65.
4. Vasan RS, Beiser A, Seshadri S, et al. Residual lifetime risk for developing hypertension in middle-aged women and men: the Framingham Heart Study. JAMA 2002;287:1003–10.
5. National High Blood Pressure Education Program Working Group. National High Blood Pressure Education Program Working Group report on hypertension in the elderly. Hypertension 1994;23(3):275–85.
6. Staessen JA, Gasowski J, Wang JG, et al. Risks of untreated and treated isolated systolic hypertension in the elderly: meta-analysis of outcome trials. Lancet 2000;355:865–72.
7. Pastor-Barriuso R, Banegas JR, Damian J, et al. Systolic blood pressure, diastolic blood pressure, and pulse pressure: an evaluation of their joint effect on mortality. Ann Intern Med 2003;139:731–9.
8. Psaty BM, Furberg CD, Kuller LH, et al. Association between blood pressure level and the risk of myocardial infarction, stroke, and total mortality. Arch Intern Med 2001;161:1183–92.
9. Domanski MJ, Davis BR, Pfeffer MA, et al. Isolated systolic hypertension: prognostic information provided by pulse pressure. Hypertension 1999;34:375–80.
10. Franklin SS, Larson MG, Khan SA, et al. Does the relationship of blood pressure to coronary heart disease risk change with aging? The Framingham Heart Study. Circulation 2001;103(9):1245–9.
11. Franklin SS, Lopez VA, Wong ND, et al. Single versus combined blood pressure components and risk for CVD. The Framingham Heart Study. Circulation 2009;119:243–50.
12. Dao HH, Essalihi R, Bouvet C, et al. Evolution and modulation of age-related medial elastocalcinosis: impact on large artery stiffness and isolated systolic hypertension. Cardiovasc Res 2005;66:307–17.
13. Mitchell GF, Parise H, Benjamin EJ, et al. Changes in arterial stiffness and wave reflection with advancing age in healthy men and women: the Framingham Heart Study. Hypertension 2004;43:1239–45.
14. Nichols WW, O'Rourke MF. Wave reflections. McDonald's blood flow in the arteries. London: Hodder Headline Group; 2005. p. 193.
15. Schriffin EL. Vascular stiffening and arterial compliance. Am J Hypertens 2004;17:39S–48S.
16. Wang X, Keith JC, Struthers AD, et al. Assessment of arterial stiffness, a translational medicine biomarker system for evaluation of vascular risk. Cardiovasc Ther 2008;26:214–23.
17. Laurent S, Boutouyrie P, Asmar R, et al. Aortic stiffness is an independent predictor of all-cause and cardiovascular mortality in hypertensive patients. Hypertension 2001;37:1236–41.

18. Sutton-Tyrrell K, Najjar SS, Boudreau RM, et al. Elevated aortic pulse wave velocity, a marker of arterial stiffness, predicts cardiovascular events in well-functioning older adults. Circulation 2005;111:3384–90.
19. Taddei S, Virdis A, Mattei P, et al. Aging and endothelial function in normotensive subjects and essential hypertensive subjects. Circulation 1995;91:1981–7.
20. Walsh MB, Donnelly T, Lyons D. Impaired endothelial nitric oxide bioavailability: a common link between aging, hypertension and atherogenesis? J Am Geriatr Soc 2009;57:140–5.
21. Wallace SML, Yasmin, McEniery CM, et al. Isolated systolic hypertension is characterized by increased aortic stiffness and endothelial dysfunction. Hypertension 2007;50:228–33.
22. Epstein M, Hollenberg NK. Age as a determinant of renal sodium conservation in normal man. J Lab Clin Med 1976;87:411–7.
23. Zemel MB, Sowers JR. Salt sensitivity and systemic hypertension in the elderly. Am J Cardiol 1988;61(16):7H–12H.
24. Anderson DE, Fedorova OV, Morrell CH, et al. Endogenous sodium pump inhibitors and age-associated increases in salt sensitivity of blood pressure in normotensives. Am J Physiol Regul Integr Comp Physiol 2008;294: R1248–54.
25. Luft FC, Miller JZ, Weinberger MH, et al. Genetic influences on the response to dietary sodium reduction, acute salt loading, or salt depletion in humans. J Cardiovasc Pharmacol 1988;12(3):S49–55.
26. Dengel DR, Brown MD, Ferrell RE, et al. Role of angiotensin converting enzyme genotype in sodium sensitivity in older hypertensives. Am J Hypertens 2001;14: 1178–84.
27. Colylewright M, Reckelhoff JE, Ouyang P. Menopause and hypertension an age-old debate. Hypertension 2008;51:952–9.
28. Weidmann P, De Mytternere-Burstein S, Maxwell MH, et al. Effect of aging on plasma renin and aldosterone in normal men. Kidney Int 1975;8:325–33.
29. Wilson TW, McCaulay FA, Waslen TA. Effects of aging on responses to furosemide. Prostaglandins 1989;38:675–87.
30. Epstein M. Aging and the kidney. J Am Soc Nephrol 1992;43(7):1100–22.
31. Seals DR, Esler MD. Human ageing and the sympathoadrenal system. J Physiol 2000;528(3):407–17.
32. Chobanian AV, Bakris GL, Black HR, et al. Seventh report of the Joint National Committee on prevention, detection, evaluation, and treatment of high blood pressure. Hypertension 2003;42:1206–52.
33. Klag MJ, Whelton PK, Randall BL, et al. Blood pressure and end-stage renal disease in men. N Engl J Med 1996;334:13–8.
34. Young JH, Klag MJ, Muntner P, et al. Blood pressure and decline in kidney function: findings from the Systolic Hypertension in the Elderly Program (SHEP). J Am Soc Nephrol 2002;13:2776–82.
35. De Leeuw PW, Lutgarde T, Birkenhager WH, et al. Prognostic significance of renal function in elderly patients with isolated systolic hypertension: results from the Syst-Eur trial. J Am Soc Nephrol 2002;13:2213–22.
36. Verhave JC, Fesler P, du Cailar G, et al. Elevated pulse pressure is associated with low renal function in elderly patients with isolated systolic hypertension. Hypertension 2005;45:586–91.
37. Cheng L, Gao Y, Gu Y, et al. Stepwise increase in the prevalence of isolated systolic hypertension with the stages of chronic kidney disease. Nephrol Dial Transplant 2008;23:3895–900.

38. Turnbull F, et al. Blood Pressure Lowering Trialists' Collaboration. Effects of different regimens to lower blood pressure on major cardiovascular events in older and younger adults: meta-analysis of randomized trials. BMJ 2008;336: 1121–3.
39. SHEP Cooperative Research Group. Prevention of stroke by antihypertensive drug treatment in older persons with isolated systolic hypertension: final results of the Systolic Hypertension in the Elderly Program (SHEP). JAMA 1991;265: 3255–64.
40. Staessen JA, Fagard R, Thijs L, et al. Randomised double-blind comparison of placebo and active treatment for older patients with isolated systolic hypertension. Lancet 1997;350:757–64.
41. Liu L, Wang JG, Gong L, et al. Comparison of active treatment and placebo in older Chinese patients with isolated systolic hypertension. J Hypertens 1998; 16:1823–9.
42. Lithell H, Hansson L, Skoog I, et al. The Study on Cognition and Prognosis in the Elderly (SCOPE): principal results of a randomized double-blind intervention trial. J Hypertens 2003;21:875–86.
43. Ungar A, Pepe G, Lambertucci L, et al. Low diastolic ambulatory blood pressure is associated with greater all-cause mortality in older patients with hypertension. J Am Geriatr Soc 2009;57:291–6.
44. Cushman WC, Cutler JA, Hanna E, et al. Prevention and Treatment of Hypertension Study (PATHS): effects of an alcohol treatment program on blood pressure. Arch Intern Med 1998;58:1197–207.
45. Whelton PK, Appel LJ, Espeland MA, et al. Sodium reduction and weight loss in the treatment of hypertension in older persons. JAMA 1998;279:839–46.
46. Cappuccio FP, Markandu ND, Carney C, et al. Double blind randomised trial of modest salt restriction in older people. Lancet 1997;350:850–4.
47. Westhoff TH, Franke N, Schmidt S, et al. Too old to benefit from sports? The cardiovascular effects of exercise training in elderly subjects treated for isolated systolic hypertension. Kidney Blood Press Res 2007;30:240–7.
48. Cook NR, Cutler JA, Obarzanek E, et al. Long-term effects of dietary sodium reduction on cardiovascular disease outcomes: observational follow-up of the Trials Of Hypertension Prevention (TOHP). BMJ 2007;334:885.
49. Cook NR, Obarzenek E, Cutler JA, et al. Joint effects of sodium and potassium intake on subsequent cardiovascular disease. Arch Intern Med 2009;169(1): 32–40.
50. Grobbee DE, Hofman A. Does sodium restriction lower blood pressure? Br Med J 1986;293:27–30.
51. Gates PE, Tanaka H, Hiatt WR, et al. Dietary sodium restriction rapidly improves large elastic artery compliance in older adults with systolic hypertension. Hypertension 2004;44:35–41.
52. Appel LJ, Moore TJ, Obarzanek E, et al. A clinical trial of the effects of dietary patterns on blood pressure. N Engl J Med 1997;336:1117–24.
53. Appel LJ on behalf of the American Society of Hypertension Writing Group. ASH Position Paper on dietary approaches to prevent and treat hypertension. J Clin Hypertens, Accessed June 18, 2009. DOI 10.1111/j.1751-7176.2009.00136.X.
54. Applegate WB, Miller ST, Elam JT, et al. Nonpharmacologic intervention to reduce blood pressure in older patients with mild hypertension. Arch Intern Med 1992;152:1162–6.
55. Patel AB, Kostis JB, Wilson AC, et al. Fourteen-year follow-up of the Systolic Hypertension in the Elderly Program. Stroke 2008;39:1084–9.

56. Staessen JA, Thijs L, Fagard R, et al. Effects of immediate versus delayed antihypertensive therapy on outcome in the Systolic Hypertension in Europe Trial. J Hypertens 2004;22:847–57.
57. Furberg CD, Wright JT, Davis BR, et al, for the ALLHAT Officers and Coordinators for the ALLHAT Collaborative Research Group. Major outcomes in high-risk hypertensive patients randomized to angiotensin-converting enzyme inhibitor or calcium channel blocker versus diuretic. JAMA 2002;288:2981–97.
58. Costanzo LS. Localization of diuretic action in microperfused rat distal tubules: Ca and Na transport. Am J Physiol 1985;248:F527–35.
59. Ray WA, Griffin MR, Downey W, et al. Long-term use of thiazide diuretics and risk of hip fracture. Lancet 1989;1:687–90.
60. Wanich R, Davis J, Ross P, et al. Effects of thiazides on rates of bone mineral loss: a longitudinal study. Br Med J 1990;310:1303–5.
61. Reid IR, Ames IW, Orr-Walker BJ, et al. Hydrochlorothiazide reduces loss of cortical bone in normal post-menopausal women: a randomized controlled trial. Am J Med 2000;109:362–70.
62. Poon IO, Braun U. High prevalence of orthostatic hypotension and its correlation with potentially causative medications among elderly veterans. J Clin Pharm Ther 2005;30:173–8.
63. Lind L, Pollare T, Berne C, et al. Long-term metabolic effects of hypertensive drugs. Am Heart J 1994;128:1177–83.
64. Black HR, Davis B, Barzilay J, et al. Metabolic and clinical outcomes in nondiabetic individuals with the metabolic syndrome assigned to chlorthalidone, amlodipine or lisinopril as initial treatment for hypertension. Diabetes Care 2008;31: 353–60.
65. Barzilay JI, Davis BR, Cutler JA, et al. Fasting glucose levels and incident diabetes mellitus in older nondiabetic adults randomized to receive 3 different classes of antihypertensive treatment. Arch Intern Med 2006;166:2191–201.
66. Kostis JB, Wilson AC, Freudenberger RS, et al. Long-term effect of diuretic-based therapy on fatal outcomes in subjects with isolated systolic hypertension with and without diabetes. Am J Cardiol 2005;95:29–35.
67. Gianni M, Bosch J, Pogue J, et al. Effects of long-term ACE inhibitor therapy in elderly vascular disease patients. Eur Heart J 2007;28:1382–8.
68. Dahlof B, Devereux RB, Kjeldsen SE, et al. Cardiovascular morbidity and mortality in the Losartan Intervention For Endpoint reduction in hypertension study (LIFE): a randomized trial against atenolol. Lancet 2002;359:995–1003.
69. Bang LE, Winberg N, Wachtell K, et al. Losartan versus atenolol on 24-hour ambulatory blood pressure. A LIFE substudy. Blood Press 2007;16:392–7.
70. Dahlof B, Sever PS, Poulter NR, et al. Prevention of cardiovascular events with an antihypertensive regimen of amlodipine adding perindopril as required versus atenolol adding benzoflumethiazide as required, in the Anglo-Scandinavian Cardiac Outcomes Trial – Blood Pressure Lowering Arm (ASCOT-BPLA): a multicentre randomized controlled trial. Lancet 2005;366:895–906.
71. Jamerson K, Weber MA, Bakris GL, et al. Benazepril plus amlodipine or hydrochlorothiazide for hypertension in high-risk patients. N Engl J Med 2008;359(23): 2417–28.
72. Jamerson KA, Weber MA. Benazepril plus amlodipine or hydrochlorothiazide for hypertension. N Engl J Med 2009;360:1147–50, Correspondence.
73. Lindholm LH, Carlberg B, Samuelsson O. Should β-blockers remain first choice in the treatment of primary hypertension? A meta-analysis. Lancet 2005;366: 1545–53.

74. Messerli FH, Grossman E, Goldbourt U. Are beta-blockers efficacious as first-line therapy for hypertension in the elderly? A systematic review. JAMA 1998; 279(23):1903–7.

75. Dhakam Z, Yasmin, McEniery CM, et al. A comparison of atenolol and nebivolol in isolated systolic hypertension. J Hypertens 2008;26(2):351–6.

76. Jawa A, Nachimuthu S, Pendergrass M, et al. Beta blockers have a beneficial effect upon endothelial function and microalbuminuria in African American subjects with diabetes and hypertension. J Diabet Complications 2008;22(5): 303–8.

77. Bakris GL, Fonseca V, Katholi RE, et al. Metabolic effects of carvedilol versus metoprolol in patients with type 2 diabetes and hypertension. JAMA 2004;292: 2227–36.

78. Oparil S, Weber M. Angiotensin receptor blocker and dihydropyridine calcium channel blocker combinations: an emerging strategy in hypertension therapy. Postgrad Med 2009;121:25–39.

79. Dickson M, Plauschinat CA. Compliance with antihypertensive therapy in the elderly. Am J Cardiovasc Drugs 2008;8(1):45–50.

80. Ernst ME, Carter BL, Goerdt CJ, et al. Comparative antihypertensive effects of hydrochlorothiazide and chlorthalidone on ambulatory and office blood pressure. Hypertension 2006;47:352–8.

81. Bartsch GE, Broste SK, Grandits GA, et al. Hydrochlorothiazide, chlorthalidone and mortality in the Multiple Risk Factor Intervention Trial. Circulation 1984; 70(Suppl II):II–360.

82. Multiple Risk Factor Intervention Trial Research Group. Mortality after 10½ years for hypertensive participants in the Multiple Risk Factor Intervention Trial. Circulation 1990;82:1616–28.

83. Angela F, Verdecchia P, Riboldi GP, et al. Calcium channel blockade to prevent stroke in hypertension. Am J Hypertens 2004;17:817–22.

84. Wald LJ, Law MR. A strategy to reduce cardiovascular disease by more than 80%. BMJ 2003;326:1419.

85. Yusuf S, Pais P, Afzal R, et al. Effects of a polypill (Polycap) on risk factors in middle aged individuals without cardiovascular disease (TIPS): a phase II, double blind, randomized trial. Lancet 2009;373:1341–51.

86. Dahlof B, Hansson L, Lindholm LH, et al. Morbidity and mortality in the Swedish Trial in Old Patients with Hypertension (STOP-Hypertension). Lancet 1991;338: 1281–5.

87. Gueyffier F, Bulpitt C, Boissel J, et al. Antihypertensive drugs in very old people: a subgroup meta-analysis of randomised controlled trials. Lancet 1999;353: 793–6.

88. Beckett NS, Peters R, Flaetcher AE, et al. Treatment of hypertension in patients 80 years of age or older. N Engl J Med 2008;358(18):1887–98.

89. DiMatteo MR. Variations in patients' adherence to medical recommendations: a quantitative review of 50 years of research. Med Care 2004;42:200–9.

90. Kripalani S, Yao X, Haynes RB. Interventions to enhance medication adherence in chronic medical conditions. A systematic review. Arch Intern Med 2007;167: 540–50.

91. Chapman RH, Petrilla AA, Benner JS, et al. Predictors of adherence to concomitant antihypertensive and lipid-lowering medications in older adults: a retrospective, cohort study. Drugs Aging 2008;25(10):885–92.

92. Bangalore S, Kamalakkannan G, Parkar S, et al. Fixed-dose combinations improve medication compliance: a meta-analysis. Am J Med 2007;120(8):713–9.

93. Banning M. Older people and adherence to medication: a review of the literature. Int J Nurs Stud 2008;45:1550–61.

94. Frishman WH. Effects of nonsteroidal antiinflammatory drug therapy on blood pressure and peripheral edema. Am J Cardiol 2002;89:18D–25D.

95. Ishiguro C, Fukita T, Omori T, et al. Assessing the effects of nonsteroidal antiinflammatory drugs on antihypertensive drug therapy using post-marketing surveillance database. J Epidemiol 2008;18(3):119–24.

96. Pavlicevic I, Kuzmanic M, Rumboldt M, et al. Interaction between antihypertensives and NSAIDS in primary care: a controlled trial. Can J Clin Pharmacol 2008; 15(3):e372–82.

97. Wilson SL, Poulter NR. The effect of nonsteroidal antiinflammatory drugs and other commonly used nonnarcotic analgesics on blood pressure levels in adults. J Hypertens 2006;24:1457–69.

98. Whelton A, White WB, Bello AE, et al. Effects of celecoxib and rofecoxib on blood pressure and edema in patients 65 years of age with systemic hypertension and osteoarthritis. Am J Cardiol 2002;90:959–63.

99. Morgan TO, Anderson A, Bertram D. Effects of indomethacin on blood pressure in elderly people with essential hypertension well-controlled with amlodipine or enalapril. Am J Hypertens 2000;13:1161–7.

100. Avancini F, Palumbo G, Alli C, et al. Effects of low-dose aspirin on clinic and ambulatory blood pressure in treated hypertensive patients. Am J Hypertens 2000;13:611–6.

101. Beckett NS, Connor M, Sadler JD, et al. Orthostatic fall in blood pressure in the very elderly hypertensive: results from the Hypertension in the Very Elderly Trial (HYVET)—pilot. J Hum Hypertens 1999;13:839–40.

102. Hiitola P, Enlund H, Kettunen R, et al. Postural changes in blood pressure and the prevalence of orthostatic hypotension among home-dwelling elderly aged 75 years or older. J Hum Hypertens 2009;23:33–9.

103. Cohen I, Rogers P, Burke B, et al. Predictors of medication use, compliance and symptoms of hypotension in a community-based sample of elderly men and women. J Clin Pharm Ther 1998;23:423–32.

104. Rutan GH, Hermanson B, Bild DE, et al. Orthostatic hypotension in older adults. The Cardiovascular Health Study. Hypertension 1992;19:508–19.

105. Kaplan DT, Furman MI, Pincus SM, et al. Aging and the complexity of cardiovascular dynamics. Biophys J 1991;59:945–9.

106. Shi X, Wray W, Formes KJ, et al. Orthostatic hypotension in aging humans. Am J Physiol Heart Circ Physiol 2000;279:H1548–54.

107. Fratiglioni L, De Ronchi D, Agüero-Torres H. World-wide prevalence and incidence of dementia. Drugs Aging 1999;15:365–75.

108. Launer L, Masaki K, Petrovitch H, et al. The association between midlife blood pressure levels and late-life cognitive function. JAMA 1995;274:1846–51.

109. Qiu C, Winblad B, Fratiglioni L. The age-dependent relation of blood pressure to cognitive function and dementia. Lancet Neurol 2005;4:487–99.

110. Forette F, Seux M, Staessen J, et al. Prevention of dementia in a randomised double blind placebo controlled Systolic Hypertension in Europe (Syst-Eur) trial. Lancet 1998;352:1347–51.

111. Peters R, Beckett N, Forette F, et al. Incident dementia and blood pressure lowering in the Hypertension in the Very Elderly Trial cognitive function assessment (HYVET-COG): a double-blind, placebo controlled trial. Lancet Neurol 2008;7:683–9.

Glomerular Disease in the Elderly

Richard J. Glassock, MD, MACP

KEYWORDS

- Glomerulonephritis • Nephrotic syndrome
- Immunosuppressive therapy • Primary glomerular disease
- Secondary glomerular disease

It is widely recognized that acute and chronic glomerular disease is a common cause of disability and mortality in the elderly population.[1,2] The underlying cause of the glomerular disease in this population is diverse but can generally be divided into those that affect the kidneys primarily (primary glomerular disease) and those in which the kidney damage is a part of a system-wide process (secondary glomerular disease). Regardless of the underlying cause, the clinical features can be condensed into a few "clinical syndromes." The comorbid features associated with advancing age have important modifying influences on the clinical presentation and course of glomerular disease. This article briefly outlines the common presentations of glomerular disease in the elderly and discusses the clinical features, prognosis, and management of the primary and secondary glomerular diseases in this population of patients.

CLINICAL PRESENTATION

The common clinical syndromes at presentation for glomerular disease are given in **Box 1**.

Acute nephritic syndrome (ANS) is characterized by the abrupt onset of hematuria and proteinuria often accompanied by edema, hypertension, and reduced renal function (impaired glomerular filtration rate or GFR). In the elderly, due to concomitant chronic ischemic heart disease or preexisting hypertensive cardiomyopathy, marked fluid retention with acute congestive heart failure (pulmonary edema) may be a presenting finding in ANS. There is a tendency for spontaneous recovery, although this is much less evident in the elderly than in much younger persons. A preceding streptococcal (throat or skin) or a staphylococcal (skin or soft tissue) infection may be documented (poststreptococcal or poststaphylococcal glomerulonephritis).

Rapidly progressive glomerulonephritis (RPGN) presents in a more insidious fashion also with hematuria and proteinuria, but with a progressive and relentless (if untreated)

The David Geffen School of Medicine at UCLA, 8 Bethany, Laguna Niguel, Los Angeles, CA 92677, USA
E-mail address: glassock@cox.net

Clin Geriatr Med 25 (2009) 413–422
doi:10.1016/j.cger.2009.06.006
0749-0690/09/$ – see front matter
geriatric.theclinics.com

Box 1
The common clinical syndromes of glomerular disease

Acute nephritic syndrome

Rapidly progressive glomerulonephritis

Nephrotic syndrome

"Asymptomatic" hematuria and/or proteinuria

Chronic glomerular disease

---

loss of renal function, and much less evidence of edema and hypertension. Progression to end-stage renal disease (ESRD) may occur in a matter of days or weeks. Although a presenting infection may also be present, more often than not such features are absent, especially in the elderly.

Nephrotic syndrome (NS) is characterized by the abrupt or insidious onset of marked proteinuria (usually more than 3.5 g/d), with or without hematuria, but with a prominent tendency for edema (face and legs), hypoalbuminemia, and hyperlipidemia. Renal function may be normal or abnormal. In the elderly the peripheral edema may be quite severe if there is concomitant congestive heart failure or venous insufficiency.

Asymptomatic hematuria and/or proteinuria (ASHP) is characterized by "symptom-free" (eg, no lower urinary tract symptoms such as dysuria or frequency) excretion of abnormal numbers of erythrocytes or increased amounts of protein (albumin) in association with normal renal function, normal blood pressure (adjusted for age), and absence of edema. This presentation is often discovered serendipitously during a routine urinalysis, although at times the hematuria may be episodic and "gross" or macroscopic, bringing the patient to the physician's attention. More often than not the hematuria is microscopic.

Chronic glomerular disease (CGN) can be said to be present when any of the conditions causing glomerular injury have progressed slowly to definitely impaired renal function (usually a GFR <45 ml/min/1.73 m^2 in the elderly), nearly always with an elevated serum creatinine (Scr) concentration. Some degree of proteinuria and hypertension is also nearly always present.

One feature that links all of the "glomerular disease syndromes" is the nearly universal excretion of increased numbers of abnormally shaped, smaller than normal (microcytic), poorly hemoglobinized (hypochromic) erythrocytes in the urine,[3] also known as "dysmorphic" or glomerular hematuria. This condition is an extremely valuable diagnostic tool that requires careful microscopic examination of the urinary sediment (using specials stains or a phase-contrast microscope). When present in larger than normal numbers (>10,000/mL of uncentrifuged urine or >80% of the erythrocytes in a spun urinary sediment), these "dysmorphic" erythrocytes are virtually diagnostic of an underlying glomerular disease. Acanthocyturia (erythrocytes with multiple bubble-like projections of the cell-membrane) are pathognomonic of glomerulonephritis.

Renal biopsy is often employed for definitive diagnosis of the underlying disease process. The spectrum of renal diseases encountered in the clinical syndromes described here are substantially different in the elderly and the very elderly compared with a younger group of patients. **Box 2** summaries the frequency of the more

---

Box 2
Renal biopsy diagnosis in the very elderly (older than 80 years of age)

Pauci-immune crescentic glomerulonephritis: 18%

Hypertensive nephrosclerosis/focal and segmental glomerulosclerosis: 7%

Hypertensive nephrosclerosis: 7%

IgA nephropathy: 7%

Membranous nephropathy: 7%

Amyloidosis: 6%

Minimal change disease: 4%

Myeloma cast nephropathy: 4%

Data from Moutzouris D-A, Herlitz L, Appel GA, et al. Renal biopsy in the very elderly. Clin J Am Soc Nephrol 2009;4:1073–82.

---

common lesions encountered in the very elderly (older than 80 years of age) when renal biopsies are performed to evaluate clinical renal disease.

PRIMARY GLOMERULAR DISEASE

The lesions that underlie primary glomerular disease are diverse.[4] The relative frequency of the individual glomerular lesions falling within the spectrum of primary glomerular disease is different in the elderly than in the younger patient (see **Box 3**).[5,6] A step-wise approach to diagnosis of the underlying condition is needed, but renal biopsy is often required for definitive diagnosis[5,6] Five lesions account for more than 80% of the lesions of primary glomerular disease in the elderly: membranous nephropathy (MN), mesangial, endocapillary, or focal proliferative glomerulonephritis (PGN, MesGN, including IgA nephropathy), focal and segmental glomerulosclerosis (FSGS), crescentic glomerulonephritis (CrGN), and minimal change disease (MCD). Membranoproliferative glomerulonephritis (MPGN) is relatively

---

Box 3
The frequency of primary glomerular lesions in the elderly (according to renal biopsy series)

Membranous nephropathy: 28%

Mesangial proliferative GN[a]: 24%

Crescentic glomerulonephritis (pauci-immune): 13%

Minimal change disease: 10%

Focal and segmental glomerulosclerosis: 9%

Membranoproliferative glomerulonephritis: 8%

Endocapillary (acute) proliferative glomerulonephritis: 4%

"Chronic" glomerulonephritis (not otherwise specified): 4%

[a] Including IgA nephropathy and pure mesangial proliferative glomerulonephritis.
Data from Faubert PF, Porush JG. Primary glomerular disease. In: Renal disease in the elderly, 2nd edition. New York: Marcel Dekker; 1998. p. 129–73.

---

uncommon in the elderly, and is most commonly found to underlie a systemic disease (such as a monoclonal gammopathy).

Idiopathic membranous nephropathy is the most commonly encountered glomerular lesion in the elderly with primary glomerular disease (it is found in 20%–30% of renal biopsies performed for diagnostic purposes in this age group).[1,5–7] Most patients with MN have NS (>80%), but a few present with asymptomatic proteinuria. Persistence of proteinuria is the rule, but spontaneous remissions do occur in 15% to 20% of patients. Continuing nephrotic-range proteinuria, particularly more than about 6 to 8 g/d, is often associated with a slowly progressive course to ESRD over many years. Hyperlipidemia may aggravate an underlying tendency to progressive atherosclerosis. There is also a marked tendency to thromboembolic diseases. Conservative management (salt restriction, loop-acting diuretics, antihypertensives—mainly angiotensin-converting enzyme inhibitors [ACEi], angiotensin receptor blockers [ARB], or direct renin inhibitors [DRI]) is indicated when proteinuria is modest (<5 g/d), the symptoms of NS are tolerable and manageable, and features suggesting progressive disease (declining GFR) are absent. Concomitant therapy with a "stain" to help reduce the hypercholesterolemia is often indicated. Prophylactic anticoagulants may be indicated when the serum albumin level is very low (<2.5 g/dL), or if the patient has had a prior thromboembolic event or has another thrombophilic disorder.[8] Patients with marked proteinuria (>5 g/d for 6 months or longer), and those with severe symptomatic NS or progressive renal disease (Scr 1.5–2.5 mg/dL) are candidates for specific therapy.[7] Several choices are available for initial therapy and the selection of one depends very much on individual preferences and the importance of side effects. Two regimens are commonly considered. First, cyclical oral cyclophosphamide and glucocorticoids for 6 months (the Ponticelli regimen) may be used (Evidence Grade A). This regimen has a high success rate (complete or partial remissions in more than 80%) and definitely delays the onset of progressive renal failure. However, in the elderly it may be associated with a somewhat higher risk of leukopenia and viral infections (eg, herpes zoster). Concomitant elevation of Scr greatly increases this risk and lower doses of cyclophosphamide (50%–75% of the usual recommended dose) are used in the regimen. Relapses occur in about 30% of patients after initial success. The regimen may be repeated, but usually no more than once. Alternatively, treatment may be initiated with a calcineurin inhibitor (CNI; cyclosporine or tacrolimus), alone as monotherapy or combined with low-dose steroids for 4 to 6 months (Evidence Grade A). The success rate with CNI is about equivalent to the Ponticelli regimen, but relapses are much higher (around 60%–70%) when the therapy is tapered or discontinued, and treatment must be prolonged to maintain remission, exposing the patient to the potential of nephrotoxicity of these agents. Many patients become CNI-dependent. Tacrolimus may produce somewhat more stable remissions. Alternative agents, not yet fully evaluated for long-term benefits and risks, include synthetic depot corticotropin (twice weekly for 6 months to 1 year) (Evidence Grade B); intravenous courses of rituximab (a monoclonal anti-CD20 B-cell antibody) (Evidence Grade C), and mycophenolate mofetil (MMF) plus steroids (Evidence Grade C). Failure to respond to the Ponticelli regimen or to CNI is a common indication for these second-line therapies, but the response is difficult to predict. Concomitant use of Rituximab and a CNI (in CNI-dependent patients) has produced long-term remission free of relapse, but this has not yet been evaluated in a suitable randomized clinical trial[9] (Evidence Grade C). Complete or partial remissions are associated with marked protection from ESRD. Recurrences of MN in renal transplants can develop in 15% to 20% of cases, but few elderly patients will be candidates for such a procedure.

Mesangial, endocapillary, or focal proliferative glomerulonephritis is most commonly a manifestation of an underlying streptococcal or staphylococcal infection or a viral infection.[10] Poststreptococcal GN (PSGN) is not a benign disease in the elderly. PSGN may provoke a fatal bout of acute congestive heart failure. Treatment is primarily supportive with diuretics, bed rest, and salt restriction. Poststaphylococcal GN may be associated with IgA deposits in the glomeruli and has a poor prognosis, especially in the concomitant presence of diabetes. IgA nephropathy is not uncommon in the elderly (accounting for about 15% of diagnoses of primary glomerular disease).[5,11] The prognosis and treatment of PSGN in the elderly are largely unknown. Too few elderly patients have been included in randomized trials to help guide treatment decisions. The standard therapy is maximum dosages of an ACEi/ARB or DRI (Evidence Grade A-B). Patients with persistent proteinuria of more than 1.0 g/d and Scr <1.5 mg/dL can be treated with cyclical oral and intravenous prednisone (Pozzi Regmen)[11] (Evidence Grade A). Patients with progressive disease can be treated with low-dose sequential cyclophosphamide-azathioprine and glucocorticoids (Ballardie-Roberts regimen)[11] (Evidence Grade A-B), but the safety and efficacy of this approach in the elderly is unknown. IgA nephropathy frequently recurs in the renal allograft but this does not have a major effect on graft or patient survival.

Focal and segmental glomerulosclerosis is a relatively common lesion found to underlie proteinuria and the NS in the geriatric population.[1,5,12] It may be difficult to clearly separate this lesion from MCD on pathologic grounds alone, due to the very common superimposition of global glomerulosclerosis, and vascular lesions in the elderly kidney. Patients with FSGS tend to have an insidious onset of NS, have some degree of renal impairment, and more frequent hypertension. This lesion tends to be uncommon in the very elderly (>80 years of age).[5] Proteinuria may be marked (as much as 20 g/d) and progressive renal failure is common if marked proteinuria persists. Patients with nonnephrotic proteinuria largely have a benign evolution and can be managed conservatively with diuretics and ACEi/ARB/DRI. Management is problematic for those with persistent nephrotic-range proteinuria because there are few randomized controlled trials that have included elderly patients to help in decision making. A prolonged course of oral glucocorticoids (4–6 months) is often used (Evidence Grade C), but side effects are frequent, especially in the elderly (osteoporosis, diabetes, sleep disturbances, easy bruising, myalgias, fatigue). For this reason, some prefer to initiate therapy with a combination of a CNI (cyclosporine or tacrolimus) and low-dose alternate-day oral steroids (along with concomitant maximum-dose ACEi/ARB/DRI) (Evidence Grade A-B). Treatment is often complicated by further impairment of renal function and dosage of CNI frequently needs to be adjusted. Alkylating agents (cyclophosphamide or chlorambucil) are of no value and should be avoided. Oral MMF, given with steroids, has been helpful in some situations, but there are no controlled trials and the long-term benefits are unknown. Combinations of MMF and a CNI have been used on an anecdotal basis. Ritiximab has shown some limited benefit, but no controlled trails are yet available. Patients refractory to treatment generally progress to ESRD over 2 to 4 years. The subvariant of FSGS known as collapsing glomerulopathy has a poorer prognosis and tends to be less responsive to treatment when glomerular involvement is severe (>25% of glomeruli involved with collapsing lesions). The disease may recur in the transplanted kidney in up to 40% of cases.

Crescentic glomerulonephritis is one of the more common primary glomerular lesions found in elderly subjects (40%–50% in some series).[1,5,13] This lesion is also known a "pauci-immune" necrotizing and crescentic glomerulonephritis (PICrGN) to emphasize the relative lack of immunoglobulin deposition in glomeruli. This condition is frequently (>80%) associated with circulating antineutrophil cytoplasmic autoantibodies (ANCA) directed to myeloperoxidase or proteinase-3 in the azurophilic granules of leukocytes. This lesion frequently is associated with the syndrome of rapidly progressive glomerulonephritis. The diagnosis should always be suspected when hematuria and proteinuria are found and the Scr is rising rapidly. Urgent diagnosis by serology or renal biopsy is indicated. In the absence of early and aggressive therapy, most patients either die or develop irreversible ESRD. Renal biopsies showing few normal glomeruli suggest an adverse prognosis for eventual recovery. The treatment needs to be initiated early for maximal benefit. Induction therapy consists of oral or intravenous glucocorticoids, oral or intravenous cyclophosphamide, and in some cases intensive plasma exchange (Evidence Grade A). After induction of remission, the intensity of treatment may be diminished and maintenance of remission with oral azathioprine or MMF and low-dose glucocorticoids may be sufficient. Relapses are common, particularly in the variety associated with antibodies to proteinase-3. The overall response rate to this therapy following induction regimens is about 80% to 90%, but complications are frequent and the mortality rate remains high (more than 20%). The elderly are especially vulnerable to complications. If the burden of side effects is too high, it is better to withhold therapy and plan for dialysis. Intensive plasma exchange (seven treatments of more than 10 days) can be given when the presentation is acute renal failure requiring dialysis for less than 2 weeks. PICrGN occasionally recurs in the renal allograft.

Minimal change disease in many ways is the most difficult lesion to identify with certainty as a cause for NS in the elderly.[1,2,5,14] The lesions of arteriolo-nephrosclerosis, so common in the aged kidney, may result in imprecision, when rendering diagnosis of MCD by light microscopy alone. However, using electron microscopy the signpost of MCD, namely, diffuse foot process effacement of the visceral epithelial cells (podocytes) of the glomeruli, become evident. In the elderly, MCD is a fairly common cause of the idiopathic NS, accounting for about 10% to 15% of all cases, diminishing with even more advancing age. A characteristic feature of MCD in the elderly is its common association with acute, mostly reversible acute renal failure (ARF). Episodes of ARF develop in about one-third of cases, often at the onset of disease. The ARF is commonly spontaneously reversible, but permanent renal failure has also been observed. The reasons underlying this propensity for ARF with MCD in the elderly (and older adults as well) is not well understood. Except for this tendency, MCD in the elderly is very similar to that found in younger subjects in terms of presentation and course. Spontaneous remissions are uncommon. The treatment is not well known, again because of a paucity of randomized controlled trials in the aged. However, if the NS is severe, treatment with oral glucocorticoids, once daily or every other day at a dosage of 1 mg/kg/d, are usually given (Evidence Grade C). Treatment must be prolonged in many cases, for 16 to 20 weeks, to achieve a remission or relapses may develop, although relatively infrequently in the elderly compared with younger persons. Adjunctive use of short-term oral cyclophosphamide (for 8–10 weeks) or a CNI regimen (similar to that used in FSGS) can be offered for those few patients with frequent recurrences, but are not without side effects and potential risks. Overall, the prognosis for maintenance of good renal function is reasonably good for MCD in the elderly, except if ARF supervenes.

SECONDARY GLOMERULAR DISEASE

The secondary glomerular diseases afflicting the elderly are extraordinarily diverse (**Box 4**).[1,2,15] These diseases may produce any or all of the clinical syndromes outlined

---

Box 4
Common secondary glomerular diseases in the elderly

Diabetic glomerulosclerosis (diffuse and nodular types)

Systemic necrotizing and crescentic glomerulonephritis

(Antineutrophil cytoplasmic autoantibody positive)

Systemic amyloidosis

(AL type, primary and secondary to multiple myeloma)

Nonamyloid monoclonal immunoglobulin deposition diseases

(Light chain, heavy chain, light-heavy chain, Cryoglobulinemia)

Idiopathic (nondiabetic) nodular glomerulosclerosis

Malignancy-related glomerulopathy

(Membranous nephropathy, focal and segmental glomerulosclerosis, minimal change disease)

Drug-related glomerular disease

(Nonsteroidal anti-inflammatory agents, cancer chemotherapeutic agents, pamidronate)

---

above. Often their systemic features give clues to the correct diagnosis, but in many cases the clues are nonspecific and of little diagnostic help. Because renal biopsies are only done for diagnosis when the causes of the clinical syndrome are not immediately self-evident, the frequency of secondary lesions among renal biopsy series gives a distorted view of their true prevalence. For example, diabetic glomerulosclerosis (both diffuse and nodular) (DGS, described elsewhere in this issue), due to Type 2 diabetes mellitus, is among the most common causes of a glomerulopathy in the elderly, but is much less common (usually about 5%–10%) in renal biopsy series. In addition, DGS may also be associated (superimposed upon) with other primary or secondary glomerular diseases. The most important causes of secondary glomerular disease, those that are much more common in the elderly than in younger subjects, are: amyloidosis, nonamyloid monoclonal immunoglobulin deposition diseases, nondiabetic nodular glomerulosclerosis, Goodpasture disease (anti-GBM antibody nephritis), and systemic necrotizing polyangiitis. Lupus nephritis is uncommon in the elderly. Membranous nephropathy, and to a lesser extent FSGS and MCD, may also develop as a consequence of malignancies in older individuals.[16] Indeed, about 25% of patients with MN diagnosed after the age of 65 years have an underlying malignancy, most often a carcinoma (breast, stomach, lung, or colon). Hodgkins disease, thymomas, and lymphomas, and other solid malignancies or leukemias may be associated with MCD or FSGS. Drugs, such as nonsteroidal anti-inflammatory agents, consumed more commonly by the elderly for a variety of symptoms, can also evoke glomerular disease (MCD and MN). Therapeutic agents such as interferon or pamidronate, used in the treatment of cancer and its complications in the elderly, can also induce glomerular lesions (MCD and collapsing FSGS). Viral infections such as HIV, hepatitis B, and hepatitis C, though they cause glomerular lesions such as MN and membranoproliferative glomerulonephritis, are more common in younger than in older subjects. However, chronic hepatitis C infection is a not uncommon cause of mixed IgG/IgM cryoglobulinemia in elderly patients, particularly women.

Amyloidosis is a cause of the NS in about 10% of elderly subjects.[17] Amyloidosis may present as a renal disease (nephrotic syndrome most commonly) but without any extrarenal manifestations, but more frequently some clues to the correct diagnosis are present; such as carpal tunnel syndrome, macroglossia, easy bruising, postural hypotension, and organomegaly. In the elderly, AL amyloidosis is the most common disease, but rarely AA amyloidosis or even hereditary amyloidosis (fibrinogen mutations) may be the cause. The Congo-Red stain is positive and 10- to 12-nm non-branching fibrils are found on electron microscopy. Marked proteinuria (even up to 20 g/d) and some impairment of renal function with mild hypertension is the rule. Plasma levels of free monoclonal immunoglobulin light chains (λ) are very frequently elevated (>80%) and a monoclonal paraprotein can often be found in the urine (λ light chains most often). About 1% to 15% of patients will be found to have a frank multiple myeloma on bone marrow examination or bone survey. Nephrotic syndrome and reduced renal function are ominous prognostic signs and in the absence of therapy, nearly all patients die or progress to ESRD in a matter of a few years from discovery. Although the elderly have a high risk of serious side effects and complications, an attempt at therapy is usually warranted. This therapy includes high-dose melphalan plus steroids, or bortezomide and lenolinamide (a congener of thalidomide). Autologous bone marrow (or peripheral stem cell) transplantation is poorly tolerated in the elderly, especially if cardiac involvement is present, and this approach (although curative) may be too risky to be applied to the elderly population with renal amyloidosis.

Nonamyloid monoclonal immunoglobulin deposition diseases (MIDD) are also a common cause of renal disease in they older population.[18] Collectively they may account for 5% to 10% of cases. The diseases consist of light chain MIDD (usually κ light chain), heavy chain MIDD, light-heavy chain MIDD, IgG MIDD, monoclonal cryoglobulinemia, crystal cryoglobulinemia, and immunotactoid glomerulopathy. These diseases share in common the deposition of a monoclonal protein (Congo-Red stain negative) in the glomerular capillaries, without the formation of typical amyloid fibrils (the β-pleated sheet conformation), causing structural and functional deficits including NS and progressive renal failure. Identification of the offending monoclonal protein by immunochemical means is essential for the correct diagnosis, and chemotherapy is needed to reduce the production of the abnormal protein from a neoplastic clone of B cells or plasma cells.

Idiopathic (nondiabetic) nodular glomerulosclerosis is a recently described condition in which the pathologic findings of nodular DGS are found in patients who have no evidence of diabetes mellitus.[19] The patients tend to be elderly women with a marked history of smoking and hypertension. The pathogenesis is unknown and the prognosis is poor. No effective treatment, other than control of blood pressure and stopping smoking, is available.

Goodpasture disease (antiglomerular basement membrane[GBM] nephritis) is an uncommon disorder characterized by crescentic GN and circulating antibodies to GBM.[13] In the elderly it is chiefly found in women and may not have overt pulmonary hemorrhage. With extensive crescents the prognosis for recovery is poor without aggressive therapy. Treatment consists of oral cyclophosphamide (in reduced dosage), oral and intravenous glucocorticoids, and aggressive plasma exchange (14 sessions for several weeks) (Evidence Grade C). Circulating antibody levels decrease quickly but renal recovery depends on the extent of damage at the time treatment is begun. Dialysis-dependent patients with Scr of more than 7 mg/dL have only a 10% chance of recovery. If life-threatening pulmonary hemorrhage is also present, plasma exchange may be life-saving.

Systemic "pauci-immune" necrotizing and crescentic polyangiitis is among the most common secondary glomerular diseases affecting the elderly.[13] This condition is similar to the "renal-limited" form (discussed above in the Primary Glomerular Disease section) and comes in two forms: Wegener granulomatosus (WG) or granulomatous polyangiitis affecting the kidneys, lungs, upper airways, sinuses, sclera, and auditory canal; and microscopic polyangiitis (MPA), also affecting the kidneys, lungs, skin, and joints, but without tissue granulomas. Both diseases are strongly associated (>90%) with ANCA—mostly antiproteinase-3 in WG and antimyeloperoxidase in MPA. Systemic features of fever, cough, myalgias, pulmonary hemorrhage, cutaneous angiitis, sinusitis, and upper and lower airway disease can be present. The treatment is identical to that described for "renal-limited" necrotizing and crescentic glomerulonephritis (Evidence Grade A-B), but the prognosis may be poorer because of the multiorgan involvement. Patients who are dialysis dependent for less than 2 weeks will likely benefit from the addition of intensive plasma exchange but the risk of complications is great, especially in the elderly infirm. Courses of rituximab are emerging as an alternative to cyclophosphamide-glucocorticoid regimens (Evidence Grade C), but the benefits and hazards of this approach in the elderly are not well understood as yet. Rarely CNI or MMF may be useful, but only anecdotal evidence is available to guide decisions in this area.

SUMMARY

This brief recapitulation of the major features of glomerular disease in the geriatric population provides several lessons. The importance of careful examination of the urinary sediment for dysmorphic erythrocytes as a diagnostic tool in glomerular disease needs to be emphasized. A high degree of suspicion for underlying glomerular disease needs to be present when hematuria and proteinuria are present concomitantly, and a rising serum creatinine level should be viewed with a sense of urgency. The atypical clinical features of acute and chronic glomerular disease in the elderly should be borne in mind. The common causes of nephrotic syndrome, such as MN, focal and segmental glomerulosclerosis, MCD, and amyloidosis need to be considered in patients with edema and marked proteinuria. The unusual predilection of the elderly to develop rapidly progressive glomerulonephritis due to both renal-limited and systemic forms of necrotizing and crescentic glomerulonephritis (often antineutrophil cytoplasmic autoantibody positive) needs to be appreciated. The development of glomerular disease due to an underlying neoplastic process, such as monoclonal immunoglobulin deposition disease or a carcinoma, also needs to be needs to be remembered. Finally, the fact that many clinical trials have failed to include sufficient numbers of elderly persons makes it difficult to translate therapeutic recommendations from the young to the old. In addition, the risks of aggressive treatment of glomerular disease may be enhanced in older persons and this needs to be recognized in therapeutic decision making. However, many effective and reasonably safe treatment regimens are available to ameliorate the adverse consequences of acute, progressive, and chronic glomerular disease in the geriatric population. These treatments must be used with care, and with full recognition of their potential benefits and hazards in this uniquely vulnerable population.

REFERENCES

1. Faubert PF, Porush JG. Primary glomerular disease. In: Renal disease in the elderly. 2nd edition. New York: Marcel Dekker, Inc.; 1998. p. 129–73.
2. Glassock RJ. Glomerular disease in the elderly population. In: Oreopoulos DG, Hazzard WR, Luke R, editors. Nephrology and geriatrics integrated. Dodrecht: Kluwer Academic Publishers; 2000. p. 57–66.
3. Becker GJ, Fairley KF. Urinalysis. In: Textbook of nephrology, Massry S, Glassock R, 4th edition. Philadelphia: Lippincott, Williams and Wilkins; p. 1765–83

4. Ponticelli C, Glassock RJ. Treatment of primary glomerulonephritis. 2nd edition. Oxford: Oxford University Press; 2009. p. 1–476.
5. Moutzouris D-A, Herlitz L, Appel GA, et al. Renal biopsy in the very elderly. Clin J Am Soc Nephrol 2009;4:1073–82.
6. Vendemia F. The diagnosis of renal disease in elderly patients. What role is there for renal biopsy? In: JFM Nunez, JS Cameron, DG Oreopoulos, editors. The aging kidney in health and disease, New York: Springer; 2008. p. 307–28.
7. Passerini P, Ponticelli C. Membranous nephropathy. In: Ponticelli C, Glassock R, editors. Treatment of primary glomerular disease. 2nd edition. Oxford: Oxford University Press; 2009. p. 261–312.
8. Glassock RJ. Prophylactic anti-coagulation in nephrotic syndrome: a clinical conundrum. J Am Soc Nephrol 2007;18:2221–5.
9. Segarra A, Praga M, Ramos N, et al. Successful treatment of membranous glomerulonephritis with rituximab in calcineurin inhibitor-dependent patients. Clin J Am Soc Nephrol 2009;4:1083–8.
10. Moroni G, Ponticelli C. Acute post-infectious glomerulonephritis. In: Ponticelli C, Glassock R, editors. Treatment of primary glomerular disease. 2nd edition. Oxford: Oxford University Press; 2009. p. 153–78.
11. Glassock RJ, Lee G. Immunoglobulin A nephropathy. In: Ponticelli C, Glassock R, editors. Treatment of primary glomerular disease. 2nd edition. Oxford: Oxford University Press; 2009. p. 313–74.
12. Scolari F, Ponticelli C. Focal and segmental glomerulosclerosis. In: Ponticelli C, Glassock R, editors. Treatment of primary glomerular disease. 2nd edition. Oxford: Oxford University Press; 2009. p. 215–60.
13. Nachman P, Glassock R. Crescentic glomerulonephritis. In: Ponticelli C, Glassock R, editors. Treatment of primary glomerular disease. 2nd edition. Oxford: Oxford University press; 2009. p. 399–434.
14. Coppo R, Ponticelli C. Minimal change nephropathy. In: Ponticelli C, Glassock R, editors. Treatment of primary glomerular disease. 2nd edition. Oxford: Oxford University Press; 2009. p. 179–214.
15. Faubert PF, Porush JG. Renal involvement in systemic disease. In: Renal disease in the elderly. 2nd edition. New York: Marcel Dekker, Inc; 1998. p. 175–237.
16. Bjoneklett R, Vikse BE, Svarstad E, et al. Long-term risk of cancer in membranous nephropathy patients. Am J Kidney Dis 2007;50:396–403.
17. Dember LM. Amyloidosis-associated kidney disease. J Am Soc Nephrol 2006;17: 3458–71.
18. Lin J, Markowitz GA, Valeri AM, et al. Renal immunoglobulin deposition disease: the clinical spectrum. J Am Soc Nephrol 2001;12:1482–92.
19. Nasr SH, D'Agati VD. Nodular glomerulosclerosis in the nondiabetic smoker. J Am Soc Nephrol 2007;18:2032–6.

Urinary Tract Infections in the Elderly

L.E. Nicolle, MD, FRCPC[a,b]

KEYWORDS

- Urinary infection • Cystitis • Pyelonephritis
- Asymptomatic bacteriuria • Elderly • Long-term care facility

Urinary tract infection is the most common bacterial infection occurring in older populations. Asymptomatic infection is identified when bacteria or yeast are isolated in appropriate quantitative counts from a urine culture without accompanying signs or symptoms attributable to the genitourinary tract.[1] In this article, the terms asymptomatic bacteriuria and asymptomatic urinary tract infection are used interchangeably. Symptomatic urinary tract infection presents along a continuum of clinical signs and symptoms from minor, irritative lower tract symptoms to septic shock. The site of infection may be the bladder (acute cystitis or acute lower tract infection) or kidney (acute pyelonephritis or acute upper tract infection). For men, acute or chronic bacterial prostatitis is another presentation of urinary tract infection.[2] Urinary infection in women with a normal genitourinary tract is called acute uncomplicated urinary tract infection. Complicated urinary tract infection occurs in patients with underlying functional or structural abnormalities of the genitourinary tract.[3]

Urinary infection is an important clinical problem in older populations across the full spectrum of functional capacity, from well, elderly men and women living independently in the community to the highly functionally impaired nursing home resident with multiple comorbidities. This article addresses urinary tract infection for the community and for long-term care facility populations. In addition, individuals with voiding managed with a chronic indwelling urethral catheter have unique considerations with respect to the diagnosis, complications, and management of urinary tract infection.[4] This article is relevant to individuals without a chronic indwelling catheter, unless it is specifically noted that the catheterized patient is being addressed.

---

[a] Department of Internal Medicine, Health Sciences Centre, University of Manitoba, Room GG443, 820 Sherbrook Street, Winnipeg, Manitoba, R3A 1R9, Canada
[b] Department of Medical Microbiology, Health Sciences Centre, University of Manitoba, Room GG443, 820 Sherbrook Street, Winnipeg, Manitoba, R3A 1R9, Canada
E-mail address: lnicolle@hsc.mb.ca

Clin Geriatr Med 25 (2009) 423–436
doi:10.1016/j.cger.2009.04.005
0749-0690/09/$ – see front matter © 2009 Elsevier Inc. All rights reserved.

EPIDEMIOLOGY
Community Populations

In women, asymptomatic bacteriuria increases with increasing age, reaching a prevalence of 20% in those older than 80 years. For healthy men, asymptomatic bacteriuria is unusual until beyond 60 years of age; 5% to 10% of men older than 80 years are bacteriuric.[1,5] Asymptomatic bacteriuria in older populations is benign. Individuals with bacteriuria are at increased risk for symptomatic infection, but episodes of symptomatic infection are not attributable to bacteriuria. Longer-term negative outcomes such as renal failure or hypertension are not associated with bacteriuria, and survival is similar for bacteriuric and nonbacteriuric subjects when stratified by other risk factors for mortality.[1]

Estimates of the burden of illness attributable to symptomatic urinary infection in older community populations have been developed using administrative databases or in prospective studies in selected populations (**Table 1**).[6–11] Older women experience a higher frequency of symptomatic infection than men, but the magnitude of the gender difference is less than in younger populations. Hospitalization for acute pyelonephritis increases with age, with the highest rates in the highest age groups.[10,11] Episodes of symptomatic urinary infection in well older individuals are usually accompanied by limited morbidity. More severe presentations require hospitalization, but mortality directly attributable to urinary infection is uncommon.[7] Frequent recurrent infection may be problematic for some older persons, particularly those with underlying urologic abnormalities.

Institutionalized Populations

A remarkable aspect of the long-term care facility population is the high prevalence of asymptomatic bacteriuria: from 25% to 50% of women and 15% to 40% of men.[1,12,13] A high "turnover" of bacteriuria has been described, with about one third of bacteriuric individuals developing negative urine cultures by 3 to 6 months, and a further one third

Table 1 Occurrence of asymptomatic bacteriuria and symptomatic urinary infection in older populations		
Community	**Asymptomatic**	**Symptomatic**
Women		
>80 years	20%[5]	–
55–75 years	–	7/100 patient years[6]
Hospitalization/pyelonephritis >60 years	–	1.4–2.3/10,000[7]
Men		
>80 years	5%–10%[5]	0–17/1000 d[8]
75–84 years	–	2.8–6.7/1000 population[9]
>85 years	–	4.3–7.8/1000 population[9]
Hospitalization, pyelonephritis >60 years	–	0.6–1.3/10,000 population[7]
Women and men		
Pyelonephritis hospitalization >70 years	–	1.0–1.5/10,000[10]
Long-term care	15%–50%[1]	0.57/1000 d[11]
Chronic indwelling catheter	100%	3.2/1000 catheter days[11]

of individuals without bacteriuria becoming bacteriuric in the same timeframe.[14] Bacteriuria persists for years in many residents, often with the same organism. Asymptomatic bacteriuria is not associated with negative outcomes.[1] The decreased survival of bacteriuric institutionalized residents reported in early studies was not confirmed in subsequent studies stratified by potential confounders for mortality. One adverse outcome of bacteriuria is inappropriate antimicrobial use; unnecessary treatment is frequently given for asymptomatic bacteriuria, contributing to resistance development and adverse drug effects.[1]

Symptomatic urinary tract infection is second only to pneumonia as a cause of infections in residents. The reported incidence varies from 0.1 to 2.4/1000 resident days[12] and 0 to 2.31/1000 resident days.[11] Urinary tract infection is a common reason for transfer of residents to an acute care facility in American nursing homes, but is seldom a direct cause of mortality.[12] From 45% to 56% of bacteremia episodes in long-term care facilities are from a urinary source, but these are predominantly in residents with chronic indwelling catheters.[12,15]

Chronic Indwelling Catheter

Individuals with voiding managed by a chronic indwelling catheter are always bacteriuric.[16] The incidence of infection with a new organism in individuals with a catheter is 3% to 7% per day. There is substantially higher morbidity attributed to urinary infection in residents with catheters compared with bacteriuric residents without a catheter. The incidence of symptomatic catheter-associated urinary infection was 0 to 7.43/1000 catheter days (mean 3.2/1000) in Idaho long-term care facilities, compared with 0 to 2.28/1000 (mean 0.57/1000) for all residents.[11] Fever from a urinary source is three times more frequent in subjects with a chronic catheter, evidence of acute pyelonephritis at autopsy is eight times more frequent, and bacteremia from a urinary source is three to 39 times more frequent.[16–19] Increased mortality has been reported in elderly residents with chronic indwelling catheters.[20] However, these residents have greater functional impairment and more comorbidities, so decreased survival is expected. The excess mortality is not attributable to urinary infection.

PATHOGENESIS
Community Populations

Host determinants are similar for asymptomatic and symptomatic urinary infection. For postmenopausal women, recurrent urinary infection is most strongly associated with a history of urinary tract infection at a younger age.[6,21] Thus, genetic determinants for acute uncomplicated urinary infection remain important in the postmenopausal period. Being a nonsecretor of the blood group substances is one genetic association,[21] and there are likely others not yet characterized. Sexual intercourse is not associated with urinary infection in most studies,[6,22] although a recent study in younger postmenopausal women reported an association of symptomatic infection with intercourse, but within a 2-day timeframe only.[23]

Lactobacilli maintain the acid pH of the vagina, and are the predominant vaginal flora of premenopausal women. They are less common in the vaginal flora of postmenopausal women, and their absence is accompanied by a higher vaginal pH. The increased vaginal pH allows colonization with uropathogens including *Escherichia coli* and enterococcus species, and it is proposed that this facilitates urinary infection.[24,25] Estrogen replacement therapy restores the lactobacillus flora and re-establishes the acid pH of the vagina.[26,27] However, nonrandomized studies in postmenopausal women consistently report that systemic or topical estrogen therapy is not associated with a decreased incidence of symptomatic urinary tract infection (Table 2).[6,21,28–30] A recent Cochrane review summarized results of prospective clinical trials of estrogen therapy to prevent recurrent urinary infection in women.[29] Four trials uniformly reported no impact of oral estrogen on the frequency of urinary infection; two small trials of topical vaginal estrogen reported a decreased frequency of urinary infection;[26,31] and one comparative study reported an estrogen-containing pessary was less effective than nitrofurantoin.[32] Thus, the association of postmenopausal estrogen deficiency with urinary infection is not straightforward.

Prostate hypertrophy is the most important factor contributing to urinary infection in older men. Prostate hypertrophy causes uretheral obstruction and turbulent urine flow, which facilitates ascension of organisms into the bladder. Bacteria established in the prostate of older men may persist indefinitely because of restricted diffusion of antimicrobials into the gland and the frequent presence of bacteria in prostate stones.

As normal voiding is the most important defense against urinary infection, increased postvoid residual urine volumes have been suggested to contribute to urinary tract infection with aging.[33] The mean postvoid residual volume was 257 mL (range 150–560 mL) in bacteriuric and 133 mL (10–340 mL) in nonbacteriuric ambulatory men of median age 62 years.[34] Ambulatory women with a mean age 79 years (range 62–94 years) and a prior history of urinary infection had a significantly higher mean postvoid residual volume, 70 mL versus 33 mL, compared with women without prior infection.[33] However, in another study of postmenopausal women, an association of recurrent urinary infection and increased postvoid residual volume did not persist in a multivariate analysis.[21] A prospective study in women aged 55 to 75 years reported no association of symptomatic urinary infection with postvoid residual volume stratified as less than 50 mL, 50 to 100 ML, or greater than 100 mL.[6] Thus, studies are contradictory. Any association of residual urine volume and infection may be population-specific or only relevant at high volumes.

A Swedish study of elderly persons in the community older than 80 years reported that independent risk factors for bacteriuria in women were reduced mobility, urinary incontinence, and receiving estrogen treatment; and, in men, prostatic disease, history of stroke, and living in supervised housing.[30] Urinary incontinence is a consistent association of symptomatic and asymptomatic urinary infection in older

Table 2
Association of systemic and topical estrogen therapy with urinary infection or bacteriuria in postmenopausal women

Population	Study Design	Estrogen Delivery	Outcomes:[a] OR (95% CI)[b]
66 ± 6.9 y[21]	Matched, case control	Systemic or topical	2.14 (0.89–5.68)
55–75 y[6]	Prospective, cohort	Oral <1 mo	1.0 (0.5–1.2)
55–75 y[28]	Population-based, case control	Oral <0.625 mg/d 0.625 mg/d >0.625 mg/d	0.94 (0.69–1.27) 0.81 (0.62–1.06) 1.61 (0.99–2.63)
50–69 y[29]	Case control, administrative data	Cream, patch, or oral ≥1 y	1.1 (0.8–1.5)
>80 y[30]	Case control	Systemic or topical	2.01 (1.24–3.24) bacteriuria

[a] Symptomatic urinary infection, unless noted otherwise.
[b] Odds ratio for infection or bacteriuria in population receiving estrogen therapy (95% confidence intervals).

women.[21,30] However, incontinence is unlikely causative, as underlying genitourinary abnormalities that promote incontinence will also promote bacteriuria. Elderly women and men with genitourinary abnormalities that impair voiding, such as obstruction of the urethra or ureters, cystoceles in women, or bladder diverticuli, have an increased frequency of urinary tract infection.

Institutionalized Elderly

Asymptomatic bacteriuria in the institutionalized population is associated with increased functional impairment, incontinence of bladder and bowel, and cognitive impairment.[14] The most important contributing factor is likely voiding abnormalities accompanying chronic neurologic diseases that precipitate the need for institutional care, such as cerebrovascular disease, Parkinson disease and Alzheimer disease. The determinants of symptomatic urinary infection other than the presence of a chronic indwelling catheter are not well described. A clinical trial reported no impact of oral estrogen on the prevalence of bacteriuria or episodes of symptomatic urinary tract.[35] Increased postvoid residual urine volumes did not correlate with symptomatic or asymptomatic urinary tract infection in institutionalized men or women.[36,37] However, men with continence management using an external condom catheter have an increased prevalence of bacteriuria and frequency of symptomatic urinary infection compared with incontinent men who do not use these devices.[38]

Chronic Indwelling Catheter

Individuals with a chronic indwelling urethral catheter are always bacteriuric. Any indwelling device in the urinary tract becomes rapidly coated with biofilm.[39] Microorganisms initially adhere to a conditioning layer that forms on the device immediately following insertion, then grow along the interior and external surfaces of the catheter within an extracellular polysaccharide substance produced by the organisms. Urine components including Tamm-Horsfall protein and magnesium and calcium ions are incorporated into this biofilm. Organisms growing as microcolonies within the biofilm are in a protected environment, which restricts diffusion of antimicrobials and limits access of host defenses such as neutrophils or immunoglobulins. Biofilm formation may cause catheter encrustation and catheter obstruction. The determinants of symptomatic infection in the face of this universal bacteriuria are not well described. However, mucosal trauma or catheter obstruction may precipitate systemic infection.

Microbiology

For older men and women in the community, *E coli* remains the most common organism isolated from symptomatic infection.[40,41] Other less frequent organisms include *Klebsiella pneumoniae* and *Enterococcus* spp. Virulence determinants for *E coli* isolated from symptomatic cystitis or pyelonephritis are similar to those described for strains isolated from younger women. *E coli* remains a common infecting organism for persons with complicated urinary infection, but is less frequent. In these patients, more resistant organisms are often isolated resulting from repeated prior antimicrobial courses and health care exposures, including urologic interventions.[42,43] Other species include Enterobacteriaceae such as *K pneumoniae*, *Citrobacter* spp, *Serratia* spp, *Enterobacter* spp, and nonfermenters such as *Pseudomonas aeruginosa*. Coagulase-negative staphylococci are frequently isolated from asymptomatic men.[8] *Candida* spp are isolated occasionally, usually in patients who have diabetes, indwelling urologic devices, or are receiving broad spectrum antimicrobial therapy.

E coli remains the most common cause of asymptomatic or symptomatic urinary tract infection in women in long-term care facilities, although other Enterobacteriaceae are frequently isolated.[12,14] A wider variety of organisms are isolated from men, including *Proteus mirabilis*, *Providencia stuartii*, coagulase-negative staphylococci and *Enterococcus* spp. From 10% to 25% of noncatheterized residents have polymicrobial bacteriuria.

A wide spectrum of organisms are isolated from individuals with a chronic indwelling catheter.[16] From two to five organisms are present at any time. Urease-producing bacteria such as *P mirabilis*, *Morganella morganii*, *K pneumoniae* and *P stuartii* are particularly common.[44] There is a differential duration of species once infection is established. *Enterococcus* spp persisted for only a few weeks, whereas *P mirabilis* persisted for several months in one study.[44] *Proteus mirabilis* and other urease-producing organisms may produce larger quantities of biofilm, and are associated with an increased frequency of catheter encrustation or obstruction.

DIAGNOSIS
Clinical

Community populations
Elderly individuals in the community usually present with classic signs and symptoms of urinary tract infection. Cystitis presents with lower tract irritative symptoms including frequency, urgency, dysuria, nocturia, suprapubic discomfort and, occasionally, hematuria. Pyelonephritis presents as costovertebral angle pain or tenderness with variable lower tract symptoms and fever. Chronic bacterial prostatitis usually presents as recurrent acute cystitis.[2]

Institutionalized populations
Elderly residents of long-term care facilities may also present with these classic symptoms, but signs and symptoms are often more difficult to ascertain in this population.[45–47] Impaired communication and chronic genitourinary symptoms due to comorbid illness interfere with the identification of new or worsening symptoms. In the bacteriuric resident, any alteration in clinical status without localized findings is often interpreted as symptomatic urinary tract infection.[48] Given the high prevalence of positive urine cultures, this leads to substantial overdiagnosis. Chronic genitourinary symptoms are not attributable to bacteriuria.[14] In addition, clinical deterioration without localized genitourinary symptoms is unlikely symptomatic urinary tract infection, even in the bacteriuric resident.[49] Changes in the character of the urine such as odor, color, or turbidity are associated with bacteriuria but are usually attributed to other diagnoses such as increased incontinence or dehydration. Thus, these urinary changes are not sufficient to diagnose symptomatic urinary tract infection.

A consensus guideline addressed this diagnostic uncertainty by recommending clinical criteria for initiation of empiric antimicrobial therapy for presumed infection.[50] For the resident without an indwelling catheter, acute localized genitourinary signs or symptoms must be present before initiation of antimicrobial therapy for urinary infection. Specific clinical presentations include acute dysuria by itself, or and one of fever, acute confusion, or chills together with at least one new or worsening genitourinary symptom (urgency, frequency, suprapubic pain, gross hematuria, costovertebral angle tenderness, urinary incontinence). A prospective, randomized trial of implementation of this guideline using an algorithm, compared with standard care, reported the intervention was safe for patients and resulted in decreased antimicrobial use for urinary infection.[51]

The older resident presenting with acute confusion and without localized findings is an important diagnostic problem. This presentation is consistent with a wide spectrum of infectious and noninfectious illnesses. Urinary infection is unlikely the cause if the resident does not have a chronic catheter and there are no acute genitourinary signs or symptoms. If infection seems likely, it may be more appropriate to manage this problem as a "sepsis syndrome" of unknown cause rather than assuming urinary infection, even in the bacteriuric resident.

Chronic indwelling catheter

The most common presentation of urinary tract infection in residents with a chronic indwelling catheter is fever without localized genitourinary signs or symptoms.[16] Costovertebral angle pain or tenderness, catheter obstruction, or hematuria may also be present to support the genitourinary source. The consensus definitions for clinical presentations to initiate empiric antimicrobial therapy for residents with a chronic catheter recommend only the presence of one of fever, new costovertebral angle tenderness, rigors, or new onset delirium in the absence of an alternate source.[50]

Urine Culture

A urine culture confirms the diagnosis of urinary infection and assists antimicrobial management by identifying the specific infecting organism and susceptibilities. A urine culture should be obtained before initiating antimicrobial therapy for any older individual with suspected urinary infection. The wide variety of potential infecting organisms and increased likelihood of antimicrobial resistance in older populations makes a urine culture essential for appropriate management.[42,43] The exception to this recommendation is the healthy woman living in the community who experiences recurrent acute cystitis, for whom empiric short-course antimicrobial therapy is usually effective. However, a urine culture should also be obtained from these women if presenting symptoms are atypical so that the diagnosis is questionable, if response to empiric therapy is inadequate, or if there is early symptomatic recurrence posttherapy, suggesting infection with a resistant organism.

The urine specimen must be collected in a manner that minimizes contamination.[45] A voided clean-catch urine specimen can be obtained from most older persons. Some women residents in long-term care facilities cannot cooperate for specimen collection because of incontinence or confusion. If a urine culture is indicated for management of these women, a specimen should be obtained by in-and-out catheter. For men, urine specimens may be collected using an external condom catheter after applying a clean condom and leg bag.[47] A chronic indwelling catheter should be removed and replaced, and the urine specimen obtained through the freshly inserted catheter, before the initiation of antimicrobial therapy.[52] Urine collected through a catheter in situ for a week or more will sample biofilm as well as bladder urine. Replacing the catheter allows collection of a specimen that samples only bladder urine, and these culture results are more relevant for therapeutic decisions.

A quantitative count equal to or greater than 10^5 cfu/mL of a single organism from a urine specimen is usual for microbiologic diagnosis of urinary tract infection. Most episodes of urinary infection will meet this criterion; If lower quantitative counts are reported, the culture must be interpreted in the context of the clinical presentation. The quantitative count may not achieve 10^5 cfu/mL if diuresis or frequency limits bladder incubation time. Lower quantitative counts are isolated from as many as 10% of healthy, postmenopausal women in the community with acute uncomplicated urinary infection.[6] For men, a uropathogen count of 10^3 cfu/mL or higher from a clean-catch voided specimen is sufficient to diagnose symptomatic or asymptomatic infection.[53] If pyelonephritis is suspected, a count of 10^4 cfu/mL or higher is the proposed quantitative criterion. Any quantitative count of an organism is considered relevant if a specimen is collected by in-and-out catheter.[1] For individuals with a chronic indwelling catheter and men with a specimen collected using an external condom catheter, a quantitative count of 10^5 cfu/mL or higher is appropriate.[47]

Other Laboratory Investigations

Pyuria accompanies symptomatic and asymptomatic urinary tract infection.[1] As many as one third of long-term care facility residents who are not bacteriuric have pyuria. For residents with a chronic indwelling catheter, the degree of pyuria does not vary between asymptomatic periods and symptomatic episodes.[54] Thus, pyuria is a nonspecific finding in older populations and does not indicate symptomatic urinary infection. Absence of pyuria, however, has a high negative predictive value and is useful to exclude urinary tract infection. If a diagnosis of symptomatic urinary infection is entertained in a long-term care facility resident, it is recommended that a urine specimen be screened for pyuria. If negative, urinary infection is excluded and a urine culture should not be requested.[45]

Blood cultures should be obtained when patients present with severe sepsis or acute confusional states with or without localized symptoms. Isolation of the same organism from blood and urine usually supports a diagnosis of urosepsis.

ANTIMICROBIAL MANAGEMENT
Asymptomatic Bacteriuria

Treatment of asymptomatic bacteriuria is not indicated for either community or institutionalized older populations.[1] Antimicrobial therapy does not decrease subsequent symptomatic episodes but is associated with negative outcomes including adverse drug effects and re-infection with more resistant organisms. Treatment of asymptomatic bacteriuria in institutionalized populations also does not improve chronic genitourinary symptoms, such as incontinence. In fact, antimicrobial treatment of bacteriuria is ineffective, as recurrent bacteriuria or symptomatic urinary infection occurs early post-treatment. It follows that older populations should not be screened for asymptomatic bacteriuria.

Antimicrobial treatment of asymptomatic bacteriuria in residents with chronic indwelling catheters is also not recommended. Symptomatic episodes are not decreased with treatment, and re-infection with more resistant bacteria is significantly increased.[1]

Antimicrobial Selection

The selection of an antimicrobial regimen for the treatment of symptomatic urinary infection is similar in all populations. There is a predictable decline in creatinine clearance with aging, but age by itself does not require changes in agent or dose. A specific regimen is chosen based on efficacy, patient tolerance, clinical presentation, renal function, need for parenteral therapy, and cost. If symptoms are mild, it is preferable to delay initiation of antimicrobial therapy until urine culture results are available to avoid unnecessary treatment and facilitate optimal antimicrobial selection.

Oral therapy is usually effective (**Table 3**). First-line therapy for cystitis includes nitrofurantoin and trimethoprim/sulfamethoxazole (TMP/SMX). Nitrofurantoin is not effective for renal or prostate infection, and K pneumoniae, P mirabilis, and P aeruginosa are resistant to this agent. However, other resistant organisms such as extended spectrum β-lactamase–producing E coli and vancomycin-resistant enterococci are usually susceptible to nitrofurantoin. The fluoroquinolones (norfloxacin, ciprofloxacin, and levofloxacin) are all effective for treatment of susceptible organisms.[40,55] However, there is increasing resistance of urinary isolates to fluoroquinolones with

Table 3
Antimicrobial regimens for treatment of urinary tract infection in older persons with normal renal function[a]

Therapy	Oral	Parenteral

First-line	TMP/SMX[a] 160/800 mg twice a day
	Nitrofurantoin monohydrate/
	  macrocrystals 100 mg twice a day
	Ciprofloxacin 250–500 mg twice a day
	Norfloxacin 400 twice a day
	Levofloxacin 250–500 mg every 24 h
		Ampicillin 2 g every 6 h ± gentamicin or
		  tobramycin 5–7 mg/kg every 24 h
		Ceftriaxone 1–2 g every 24 h
		Cefotaxime 1 g every 8 h
		Ciprofloxacin 400 mg every 12 h
		Levofloxacin 500–750 mg every 24 h

Other	Amoxicillin 500 mg three times a day
	Amoxicillin/clavulanic acid 500 mg three
	  times a day or 875 mg twice a day
	Cephalexin 500 mg four times a day
	Cefuroxime axetil 500 mg twice a day
	Cefixime 400 mg once a day
	Cefpodoxime proxetil 100–200 mg
	  every 12 h
	Doxycycline 100 mg twice a day
	Trimethoprim 100 mg twice a day
		Amikacin 7.5 mg/kg every 12 h or
		  15 mg/kg every 24 h
		Cefazolin 1 g every 8 h
		Ceftazidime 1 g every 8 h
		Ertapenem 1 g once a day
		Meropenem 500 mg every 6 h or 1 g
		  every 8 h
		Piperacillin/tazobactam 3.375 g every 8 h
		Vancomycin[b] 1 g intravenously every 12 h

[a] TMP/SMX, trimethoprim/sulfamethoxazole.
[b] Gram-positive organisms only.

the intense use of this class of antimicrobials, particularly in long-term care facilities. Whenever possible, they should be reserved for treatment of individuals with severe presentations, such as pyelonephritis, or when patients have resistant organisms or are unable to tolerate other therapies. Oral cephalosporins, doxycycline, amoxicillin or amoxicillin/clavulanic acid are effective second-line oral agents for selected patients, depending on antimicrobial susceptibility and tolerance.

Parenteral therapy is indicated for patients who present with hemodynamic instability, are unable to tolerate oral therapy, have uncertain gastrointestinal absorption, or with an infecting organism known or suspected to be resistant to oral options. An aminoglycoside (gentamicin, tobramycin) with or without ampicillin, ceftriaxone or cefotaxime, or a fluoroquinolone (ciprofloxacin or levofloxacin) are recommended depending on organism susceptibility (**Table 3**). Aminoglycosides are useful agents for empiric treatment, as most gram-negative organisms remain susceptible. Parenteral therapy is usually given for the initial 48 to 72 hours, then re-evaluated after considering the initial clinical response and urine culture result. Antimicrobial therapy is usually modified to an oral or parenteral regimen based on culture results, so the aminoglycoside is not continued beyond the first few days. Toxicity is unlikely with such short-term use. If more prolonged (>7 days) aminoglycoside therapy is necessary, monitoring of drug levels and renal function is required.

Duration of Therapy

Older women in the community presenting with acute cystitis should be treated with short-course antimicrobial therapy. A prospective randomized study in women of mean age 78.5 years reported similar cure rates with 3 or 7 days ciprofloxacin, and significantly fewer adverse effects with the shorter therapy.[40] Trimethoprim/sulfamethoxazole is also likely to be effective as a 3-day regimen. Nitrofurantoin should be given as a 5-day course. Men presenting with symptoms consistent with cystitis should receive 7 days of therapy. When recurrent cystitis from chronic bacterial prostatitis is diagnosed, a 6- to 12-week course is recommended. For pyelonephritis in men or women, therapy is given for 10 to 14 days. Treatment of complicated urinary infection is individualized based on clinical presentations, underlying urologic abnormality, and response to therapy. However, 7 days is usually sufficient for patients presenting with lower tract symptoms, and 10 to 14 days for renal infection. Long-term suppressive therapy is indicated, rarely, to prevent recurrent symptomatic episodes when an underlying abnormality cannot be corrected.

The optimal duration of therapy for residents of long-term care facilities has not been determined. However, short-course therapy is likely appropriate for women presenting with cystitis and without urologic abnormalities.[40] For male residents with lower tract symptoms, 7 days of therapy is recommended. Men or women with more severe presentations or a delayed response following initiation of therapy should receive therapy for 10 to 14 days.

Chronic Indwelling Catheter

An indwelling catheter should be removed and replaced with a new catheter before initiating antimicrobial treatment of symptomatic infection. Catheter replacement allows collection of a more reliable urine specimen for culture, and also improves clinical outcomes, with a more rapid defervescence and decreased symptomatic relapse post-therapy.[52] These clinical benefits are presumed to be attributable to removal of the large numbers of organisms in the biofilm, which may not be eradicated by antimicrobial therapy. The optimal duration of therapy has not been evaluated. If there is a prompt clinical response, only 7 days is recommended to limit re-infection with more resistant organisms.

PREVENTION
Community Populations

Long-term low-dose prophylactic antimicrobial therapy can prevent recurrent, acute, uncomplicated urinary infection in older woman in the community experiencing frequent episodes (≥ 2 in 6 months). First-line regimens are nitrofurantoin 50 or 100 mg or TMP/SMX one half regular strength tablet daily or every other day, at bedtime. An initial course is usually for 6 or 12 months. Short-course self-treatment with TMP/SMX or a fluoroquinolone for 3 days is an alternative strategy, although this approach has not been evaluated in older women.

Topical vaginal estrogen decreased the frequency of recurrent infection in two prospective, randomized, placebo-controlled trials,[26,27] but was much less effective than prophylactic nitrofurantoin in a comparative trial.[22] Thus, the role of topical vaginal estrogen remains uncertain. A prospective cohort study in women aged 55 to 75 years reported no association of use of cranberry products with frequency of infection.[6] However, a prospective, randomized, placebo-controlled trial reported that daily cranberry tablets or juice decreased episodes of recurrent urinary infection by 30%. One third of women enrolled in this trial were postmenopausal, but outcomes were not stratified by age.[56] Another study reported cranberry juice was only slightly less effective than prophylactic trimethoprim in preventing urinary infection in women, but as there was no placebo arm the effectiveness of either intervention is uncertain.[57,58] There is no evidence that oral or vaginal probiotics for lactobacillus replacement of vaginal flora reduces urinary infection in older women.

For older persons with complicated urinary infection, correction of the underlying genitourinary abnormality, whenever possible, is the most important intervention to limit recurrent infection. Prophylactic antimicrobial therapy is not recommended as it does not decrease symptomatic episodes in these patients, and superinfection with resistant organisms is common.[47] Patients with asymptomatic bacteriuria who undergo a genitourinary procedure associated with mucosal bleeding (eg, TURP, ureteric stent placement) have a high risk of bacteremia and sepsis. Prophylactic antimicrobial therapy immediately before the procedure will prevent this complication.[1] The antimicrobials should not usually be continued beyond 24 hours after the procedure.

Institutionalized Populations

There are no known interventions that decrease asymptomatic or symptomatic urinary infection in institutionalized populations. Clinical trials have not reported benefits with either systemic estrogen therapy[35] or cranberry products.[47,57] Preprocedure antimicrobials to prevent bacteremia are indicated for bacteriuric residents.

Chronic Indwelling Catheters

Urinary infection can be prevented by avoiding the use of an indwelling catheter and, if a catheter is necessary, discontinuing the catheter as soon as possible.[4,47] Use of an external condom catheter for incontinence management in men may avoid an indwelling catheter and lower the risk of infection. Intermittent catheterization may be another option to avoid an indwelling catheter in selected male or female residents. A clean technique is recommended as infection rates are similar with clean or sterile techniques, and clean intermittent catheterization is less costly.[47] Appropriate catheter care to prevent trauma and early identification of obstruction will limit episodes of systemic infection. Routine catheter change, use of a specific catheter type, antimicrobial impregnated catheters, and antiseptics in the drainage bag do not decrease symptomatic urinary infection and are not recommended.[47] There is a small risk of transient bacteremia when a chronic indwelling catheter is replaced, but harmful outcomes have not been reported with this procedure, so antimicrobial prophylaxis with catheter change is not recommended.[47]

SUMMARY

Urinary infection is an important problem in older populations. Physicians who care for these patients need to understand the appropriate management of symptomatic infection and that asymptomatic bacteriuria is ubiquitous and does not require treatment. There are many areas of uncertainty relevant to urinary infections in the elderly. The role of estrogen deficiency in contributing to or preventing urinary infection in older women requires further study, as well as improved strategies for the diagnosis and treatment of chronic bacterial prostatitis in men. Reasons for the high prevalence of asymptomatic bacteriuria in residents of long-term care facilities need to be further characterized, and clinical presentations of symptomatic urinary infection in residents further defined in diagnostic and therapeutic studies. Comparative clinical trials exploring optimal agents and duration of therapy are needed for all older populations experiencing urinary infection. Finally, the ultimate solution for the problem of urinary infection in residents with chronic indwelling catheters will require advances in the development of biofilm-resistant biomaterials.

REFERENCES

1. Nicolle LE, Bradley S, Colgan R, et al. IDSA guidelines for the diagnosis and treatment of asymptomatic bacteriuria in adults. Clin Infect Dis 2005;40:643–54.

2. Schaeffer AJ. Chronic prostatitis and the chronic pelvic pain syndrome. N Engl J Med 2006;355:1690–8.

3. Nicolle LE. A practical approach to the management of complicated urinary tract infection. Drugs Aging 2001;18:243–54.

4. Nicolle LE. The chronic indwelling catheter and urinary infection in long term care facility residents. Infect Control Hosp Epidemiol 2001;22:316–21.

5. Hedin K, Peterson C, Wideback K, et al. Asymptomatic bacteriuria in a population of elderly in municipal; institutional care. Scand J Prim Health Care 2002;20:166–9.

6. Jackson SL, Boyko EJ, Scholes, et al. Predictors of urinary tract infection after menopause: a prospective study. Am J Med 2004;117:903–11.

7. Foxman B, Klemstein KL, Brown PD. Acute pyelonephritis in US hospitals in 1997: hospitalization and in-hospital mortality. Ann Epidemiol 2003;13:144–50.

8. Mims AD, Norman DC, Yamamura RH, et al. Clinically inapparent (asymptomatic) bacteriuria in ambulatory elderly men: epidemiological, clinical, and microbiological findings. J Am Geriatr Soc 1990;38:1209–14.

9. Griebling TL. Urologic diseases in America project: trends in resource use for urinary tract infections in men. J Urol 2005;173:1288–94.

10. Nicolle LE, Friesen D, Harding GKM, et al. Hospitalization from acute pyelonephritis in Manitoba, Canada during the period 1989–1992. Impact of diabetes, pregnancy, and aboriginal origin. Clin Infect Dis 1996;22:1051–6.

11. Stevenson KB, Moore J, Colwell H, et al. Standardized infection surveillance in long-term care: interfacility comparisons from a regional cohort of facilities. Infect Control Hosp Epidemiol 2005;26:231–8.

12. Nicolle LE, Strausbaugh LJ, Garibaldi RA. Infections and antibiotic resistance in nursing homes. Clin Microbiol Rev 1996;9:1–17.

13. Rodhe N, Lofgren S, Matussek A, et al. Asymptomatic bacteriuria in the elderly: high prevalence and high turnover of strains. Scand J Infect Dis 2008;40:804–10.

14. Nicolle LE. Asymptomatic bacteriuria in the elderly. Infect Dis Clin North Am 1997; 11:647–62.

15. Mylotte JM, Tayara A, Goodnough S. Epidemiology of bloodstream infection in nursing home residents: evaluation in a large cohort from multiple homes. Clin Infect Dis 2002;35:1484–90.

16. Nicolle LE. Catheter-related urinary tract infection. Drugs Aging 2005;22:627–39.

17. Warren JW. Catheter-associated urinary tract infections. Infect Dis Clin North Am 1997;11:609–22.

18. Muder RR, Brennen C, Wagener MM, et al. Bacteremia in a long term care facility: a five year prospective study of 163 consecutive episodes. Clin Infect Dis 1992; 14:647–54.

19. Rudman D, Hontanosas A, Cohen Z, et al. Clinical correlates of bacteremia in a veterans administration extended care facility. J Am Geriatr Soc 1998;36:726–32.

20. Kunin CM, Douthitt S, Dancing J, et al. The association between the use of urinary catheters and morbidity and mortality among elderly patients in nursing homes. Am J Epidemiol 1992;135:291–301.

21. Raz R, Gennesin Y, Wasser J, et al. Recurrent urinary tract infections in postmenopausal women. Clin Infect Dis 2000;30:152–6.

22. Foxman B, Somsel P, Tallman P, et al. Urinary tract infection among women aged 40 to 65: behavioral and sexual risk factors. J Clin Epidemiol 2001;54:710–8.

23. Moore EE, Howes SE, Scholes D, et al. Sexual intercourse and risk of symptomatic urinary tract infection in post-menopausal women. J Gen Intern Med 2008;23:595–9.

24. Pabich WL, Fihn SD, Stamm WE, et al. Prevalence and determinants of vaginal flora alterations in postmenopausal women. J Infect Dis 2003;188:1054–8.

25. Burton JP, Reid G. Evaluation of the bacterial vaginal flora of 20 postmenopausal women by direct (Nugent Score) and molecular (polymerase chain reaction and denaturing gradient gel electrophoresis) techniques. J Infect Dis 2002;186: 1770–80.
26. Raz R, Stamm W. A controlled trial of intra-vaginal estriol in post-menopausal women with recurrent urinary tract infections. N Engl J Med 1993;329:753–7.
27. Eriksen B. A randomized, open, parallel group study on the preventive effect of an estriol-releasing vaginal ring (Estring) on recurrent urinary tract infections in postmenopausal women. Am J Obstet Gynecol 1999;180:1072–9.
28. Hu KK, Boyko EJ, Scholes D, et al. Risk factors for urinary tract infections in post-menopausal women. Arch Intern Med 2004;164:989–93.
29. Orlander JD, Jick SS, Dean AD, et al. Urinary tract infections and estrogen use in older women. J Am Geriatr Soc 1992;40:817–20.
30. Rodhe N, Molstad S, Englund L, et al. Asymptomatic bacteriuria in a population of elderly residents living in a community setting: prevalence, characteristics, and associated factors. Fam Pract 2006;23:303–7.
31. Penrotta C, Aznar M, Mejia R, et al. Oestrogens for preventing recurrent urinary tract infections in post-menopausal women. Cochrane Database Syst Rev 2008;(2):CD005131. doi:10.1002/14651858. CD005131.pub2.
32. Raz R, Colodner R, Rohana Y, et al. Effectiveness of estriol-containing vaginal pessaries and nitrofurantoin macrocrystal therapy in the prevention of recurrent urinary tract infection in post-menopausal women. Clin Infect Dis 2003;36: 1362–8.
33. Stern JA, Hsieh V-C, Schaeffer AJ. Residual urine in the elderly female population: novel implications for oral estrogen replacement and impact on recurrent urinary tract infection. J Urol 2004;171:768–70.
34. Truzzi JCI, Almeida MR, Nunes EC, et al. Residual urinary volume and urinary tract infection – when are they linked. J Urol 2008;180:182–5.
35. Ouslander JG, Greendale GA, Uman G, et al. Effects of oral estrogen and progestin on the lower urinary tract among female nursing home residents. J Am Geriatr Soc 2001;49:803–7.
36. Omli R, Skotnes LH, Mykletun A, et al. Residual urine as a risk factor for lower urinary tract infection: a 1-year follow-up study in nursing homes. J Am Geriatr Soc 2008;56:871–4.
37. Barabas G, Molstad S. No association between elevated post-void residual volume and bacteriuria in residents of nursing homes. Scand J Prim Health Care 2005;23:52–6.
38. Ouslander JG, Greengold B, Chen S. External catheter use and urinary tract infection among incontinent male nursing home patients. J Am Geriatr Soc 1987;35:1063–70.
39. Saint S, Chenoweth CE. Biofilms and catheter-associated urinary tract infections. Infect Dis Clin North Am 2003;17:411–32.
40. Vogel T, Verreault R, Gourdeau M, et al. Optimal duration of antimicrobial therapy for uncomplicated urinary tract infection in older women: a double-blind, randomized controlled trial. Can Med Assoc J 2004;170:469–73.
41. Boyko EJ, Fihn SD, Scholes D, et al. Diabetes and the risk of acute urinary tract infection among postmenopausal women. Diabetes Care 2002;25:1778–83.
42. Wright SW, Warren KD, Haynes ML. Trimethoprim/sulfamethoxazole resistance among urinary coliform isolates. J Gen Intern Med 1999;14:606–9.
43. Colodner R, Kometiani I, Chazan B, et al. Risk factors for community-acquired urinary tract infection due to quinolone resistant E. coli. Infection 2008;36:41–5.

44. Warren JW, Tenney JH, Hoopes JM, et al. A prospective microbiologic study of bacteriuria in patients with chronic indwelling urethral catheters. J Infect Dis 1982;146:719–23.

45. High KP, Bradley SF, Gravenstein S, et al. Clinical practice guideline for the evaluation of fever and infection in older adult residents of long-term care facilities. Clin Infect Dis 2009;48:149–71.

46. Nicolle LE. Consequences of asymptomatic bacteriuria in the elderly. Int J Antimicrob Agents 1994;4:107–12.

47. Nicolle LE, SHEA Long Term Care Committee. Urinary tract infections in long term care facilities. Infect Control Hosp Epidemiol 2001;22:167–75.

48. Juthani-Mehta M, Quagliarello V, Perrelli E, et al. Clinical features to identify UTI in nursing home residents: a cohort study. J Am Geriatr Soc 2009;57:963–70.

49. Orr P, Nicolle LE, Duckworth H, et al. Febrile urinary infection in the institutionalized elderly. Am J Med 1996;100:71–7.

50. Loeb M, Bentley DW, Bradley S, et al. Development of minimum criteria for the initiation of antibiotics in residents of long term care facilities: results of a consensus conference. Infect Control Hosp Epidemiol 2001;22:120–4.

51. Loeb M, Brazil K, Lohfeld L, et al. Effect of a multifaceted intervention on number of antimicrobial prescriptions for suspected urinary tract infections in residents of nursing homes: cluster randomized controlled trial. BMJ 2005;331(7518):669.

52. Raz R, Schiller D, Nicolle LE. Chronic indwelling catheter replacement prior to antimicrobial therapy for symptomatic urinary infection. J Urol 2000;164:1254–8.

53. Lipsky BA. Urinary tract infections in men. Epidemiology, pathophysiology, diagnosis and treatment. Ann Intern Med 1989;110:138–50.

54. Steward DK, Wood GL, Cohen RL, et al. Failure of the urinalysis and quantitative urine culture in diagnosing symptomatic urinary tract infections in patients with long-term urinary catheters. Am J Infect Control 1995;13:154–60.

55. Gomolin IH, Siami PF, Reuning-Scherer J, et al. Efficacy and safety of oral ciprofloxacin suspension versus trimethoprim-sulfamethoxazole oral suspension for treatment of older women with acute urinary tract infection. J Am Geriatr Soc 2001;49:1606–13.

56. Stothers L. A randomized trial to evaluate effectiveness and cost effectiveness of naturopathic cranberry products as prophylaxis against urinary tract infection in women. Can J Urol 2002;9:1558–62.

57. McMurdo ME, Argo I, Phillips G, et al. Cranberry or trimethoprim for the prevention of recurrent urinary tract infections? A randomized controlled trial in older women. J Antimicrob Chemother 2009;63:389–95.

58. McMurdo ME, Bissett LY, Price RJ, et al. Does ingestion of cranberry juice reduce symptomatic urinary tract infections in older people in hospital? A double-blind, placebo-controlled trial. Age Ageing 2005;34:256–61.

Obstructive Uropathy

Timothy Y. Tseng, MD, Marshall L. Stoller, MD*

KEYWORDS

- Uropathy • Urinary tract • Obstruction
- Postobstructive diuresis • Benign prostatic hyperplasia

Obstructive uropathy is a relatively common condition in which an anatomic or functional problem causes obstruction to normal urinary flow. The clinical manifestations of obstructive uropathy range from little or no symptoms to florid acute renal failure. Because its prevalence increases with increasing age, the diagnosis and management of obstructive uropathy is particularly relevant to the geriatric population.

EPIDEMIOLOGY

Hydronephrosis, although indicative only of urinary tract dilation, can be a useful surrogate marker suggestive of obstruction. In a series of 59,064 autopsies, Bell[1] found the overall incidence of hydronephrosis in the general population to be 3.1%. When limited to patients aged 60 years or older, the incidence increased to 5.1%. Most of these cases occurred in men with an overall incidence of 6.2% compared with 2.9% in women and this was attributed to the increased incidence of benign prostatic hyperplasia (BPH) in this age group. When one considers the population of patients with acute renal failure, the incidence of obstructive uropathy further increases. McInnes and colleagues[2] found that among 4001 patients admitted to the geriatric units in 3 British hospitals, 6.8% were diagnosed with acute renal failure, of whom 9.5% were determined to have obstructive uropathy as the cause of their renal failure.

The US Nationwide Inpatient Sample (NIS) in 2006 recorded 343,187 discharge diagnoses of hydronephrosis, hydroureter, and/or urinary obstruction amounting to 0.9% of all discharges. Excluding diagnoses of hydronephrosis and hydroureter, which are not necessarily due to obstruction, the NIS recorded 41,144 discharge diagnoses of urinary obstruction alone. This amounted to 0.1% of all discharge diagnoses. Patients over the age of 65 years accounted for 70% of the diagnoses of urinary obstruction and men, in particular, accounted for 77% of these diagnoses.[3]

Department of Urology, University of California San Francisco, Box 0738, 400 Parnassus Avenue, UC Clinics A-638, San Francisco, CA 94143-0738, USA
* Corresponding author.
E-mail address: mstoller@urology.ucsf.edu (M.L. Stoller).

Clin Geriatr Med 25 (2009) 437–443
doi:10.1016/j.cger.2009.06.003
0749-0690/09/$ – see front matter © 2009 Elsevier Inc. All rights reserved.

ETIOLOGY

Urinary tract obstruction can occur at any point in the urinary tract and is classified by the level of obstruction and whether the cause is intrinsic or extrinsic to the urinary tract (**Table 1**). Renal obstruction in the elderly can be due to benign conditions such as renal cystic or calculous disease or malignant conditions such transitional cell carcinoma of the renal pelvis. Rarely, congenital megaureter and ureteropelvic junction (UPJ) obstruction, either intrinsic to the UPJ or due to extrinsic compression by a crossing vessel, can have their initial presentation at an advanced age. Along the course of the ureters, intrinsic causes for obstruction include calculi, ureteral strictures, and neoplasms of the transitional cell epithelium. Extrinsic compression can be due to vascular lesions such as aortic or iliac artery aneurysms, retroperitoneal malignancies such as colon cancer or metastatic bladder cancer, or inflammatory conditions such as retroperitoneal fibrosis. Although less common in elderly women, gynecologic malignancies may also be a source of urinary tract obstruction.

In the lower urinary tract, the most common reason for obstruction is BPH. Other causes include bladder calculi, urethral stricture, and neoplasms of the bladder, prostate, or urethra. In women, prolapse of pelvic organs such as the bladder, rectum, or small bowel through the vagina can also lead to functional outlet obstruction through kinking or compression of the urethra.[4] Iatrogenic injuries such as bladder neck contractures secondary to radical prostatectomy and urethral strictures secondary to urethral instrumentation are also possibilities.[5,6] Finally, indwelling urethral catheters, suprapubic catheters, or percutaneous nephrostomy tubes may become dislodged or kinked resulting in obstruction to urinary outflow.

Table 1 Causes of urinary tract obstruction in the elderly		
	Intrinsic	**Extrinsic**
Kidney	Calculous disease Cystic disease Renal cell carcinoma Transitional cell carcinoma of the renal pelvis Obstructive pyelonephritis Congenital fibrous ureteropelvic junction obstruction	Ureteropelvic junction obstruction as a result of a crossing vessel
Ureter	Calculous disease Stricture Transitional cell carcinoma Congenital megaureter	Aortic or iliac artery aneurysm Compression because of a vascular graft Retroperitoneal malignancy Retroperitoneal fibrosis Pelvic lipomatosis Gynecologic malignancy
Bladder	Neurogenic bladder Bladder neck contracture Malignancy of the bladder or prostate Calculous disease	BPH Prostatitis Pelvic organ prolapse
Urethra	Stricture Phimosis Meatal stenosis Malignancy of the urethra	

In addition to anatomic sources of urinary tract obstruction, functional obstruction may also be caused by a neurogenic bladder. Decreased bladder contractility may occur when parasympathetic motor innervation is interrupted after severe pelvic trauma or after extensive pelvic surgery such as abdominal perineal resection for rectal cancer. A sensory neurogenic bladder occurs when the afferent nerve fibers from the bladder are damaged and is most common because of diabetes mellitus, tabes dorsalis, or pernicious anemia. In this condition, a decrease in sensation of fullness results in chronic overdistention of the bladder which can eventually lead to stretch injury and decreased contractility. Another form of neurogenic outlet obstruction occurs with discoordination between bladder contraction and urethral sphincter relaxation termed detrusor-sphincter dyssynergia. This occurs primarily with upper motor neuron diseases such as cerebrovascular accident, Parkinson's disease, and demyelinating disorders.[7]

Functional bladder outlet obstruction may also be nonneurogenic in origin. The dysfunctional elimination syndrome is characterized by bladder and bowel dysfunction. It is thought that gross fecal impaction leads to mechanical compression of the bladder and bladder neck, which results in urinary obstruction.[8] Medications may also play a role in inducing functional bladder outlet obstruction. Anticholinergic medications commonly used for the treatment of overactive bladder, such as oxybutinin, may occasionally cause urinary retention. In addition, several other classes of medications including tricyclic antidepressants such as amitriptyline, antiemetic phenothiazines such as promethazine, and the anticonvulsant carbamazepine have significant anticholinergic effects that can lead to urinary retention.

Despite the many possible causes of obstructive uropathy, in studies of elderly patients with acute renal failure, the most common cause among all patients (male and female) was BPH.[5,9] In 47 elderly patients with obstructive uropathy as the cause of their acute renal failure, Kumar and colleagues[9] found that 38% were due to BPH, 19% were due to neurogenic bladder, and 15% were due to obstructive pyelonephritis. Calculous disease and the remaining individual malignancies each accounted for less than 10% of the total.

CLINICAL PRESENTATION

The clinical presentation of obstructive uropathy varies greatly and generally reflects the source of the obstruction. Patients with upper urinary tract obstruction of the kidneys or the ureters may present with flank pain or enlarged tender kidneys. Patients with lower urinary tract obstruction may present with symptoms of urgency, frequency, decreased force of stream, or incomplete emptying of the bladder frequently associated with BPH. Recurrent or persistent urinary tract infections are commonly associated with the prolonged urinary stasis of lower urinary tract obstruction. Those patients with significant urinary retention secondary to bladder outlet obstruction or a neurogenic bladder may also have a large, palpable, distended bladder in the lower abdomen.[10] Patients may present with anuria in those cases where the obstruction is complete, such as complete occlusion of the prostatic urethra, bilateral ureteral obstruction, or unilateral ureteral obstruction of a solitary kidney.[5,11]

In many cases, however, patients may be relatively asymptomatic and present primarily with sequelae of renal insufficiency. In their series of elderly patients with obstructive uropathy, Faubert and Porush[5] found that up to 40% were clinically uremic and presented with nausea, vomiting, and/or mental status changes. In another series, Batlle and colleagues[12] found that electrolyte disturbances consisting primarily of hyperkalemia and nonanion gap acidosis were present in 70% of patients. Patients with chronic obstruction may further present with hypertension due to hypervolemia in the case of bilateral obstruction or to increased renin release in the case of unilateral obstruction.[13] Microscopic or gross hematuria may also be found in up to 30% of patients.[5]

DIAGNOSIS OF URINARY TRACT OBSTRUCTION

A careful history should be taken with an emphasis on potentially predisposing conditions. All medications with anticholinergic effects should be noted. The physical examination should evaluate costovertebral angle tenderness and the presence of a palpable bladder in the abdomen. A rectal examination should assess rectal tone and evidence for constipation. In men, a determination of prostate size should also be made on rectal examination. In women, a pelvic examination should be performed to identify potential pelvic organ prolapse.

After physical examination, the diagnosis of urinary tract obstruction should be directed toward localizing the site of obstruction. A test that can be performed at the bedside to help identify lower urinary tract obstruction is the determination of a patient's postvoid residual urine volume (PVR). This can be accomplished noninvasively with a commonly available ultrasound-based bladder scanner or through urethral catheterization after having a patient attempt to void when he or she feels the urge to void. Although an elevated postvoid residual urine volume in the asymptomatic patient does not appear to significantly predict the development of a future episode of acute urinary retention, an elevated PVR of greater than 150 mL in the appropriate setting of oliguria, anuria, or acute renal insufficiency is suggestive of anatomic or functional lower tract obstruction.[5,14]

In those patients who are relatively asymptomatic and present with renal insufficiency, renal ultrasound is the initial imaging test of choice. Renal ultrasound is used generally to identify anatomic abnormalities such as hydronephrosis or ureteral dilatation that are suggestive of upper tract obstruction.[5,6] In some patients, renal pelvis or ureteral dilatation can be chronic in nature, possibly because of a past history of obstruction, but not indicative of current obstruction. Although upper urinary tract dilatation is frequently suggestive of upper urinary tract obstruction, the presence of bilateral hydronephrosis or hydroureter should prompt consideration of a lower urinary tract source of obstruction. Ultrasound may also be able to identify causes of obstruction such as urolithiasis or soft tissue masses. However, it is generally less useful than other imaging modalities for this purpose.

In patients who present with symptoms of colicky flank or abdominal pain suggestive of urolithiasis, a noncontrast renal protocol CT scan will visualize most stones. The addition of intravenous contrast aids in the identification of malignancies as a cause of obstruction but may not be feasible in patients with renal insufficiency. Excretory phase imaging with an intravenous pyelogram (IVP) or CT-IVP may further show intraluminal masses or evidence for extrinsic compression of the ureters or renal pelvis. A benign entity, retroperitoneal fibrosis may be suggested by imaging showing proximal hydroureteronephrosis with medial deviation of the ureters.[15]

For patients who cannot receive intravenous contrast, noninvasive imaging studies may be unable to pinpoint the source of obstruction. In this situation, urological consultation is warranted for retrograde pyelography to identify potential anatomic causes of obstruction. In the event that retrograde pyelography is technically infeasible, antegrade pyelography through percutaneous access is an alternative.

A constellation of appropriate symptoms with confirmatory imaging findings is frequently sufficient to strongly suggest the diagnosis and cause of obstruction, as well as the need for intervention, such as in the case of acute obstruction due to urolithiasis. Occasionally, however, the clinical picture may be less clear. No evidence of ureteral or renal pelvis dilation is found in approximately 5% of patients with upper urinary tract obstruction. Such nondilated obstructive uropathy is found primarily in elderly patients.[16–18] In these situations, additional investigation is warranted.

Although ultrasound and CT imaging can identify anatomic abnormalities suggestive of upper tract obstruction, only a functional study can definitively diagnose obstruction. Formerly the gold standard functional test, the Whitaker test, involves infusion of fluid at a rate of 10 mL/min through a percutaneous nephrostomy. Intrarenal pelvis pressures greater than 22 cm H_2O are considered indicative of upper tract obstruction.[19] Currently, diuretic nuclear renography is the functional test of choice. After intravenous administration of radioisotope tracer, split renal function can be calculated. Following injection of furosemide, a radiotracer clearance half-time ($t_{1/2}$) of greater than 20 minutes would be considered positive for obstruction. A normal clearance $t_{1/2}$ would be less than 10 minutes.[20] In patients with renal insufficiency, however, diuretic renography may be of limited usefulness because of inadequate excretion of the tracer.

MANAGEMENT OF OBSTRUCTIVE UROPATHY

In patients in whom the obstruction may be self-limited, such as with small ureteral calculi, conservative management is appropriate. Renal colic may be managed with nonsteroidal anti-inflammatory drugs in the absence of renal insufficiency.[21] In addition, medical therapy with a-adrenergic antagonists or calcium channel antagonists may decrease the time to expulsion of ureteral calculi.[22,23] Patients may then subsequently be referred to a urologist for definitive management should they fail a period of conservative management.

If the obstruction appears to be chronic in nature, immediate intervention may also be unnecessary. Reasons for acute intervention, however, include fever, potentially undrained infection, uncontrollable renal colic, high-grade obstruction, bilateral obstruction, obstruction of a solitary kidney, and acute renal insufficiency. In the acute setting, lower urinary tract obstruction due to anatomic or functional bladder outlet obstruction is treated with simple urinary catheter placement. Upper urinary tract obstruction can be treated with either endoscopic retrograde placement of an indwelling ureteral stent or percutaneous nephrostomy. Although both interventions are well tolerated, ureteral stenting is less effective in treating obstruction due to extrinsic compression such as that caused by malignancy.[24] On the other hand, percutaneous nephrostomy is contraindicated in patients with uncorrected coagulopathy or platelet dysfunction.

Once the obstruction is relieved, approximately 90% of patients with lower tract obstruction or bilateral upper tract obstruction experience a postobstructive diuresis.[25] In most patients, this diuresis is a physiologic response to volume expansion and solute accumulation. Therefore, the large postobstructive urine volumes need not be replaced with the administration of additional intravenous fluid. In a few patients, a pathologic diuresis due to a renal concentrating defect sustained during the period of obstruction may develop. In all patients with postobstructive diuresis, a basic metabolic panel and magnesium level should be checked daily. Patients who develop mental status changes should have their serum electrolytes and urine osmolarity checked at least every 12 hours and any abnormalities should be corrected as necessary.[6]

After an acute episode of obstruction has been addressed, referral to an urologist for definitive management can be made. For upper tract obstruction, various endoscopic, laparoscopic, and open procedures are available for reconstruction. However, observations in children have shown that there is little benefit to renal-sparing interventions in kidneys providing less than 10% of global renal function. In the elderly, kidneys with such poor function may be managed expectantly if they are asymptomatic. Otherwise, such essentially nonfunctioning kidneys are generally treated with nephrectomy.[26]

For lower tract obstruction, endoscopic and open procedures may be used to treat urethral strictures, bladder neck contractures, and BPH recalcitrant to optimized medical therapy with α-adrenergic antagonists and 5-α-reductase inhibitors. Pelvic organ prolapse in women may be corrected with pessary placement or more formal surgical repair. Medications with anticholinergic effects should be discontinued as appropriate and constipation, if present, should be corrected with an appropriate bowel regimen. If there is concern for neurogenic bladder as a cause of functional lower tract obstruction, the patient may be evaluated with urodynamics and an appropriate urinary drainage or diversion regimen selected. In some patients with sensory neurogenic bladders or altered mental status, timed or prompted voiding may be sufficient to promote adequate urinary drainage. In patients with poor bladder contractility or detrusor-sphincter dyssynergia, urinary drainage with clean intermittent catheterization is appropriate. When this is not possible because of a patient's poor manual dexterity or a lack of caregiver assistance, placement of a suprapubic catheter or a more formal urinary diversion may be necessary. In general, because of the risk for urethral erosion, chronic indwelling urethral catheter placement is not advised.

SUMMARY

Obstructive uropathy is a condition that disproportionately affects elderly patients and, in particular, elderly men. The causes of urinary tract obstruction may be anatomic, neurogenic, or iatrogenic. Although most cases are as a result of lower urinary tract obstruction from BPH and neurogenic bladder, a variety of causes involving the upper and lower urinary tract are possible. Management of acute urinary tract obstruction is directed toward establishing drainage across or around the site of obstruction. Careful monitoring of postobstructive diuresis must be undertaken to prevent complications from the development of pathologic postobstructive diuresis.

REFERENCES

1. Bell ET. Obstruction of the urinary tract – hydronephrosis. In: Renal diseases. 2nd edition. Philadelphia: Lea & Febiger; 1950. p. 117–45.
2. McInnes EG, Levy DW, Chaudhuri MD, et al. Renal failure in the elderly. Q J Med 1987;64:583–8.
3. Healthcare cost and utilization project. Agency for Healthcare Research and Quality; 2009. Available at: http://hcupnet.ahrq.gov. Accessed February 22, 2009.
4. Romanzi LJ, Chaikin DC, Blaivas JG. The effect of genital prolapse on voiding. J Urol 1999;161:581–6.
5. Faubert PF, Porush JG. Renal disease in the elderly. 2nd edition. New York: Marcel Dekker; 1998. p. 441.

6. Pais VM, Strandhoy JW, Assimos DG. Pathophysiology of urinary tract obstruction. In: Wein AJ, editor. Campbell-Walsh urology, vol. 2. 9th edition. Philadelphia: Saunders; 2007. p. 1195–226.

7. Wein AJ. Pathophysiology and classification of voiding dysfunction. In: Wein AJ, editor. Campbell-Walsh urology, vol. 3. 9th edition. Philadelphia: Saunders; 2007. p. 1973–85.

8. O'Regan S, Yazbeck S, Schick E. Constipation and the urinary system. In: O'Donnell B, Koff SA, editors. Pediatric urology. Oxford: Butterworth-Heinemann; 1997. p. 245–8.

9. Kumar R, Hill CM, McGeown MG. Acute renal failure in the elderly. Lancet 1973;1: 90–1.

10. Mukamel E, Nissenkorn I, Boner G, et al. Occult progressive renal damage in the elderly male due to benign prostatic hypertrophy. J Am Geriatr Soc 1979;27: 403–6.

11. Klahr S. Obstructive nephropathy. Intern Med 2000;39:355–61.

12. Batlle DC, Arruda JA, Kurtzman NA. Hyperkalemic distal renal tubular acidosis associated with obstructive uropathy. N Engl J Med 1981;304:373–80.

13. Jones DA, George NJ, O'Reilly PH, et al. Reversible hypertension associated with unrecognised high pressure chronic retention of urine. Lancet 1987;1:1052–4.

14. Kaplan SA, Wein AJ, Staskin DR, et al. Urinary retention and post-void residual urine in men: separating truth from tradition. J Urol 2008;180:47–54.

15. Cronin CG, Lohan DG, Blake MA, et al. Retroperitoneal fibrosis: a review of clinical features and imaging findings. AJR Am J Roentgenol 2008;191:423–31.

16. Spital A, Valvo JR, Segal AJ. Nondilated obstructive uropathy. Urology 1988;31: 478–82.

17. Maillet PJ, Pelle-Francoz D, Laville M, et al. Nondilated obstructive acute renal failure: diagnostic procedures and therapeutic management. Radiology 1986; 160:659–62.

18. Naidich JB, Rackson ME, Mossey RT, et al. Nondilated obstructive uropathy: percutaneous nephrostomy performed to reverse renal failure. Radiology 1986; 160:653–7.

19. Whitaker RH. Methods of assessing obstruction in dilated ureters. Br J Urol 1973; 45:15–22.

20. Roarke MC, Sandler CM. Provocative imaging. Diuretic renography. Urol Clin North Am 1998;25:227–49.

21. Mense S. Basic neurobiologic mechanisms of pain and analgesia. Am J Med 1983;75:4–14.

22. Hollingsworth JM, Rogers MA, Kaufman SR, et al. Medical therapy to facilitate urinary stone passage: a meta-analysis. Lancet 2006;368:1171–9.

23. Parsons JK, Hergan LA, Sakamoto K, et al. Efficacy of alpha-blockers for the treatment of ureteral stones. J Urol 2007;177:983–7 [discussion: 87].

24. Yossepowitch O, Lifshitz DA, Dekel Y, et al. Predicting the success of retrograde stenting for managing ureteral obstruction. J Urol 2001;166:1746–9.

25. Nadig PW, Valk WL. Recovery from obstructive disease. J Urol 1962;88:470–2.

26. Dhillon HK. Prenatally diagnosed hydronephrosis: the Great Ormond Street experience. Br J Urol 1998;81(Suppl 2):39–44.

Urinary Incontinence in the Elderly

Tomas L. Griebling, MD, MPH

KEYWORDS

- Urinary incontinence • Bladder • Elderly
- Geriatric • Surgery • Urology

Urinary incontinence (UI), defined as the involuntary leakage of urine, is a common clinical condition that occurs frequently in older adults. Estimates suggest that at least 25% to 30% of all adults will experience UI at some point in their lives. In people older than 65 years, the estimated prevalence of UI ranges from approximately 35% for those who reside in the community to more than 60% for those who live in long-term care facilities.[1–4] Although the incidence and prevalence of incontinence are higher in elderly compared with younger people, the condition should not be considered a normal or inevitable part of the aging process.[5] The costs of UI, in terms of financial expenditures and psychosocial burdens for older adults and caregivers, are significant. It is estimated that the total cost of UI care, including evaluation, treatment, and use of absorbent products among community-dwelling individuals, was approximately $14 billion in the year 2000 in the United States.[6,7] Older adults with UI also have greater individual annual health care costs compared with nonincontinent patients of similar age.

The personal impact of UI can be significant. Multiple studies have shown that UI is associated with a dramatic reduction in overall and health-related quality of life for older adults.[8–10] This is true for people living independently in the community and for those in assisted-living and long-term care environments.[11] UI has been linked to many other important health risks, including depression and functional disability, which may result from social isolation and inability to participate in desired activities.[12] Elderly individuals with UI have a higher risk for falls and fractures compared with those who do not leak urine.[13,14] Incontinence may have a negative effect on sexual health in men and women.[15] UI may also be a marker for increased mortality risk in some patients.[16]

Disclosures: Dr Griebling has received research support from The National Institutes of Health, The American Geriatrics Society, The John A. Hartford Foundation, Pfizer, and Medtronic.
Department of Urology and The Landon Center on Aging, Mail Stop 3016, The University of Kansas, 3901 Rainbow Boulevard, Kansas City, KS 66160, USA
E-mail address: tgriebling@kumc.edu

Clin Geriatr Med 25 (2009) 445–457
doi:10.1016/j.cger.2009.06.004
0749-0690/09/$ – see front matter © 2009 Elsevier Inc. All rights reserved.

TYPES OF URINARY INCONTINENCE

Normal lower urinary tract function requires complex coordination between the central and peripheral nervous system and the neuromuscular interface of the bladder and lower genitourinary tract. The bladder must fill at low pressures with appropriate muscular compliance to adequately store urine. Micturition requires activation of the neuromuscular pathways that lead to coordinated contraction of the detrusor with relaxation of the urethral sphincter. Parasympathetic cholinergic activity mediates bladder contractility. Sphincteric relaxation is mediated by adrenergic pathways through the spinal reflex arc from the S_2–S_4 sacral nerve roots. Central coordination occurs at the level of the pons. Any alterations to this cycle caused by anatomic or physiologic changes may lead to disruption of the normal storage and voiding cycle, which may lead to problems with UI.

There are several different types of UI seen in older adults. In most cases, careful clinical evaluation can help to categorize the type of incontinence and facilitate identification of the cause of the problem. Options for treatment are based largely on the type of UI experienced by the patient. Selection of therapy is made with consideration of the patient's goals and expectations and their concomitant health conditions.[17] Two broad categories of UI seen in older adults include transient incontinence and chronic incontinence. Both can be subdivided into several additional categories.

Transient Incontinence

The term "transient incontinence" refers to UI that develops in a patient because of a temporary underlying condition, which may or may not be directly associated with the urinary system. Treatment of the inciting factor that is causing the incontinence often leads to improvement or complete resolution of symptoms. Examples of factors that can cause transient incontinence include urinary tract infections (UTIs), atrophic vaginitis, urethritis, or prostatitis. These conditions are typically associated with dysuria and urinary urgency. Some medications, particularly diuretics, may result in new onset of UI either because of increased urine production or other adverse events associated with the medication. In these cases, discontinuation of the medication often leads to resolution of symptoms.

Several physiologic conditions may lead to polyuria and UI, including diabetes insipidus, psychogenic polydipsia, hyperglycemia, and hypercalcemia. Fluid overload associated with congestive heart failure may also lead to increased urine production and transient incontinence. Delirium is a syndrome associated with acute changes in mental status characterized by a fluctuating course. Hallmark clinical features include confusion, inattention, and alterations in level of consciousness, which may manifest as either agitation or somnolence. Many patients with delirium experience associated transient UI. Fecal impaction is often associated with development of UI. This may be due in part to the space-occupying nature of the stool in the colon adjacent to the urinary bladder. Older adults with significant fecal impaction may present with complaints of constipation or abdominal pain. Some patients have significant diarrhea as a result of liquid stool from the more proximal intestine passing around the point of impaction.

Chronic Incontinence

Most UI experienced by older adults is chronic or established. This term implies that the incontinence symptoms are persistent and not caused by a temporary associated condition. There are several common types of chronic UI observed in older adults (**Table 1**).

Table 1
Types of urinary incontinence and typical associated symptoms and etiologies

Type of UI	Common Symptoms	Common Causes
Stress	Leakage with physical activities that increase abdominal pressure	Sphincteric dysfunction Urethral hypermobility Radical prostatectomy
Urge	Urgency, frequency, nocturia, urine leakage before reaching toilet	Detrusor overactivity Neurologic disorders Spinal cord injury
Overflow	Frequent small-volume leaks often not associated with activity	Detrusor failure Neurologic disorders Spinal cord injury Diabetes
Functional	Leakage symptoms are variable	Mobility impairment Cognitive impairment
Mixed	Leakage symptoms are variable	Cause is variable

Stress Incontinence

Stress incontinence is characterized by loss of urine with activities that increase intra-abdominal pressure. Examples include coughing, sneezing, lifting, or laughing. The cause is often due to inadequate closure of the external urethral sphincter. Urethral hypermobility with loss of support of the urethra is also seen in some women with stress incontinence. In men, the most common associated risk factors include a history of either radical prostatectomy for treatment of prostate cancer or transurethral resection of the prostate for treatment of benign prostatic hyperplasia. In each of these cases, the pressure inside the abdomen exceeds the closure pressure at the urethral outlet leading to leakage of urine.

Urge Incontinence

Urge incontinence is typically associated with sudden onset of a sensation of needing to void, with loss of urine occurring before the patient is able to reach toilet facilities. Symptoms include urinary urgency, frequency, and nocturia. Physiologically, these symptoms are usually caused by uninhibited contractions of the bladder detrusor muscle. The term "overactive bladder," or OAB, has also been used to describe this condition. There are two forms, including OAB-dry, which is characterized by urinary urgency and frequency but no leakage of urine, and OAB-wet, which includes UI.[18] Common causative factors include neurologic disorders, such as multiple sclerosis, Parkinson disease, stroke, spinal cord injuries, and disorders such as spinal stenosis. Dementia may also be associated with urge incontinence.

Overflow Incontinence

Overflow incontinence is typically associated with either outlet obstruction or poor detrusor contractility and incomplete bladder emptying.[19] In men, benign prostatic hyperplasia may lead to outlet obstruction and overflow incontinence. Urethral strictures are more common in men, but may also occur in women and lead to problems with overflow. Patients typically experience frequent loss of small volumes of urine, in contrast to the larger volumes of urine leakage associated with urge incontinence.

Functional Incontinence

The term "functional incontinence" refers to urinary leakage that occurs as a result of factors not directly associated with the bladder, which may prevent independent toilet use. The most common examples in older adults include limitations in either mobility or cognition. These factors may be transient as in the case of an elderly patient who has experienced a hip fracture and is not able to physically transfer on and off a toilet independently. This may be a temporary condition that will improve with resolution of the underlying mobility problem. Chronic conditions may also lead to functional incontinence. Dementia caused by Alzheimer disease or vascular disorders may lead to functional incontinence due to lack of recognition of the sensation of a full bladder.[20] In addition, dementia patients may not be able to perform the requisite tasks including manipulation of clothing or use of the toilet to remain continent.

Mixed Incontinence

Many older adults with chronic incontinence problems describe a combination of different urinary symptoms. When more than one type of UI occurs at a time, the term "mixed incontinence" is applied. A combination of stress and urge UI is extremely common. Some patients can describe the predominant symptom and this may be amenable to initial therapy.

Another unique form of mixed incontinence that is more common in older adults is termed "detrusor hyperactivity with impaired contractility (DHIC)". In this condition, patients experience urinary urgency and frequency caused by uninhibited contractions of the detrusor. However, when they try to void voluntarily, the bladder does not contract adequately, and therefore does not empty completely. This may lead to associated overflow incontinence.

Fecal Incontinence

Neuromuscular control of the distal colon and rectum is also coordinated through the S_2–S_4 reflex arc. Patients with UI, particularly urge incontinence, may also experience problems with fecal incontinence. Although a thorough discussion of fecal incontinence is beyond the scope of this article, providers should remember to ask about problems with defecation in patients with UI. Chronic constipation is a common complaint in elderly patients, and this may exacerbate UI symptoms.

EVALUATION

The clinical evaluation of the older adult with UI includes several important components. Careful evaluation is critical because the selection of treatments varies widely depending on the type of UI an older person is experiencing. In addition, the choice of treatment needs to be placed in the context of overall functional and health status and the role of other comorbid conditions.

History and Physical Examination

A good history and physical examination is critical in the clinical assessment of older adults with UI. Patients often do not volunteer information about UI symptoms, perhaps because of embarrassment or an assumption that nothing can be done to improve the condition. Health care providers need to specifically ask about incontinence symptoms as part of their routine care of older adults. A variety of questionnaires have been developed to help quantify UI and assess the impact of the condition on overall function in multiple domains. The history should seek to gather information about the nature of the leakage, the frequency and duration of symptoms, any inciting activities or factors, and any treatments or methods of control that have already been used. A careful past history is useful to determine if underlying conditions may be associated with the incontinence. This includes an obstetric history and any information about prior genitourinary surgery, radiation, or trauma.

Physical examination includes a pelvic or genital and rectal examination in both men and women. The examination can yield valuable information about bladder and urethral mobility, prostate disease, pelvic floor support, and pelvic organ prolapse. Ideally, the patient is examined with a moderate amount of urine in the bladder. Stress incontinence with urine leakage may be observed when the patient is asked to cough or perform a Valsalva maneuver. Functional assessment in older adults includes an evaluation of the ability to perform basic activities of daily living, such as bathing, dressing, grooming, eating, and toileting. Physical examination may also provide important data about an elderly patient's mobility and cognition, which can directly influence continence status.

Voiding Diaries

Completion of a voiding diary can provide valuable information for the clinician taking care of patients with UI symptoms. The time of each urination episode and any associated symptoms of incontinence are noted for three 24-hour periods. If possible, the patient can also record the amount of fluid intake and output. However, this requires more effort and may not be possible for all patients and caregivers. This information can help to identify cases of excess fluid intake with resultant polyuria. Diaries can also help to quantify the extent of UI and nocturia and may help to differentiate between the various forms of UI, based on the pattern observed.

Laboratory Tests

Urinalysis is helpful to look for UTI, hematuria, or other medical conditions that may be associated with development of UI. If UTI is suspected based on dipstick urinalysis, then a specimen should be sent for bacterial culture and antibiotic susceptibility testing. This is extremely useful to guide appropriate antibiotic therapy. The presence of persistent hematuria should prompt additional evaluation, including upper tract imaging and cystoscopy. Some patients with bladder cancers or carcinoma in situ may present with urinary urgency and urge incontinence, with hematuria as initial symptoms. Many older adults take anticoagulants, which may increase the risk for hematuria. However, evaluation may lead to identification of significant underlying urologic pathology in approximately 15% of patients.

Measurement of levels of serum electrolytes, creatinine, and calcium may be indicated in patients if there is concern for impaired renal function or in patients with polyuria, who are not taking diuretics. Blood glucose screening may be helpful in identifying patients with diabetes and associated polyuria and UI.

Measurement of postvoid residual volume is performed to exclude urinary retention as a possible contributing factor for incontinence. This can be performed either by bladder catheterization or using a portable ultrasound device designed to measure urine volume. Although the definition of an elevated postvoid volume is somewhat controversial, a volume of more than 200 mL indicates either probable bladder outlet obstruction or detrusor dysfunction. This would be an indication for additional urologic evaluation.

Urodynamic Studies

In complex clinical cases or cases associated with significant neurologic or other comorbid disease, urodynamic testing may be indicated to guide diagnosis and therapy. This may range from simple urodynamics, with measurement of bladder capacity or noninvasive uroflowmetry, to more complex multichannel studies that examine storage and emptying capabilities. The need for urodynamics should be based on what will be done with the information gathered from the evaluation and the ability of the patient to actually undergo the testing procedure. Subjects must be able to follow commands and cooperate with testing to yield useful information. To the extent possible, the goal of the urodynamic tests should be to reproduce the symptoms experienced by the patient. Simultaneous measurement of detrusor pressure and urinary flow may be particularly helpful to differentiate between outlet obstruction and detrusor insufficiency in patients with symptoms of overflow incontinence. Urodynamic tests can also be informative in patients who have not experienced significant improvement in symptoms despite prior therapy.

TREATMENT
Conservative Treatments

Most older adults prefer to start with conservative therapies before considering medications or surgery to treat their UI symptoms. Many of these treatments can yield significant improvements in UI symptoms. However, compliance may be an issue with some forms of therapy. For many older adults, multiple small improvements in various parameters associated with UI and bladder function may lead to significant subjective improvement in symptoms.

Dietary Modification and Weight Loss

Several foods and beverages may exacerbate lower urinary tract symptoms for older adults with UI. Caffeine has a direct irritant effect on the bladder mucosa and is particularly bothersome for many patients. In some cases, restriction or elimination of dietary caffeine may lead to significant improvements in bladder symptoms. Highly acidic foods and beverages, including citrus fruits and juices, may bother some patients. Alcohol is also a common inciting factor because of bladder-irritant and diuretic properties. Many patients with incontinence may try to limit overall fluid intake in an attempt to reduce bladder symptoms. However, this can be counterproductive. If a patient becomes dehydrated, the urine will become more concentrated, which in turn can lead to increased mucosal irritation, with urinary urgency and dysuria. Older adults often have alterations in their thirst mechanism, which may influence intake. Patients should be encouraged to drink adequate volumes of fluid to remain well hydrated. Fluid volumes may need to be limited in some older adults with a history of congestive heart failure and fluid overload.

The timing of fluid intake has also been examined in older adults. Many elderly patients with lower urinary tract symptoms complain of nocturia, which may disrupt sleep, leading to reduction in quality of life and functional capacity. The causes of nocturia are generally considered to be multifactorial.[21] Decreasing late-afternoon or evening fluid intake is often advocated for elderly patients with nocturia. However, the scientific rationale and clinical usefulness of this recommendation are still under investigation. Obstructive sleep apnea has been linked to reduced production of anti-diuretic hormone in older adults.[22] Correction of the sleep apnea may help to reduce nocturia symptoms. The administration of exogenous arginine vasopressin in elderly patients is controversial and still under investigation. This form of treatment may lead to severe hyponatremia and requires close monitoring, particularly in older adults.

Weight loss may also be helpful for some patients, particularly women with stress UI. Clinical trials have demonstrated that weight loss may be helpful to reduce stress incontinence symptoms in women who are moderately or severely obese.[23] The specific role of weight reduction in elderly women has not been explicitly examined. Weight reduction in elderly patients should be done in the context of overall nutritional health, and may need to be supervised by a health care provider to ensure that adequate dietary requirements are met.

Timed Voiding and Bladder Retraining

Several behavioral techniques can be useful for elderly patients with urinary urgency and urge incontinence. Timed voiding is often recommended, particularly if patients find they are unable to delay voiding and incontinence episodes at reliable time intervals.[24] Many patients only experience problems when the bladder is full, so voiding somewhat more often to prevent this urgency caused by bladder distension may reduce problems in some cases. The term "bladder retraining" is applied to a prescribed intervention in which patients are taught to delay voiding at progressively longer intervals. This may be combined with timed voiding and pelvic floor muscle exercise techniques. Patients with urinary urgency or urge incontinence are taught to focus on the sensations in the pelvis, do several pelvic floor contractions, wait until the urgency sensation subsides, then proceed to the toilet at a normal rate of speed. This is often more successful than rushing to the toilet, which may lead to additional uninhibited bladder contractions and urinary leakage. All of these methods require the patient to have sufficient cognitive awareness and function to actively participate in these forms of therapy.

Similar techniques have been used successfully in nursing home residents who may respond well to prompted toileting on a regularly scheduled time interval.[25] In older adults with cognitive or mobility impairments, simple prompting may not be sufficient, and assisted toileting programs may be necessary. In these cases, staff members physically help the older adult to use the toilet on a regular schedule.

Pelvic Floor Muscle Exercises

Originally popularized by Kegel in the 1950s, pelvic floor muscle training (PFMT) remains one of the mainstays of behavioral therapy in the treatment of UI.[26] Although perhaps most associated with the treatment of stress UI in women, there is growing evidence that PFMT is useful for the treatment of conditions in both men and women including stress incontinence, urinary urgency, and urge incontinence. It is important that patients understand how to perform the exercises correctly, with contraction of the bulbocavernosus muscle as the primary focus. Biofeedback training may be helpful in this process.[27,28] Care should be taken to avoid performing a Valsalva maneuver during the contraction, which would increase intra-abdominal pressure. This could lead to urinary leakage. Pelvic floor relaxation techniques are also an important component of PFMT, particularly in patients with urgency and urge UI. Some studies support the combined use of PFMT and medications in this patient population.[29,30] Research on the feasibility and use of PFMT in elderly patients with cognitive impairment has been limited.

Pessaries

Pessaries have been used for hundreds of years for the treatment of pelvic organ prolapse and UI in women. They offer the advantage of avoiding surgery while providing functional support that may successfully reduce or eliminate incontinence for some women. Imaging studies demonstrate that pessaries work by providing support under the bladder and urethra.[31] This may also work to correct the angles and contact between adjacent organs.

These devices come in a wide variety of shapes and sizes, and must be fitted individually for each patient. Some models are specifically designed to provide support under the urethra to reduce stress UI due to either urethral hypermobility or intrinsic sphincter deficiency. These do require careful follow-up, and patients must be taught how to remove and reinsert the pessary for routine cleaning and care. In women with severe hand arthritis, assistance from a care provider may be necessary to manipulate the pessary. Administration of topical vaginal estrogen creams may be useful to prevent tissue erosion, particularly in women with a history of atrophic vaginitis.

Pads and Absorbent Products

By the time they seek treatment from a health care provider, many older adults are already using some type of pad or absorbent product to help control their UI. Although these certainly have an important role in the management of urinary leakage for many elderly patients, they do not cure incontinence and are generally not regarded as an ideal form of therapy. Older adults should be encouraged to seek other types of treatment if appropriate and not become complacent about the use of pads and absorbent products. There have been significant improvements in the design of available products with increased absorbency and methods to control odor. In some cases, use of these products may help older adults to remain more functional and able to engage in desired activities.[17] Use must be balanced with cost, which can be significant. This includes not only the financial cost of the product but also the psychosocial cost of the need to use pads. In addition, there is an environmental cost of placing large volumes of absorbent pads and products into landfills and other waste management systems.

Pharmacologic Treatments

Medications have been used to treat various forms of UI, although most prescription medication is now used for urge incontinence. α-Adrenergic agents can theoretically increase the outlet resistance of the external sphincter. However, these drugs tend to be associated with adverse effects and generally have poor clinical efficacy for stress incontinence, which limits overall usefulness. Administration of topical vaginal estrogens may be useful in the treatment of atrophic vaginitis associated with transient incontinence. This may also improve sexual function and comfort in older women who are sexually active. However, the clinical usefulness of estrogen to improve chronic UI is limited.

The anticholinergic, antimuscarinic medications are commonly prescribed to treat urge UI.[32] These agents work by blocking cholinergic receptors in the bladder, which leads to a decrease in bladder contractility. There are a wide variety of medications in this class that can be used to treat urge UI (**Table 2**). Older medications such as oxybutynin are nonselective and tend to be associated with a higher rate of adverse events.[33] Crossreactivity with muscarinic receptors in the salivary glands and colon leads to symptoms of dry mouth and constipation. Other common side effects may include dry eyes and blurry vision. Some of the newer agents are theoretically more uroselective and preferentially bind to the muscarinic receptors in the bladder. These may be associated with lower rates of adverse effects but are generally more expensive because of the lack of generic nonbranded formulations.

Contraindications to the use of all these drugs include hypersensitivity to the agents or a history of untreated closed-angle glaucoma. Another concern is the potential for central nervous system effects that may worsen confusion in older adults, particularly those with a history of mild cognitive impairment or dementia. Cholinesterase inhibitors are often prescribed to prevent deterioration of memory function, and the

Table 2
Common pharmacologic agents used to treat urge urinary incontinence

Generic Name	Trade Name	Typical Dosage
Oxybutynin	Ditropan	2.5–5.0 mg po bid, tid
Oxybutynin (extended release)	Ditropan XL	5, 10, or 15 mg po daily
Oxybutynin (transdermal)	Oxytrol	1 topical patch, q 3 days (provides 3.9 mg/d)
Oxybutynin (transdermal)	Gelnique	10% gel once daily
Tolterodine	Detrol	1 or 2 mg po bid
Tolterodine (extended release)	Detrol LA	2 or 4 mg po daily
Solifenacin	Vesicare	5 or 10 mg po daily
Darifenacin	Enablex	7.5 or 15 mg po daily
Trospium	Sanctura	20 mg po bid
Trospium (extended release)	Sanctura XR	60 mg po daily
Fesoterodine	Toviaz	4 or 8 mg po daily

anticholinergic agents act in pharmacologic opposition.[34] A study in 2008 showed that in people taking cholinesterase inhibitors for memory problems, addition of an anticholinergic agent to treat bladder symptoms led to more pronounced and more rapid loss of cognitive function.[35]

Surgical Treatments

Surgery is also a common form of therapy for the treatment of UI in adults. Some health care providers and elderly patients may hesitate to consider surgical therapy for incontinence due to a patient's age. However, chronologic age is generally not considered to be a good predictor of outcome in terms of either morbidity or mortality in elderly surgical patients. Overall comorbidity due to chronic diseases that are common in older patients is believed to play a much more important role in this process. These conditions include hypertension, diabetes, renal insufficiency, cardiovascular disease, and pulmonary disease. Preoperative optimization of these underlying medical conditions can help to enhance surgical outcomes and improve safety.

Elderly patients should not be excluded from consideration for surgical therapy for UI based solely on age if they are otherwise appropriate candidates. Careful discussion of the potential risks and benefits of surgery must be carried out with all older patients and their families and caregivers. Informed consent with consideration of the overall goals and objectives of treatment is also essential. This discussion focuses on surgical treatments for stress UI in women, and neuromodulation for treatment of urinary urgency and urge incontinence in men and women.

Sling Procedures

In recent years, the primary form of open surgical therapy for the treatment of stress UI in women has been the sling cystourethropexy. There are several variations in surgical technique related to the exact location of the sling and the nature of the graft material used to create the sling.[36,37] Most slings are placed either at the level of the bladder neck or at the midurethra. Functionally, these act to increase the outlet resistance to prevent urine leakage during times of increased intra-abdominal pressure. Midurethral slings appear to be most effective in women who have a component of urethral hypermobility associated with stress incontinence. In women with pure intrinsic sphincter deficiency, a pubovaginal sling located at the bladder neck may be more effective. The choices for graft material include autologous fascia from the patient, with harvest of either fascia lata or rectus abdominus fascia, allograft fascia from a cadaveric donor, xenograft materials derived from animal products, or artificial mesh materials.

Sling surgeries have been used successfully in elderly women with stress incontinence. The reported initial success rates for slings range from approximately 80% to 90% of women improved or dry. As with all surgeries, these rates decrease somewhat with time. Recurrent incontinence is not uncommon and may respond to other forms of therapy or to repeat sling surgery. The main postoperative complications after sling surgery in women include UTI, new onset urinary urgency and urge incontinence, and urinary retention or incomplete bladder emptying.[38] Although the overall rates of these complications may be slightly higher in elderly women undergoing sling compared with their younger counterparts, this should not preclude consideration of sling as a viable option for some older women with stress UI.

Bulking Agent Injection Therapy

Cystoscopic injection of bulking materials under the urethral mucosa at the neck of the bladder may be helpful to treat stress UI in some elderly women. This treatment is minimally invasive and can be performed in the outpatient clinical setting with minimal anesthetic requirements. It offers the advantage of immediate results with rapid recovery time to baseline activity. Overall reported initial success is in the range of 75% to 80%. The main problem with injection therapy is that it usually needs to be repeated with time, with approximately 70% of patients who experience good clinical improvement requiring additional injections. Several different bulking agents have been used, although glutaraldehyde crosslinked bovine collagen remains the most commonly used product. This does require allergen skin testing to make sure the patient does not have a hypersensitivity to the materials. Other materials eliminate the need for allergen testing, but can be technically more challenging to administer. The overall success rates are similar for the different available products. Injection therapy may be particularly useful in elderly women who may not be candidates for a more involved surgical procedure such as a sling. In addition, injection therapy may be quite useful as an adjuvant treatment for persistent stress incontinence after previous placement of a sling.[39] Patients need to be clearly counseled about the likely need for multiple injection procedures to achieve a clinically significant improvement.

Neuromodulation

Electrical stimulation of the nerve roots involved in the coordination of micturition may be useful for the treatment of urinary urgency, urge incontinence, and some forms of idiopathic urinary retention. The electrode is connected to a programmable pulse generator that emits a signal to the selected nerve, typically the S_3 sacral nerve root. Other nerves involved in the micturition process, including the pudendal nerve, have also been examined as potential targets for this type of therapy. Studies specifically looking at the clinical use of neuromodulation in elderly patients have been limited. However, clinical experience and available data suggest that this may be successful in selected patients.[40,41] This therapy is interactive, and programming of the device is often necessary to achieve significant improvement. Successful therapy may require multimodal therapy with continuation of pelvic floor exercise, behavioral therapy, or medications. The main risks and complications associated with neuromodulation include pain at the generator site or device infection, which can necessitate surgical removal. Because of the cost associated with the implanted materials, this therapy is expensive, and most elderly patients will try other forms of therapy before selecting neuromodulation.

PREVENTION AND CONTINENCE PROMOTION

There is increased interest in the role of targeted intervention in the prevention of UI in men and women. A National Institutes of Health consensus conference examined this topic from a multidisciplinary perspective.[42] Additional research will help to elucidate the role of various forms of treatment in the prevention of incontinence in the elderly population. The role of continence promotion and education cannot be underestimated.[43] Increased public awareness of the problem of UI, particularly in elderly patients, may lead to increased use of health care resources for the evaluation and treatment of the condition. Older adults need to understand that they do not need to suffer in silence, and that help is available to eliminate or manage symptoms for most patients.

SUMMARY

UI is a highly prevalent syndrome among older adults. The condition is often underreported, and many elderly patients suffer needlessly with symptoms that negatively affect life in general and specific activities. Continence promotion efforts need to continue to work to dispel the myth among both patients and health care providers that UI is a normal and inevitable part of the aging process. In many cases, UI may be curable with treatment or can at least be made more manageable for patients and caregivers. This can significantly improve care and quality of life for those affected by UI.

REFERENCES

1. Anger JT, Saigal CS, Stothers L, et al. The prevalence of urinary incontinence among community dwelling men: results from the National Health and Nutrition Examination Survey. J Urol 2006;176:2103–8.
2. Tennstedt SL, Link CL, Steers WD, et al. Prevalence of and risk factors for urinary leakage in a racially and ethnically diverse population of adults. Am J Epidemiol 2008;167:390–9.
3. Song HJ, Bae JM. Prevalence of urinary incontinence and lower urinary tract symptoms for community-dwelling elderly 85 years of age and older. J Wound Ostomy Continence Nurs 2007;34:535–41.
4. Goode PS, Burgio KL, Redden DT, et al. Population based study on incidence and predictors of urinary incontinence in black and white older adults. J Urol 2008;179:1449–54.
5. DuBeau CE. The aging lower urinary tract. J Urol 2006;175:S11–5.
6. Stothers L, Thom D, Calhoun E. Urologic diseases in America project: urinary incontinence in males: demographics and economic burden. J Urol 2005;173:1302–8.
7. Thom DH, Nygaard IE, Calhoun EA. Urologic diseases in America project: urinary incontinence in women – national trends in hospitalizations, office visits, treatment and economic impact. J Urol 2005;173:1295–301.
8. Ko Y, Lin SJ, Salmon JW, et al. The impact of urinary incontinence on quality of life of the elderly. Am J Manag Care 2005;11:S103–11.
9. Teunissen D, van den Bosch W, van Weel C, et al. "It can always happen": the impact of urinary incontinence on elderly men and women. Scand J Prim Health Care 2006;24:166–73.

10. DuBeau CE, Kuchel GA, Johnson T, et al. Incontinence in the frail elderly. Chapter 11. In: Abrams P, Cardozo L, Khoury S, et al, editors. 4th International consultation on Incontinence. Paris: Health Publication Ltd; 2009. p. 961–1024.

11. DuBeau CE, Simon SE, Morris JN. The effect of urinary incontinence on quality of life in older nursing home residents. J Am Geriatr Soc 2006;54:1325–33.

12. Huang AJ, Brown JS, Thom DH, et al. Urinary incontinence in older community-dwelling women: the role of cognitive and physical function decline. Obstet Gynecol 2007;109:909–16.

13. Brown JS, Vittinghoff E, Wyman JF, et al. Urinary incontinence: does it increase risk for falls and fractures? Study of Osteoporotic Fractures Research Group. J Am Geriatr Soc 2000;48:721–5.

14. Morris V, Wagg A. Lower urinary tract symptoms, incontinence and falls in elderly people: time for an intervention study. Int J Clin Pract 2007;61:320–3.

15. Griebling TL. The impact of urinary incontinence on sexual health in older adults. J Am Geriatr Soc 2006;54:1290–2.

16. Holroyd-Leduc JM, Mehta KM, Covinsky KE. Urinary incontinence and its association with death, nursing home admission, and functional decline. J Am Geriatr Soc 2004;52:712–8.

17. Pfisterer MH, Johnson TM II, Jenetzky E, et al. Geriatric patients' preferences for treatment of urinary incontinence: a study of hospitalized, cognitively competent adults aged 80 and older. J Am Geriatr Soc 2007;55:2016–22.

18. Wagg AS, Cardozo L, Chapple C, et al. Overactive bladder syndrome in older people. BJU Int 2007;99:502–9.

19. Taylor JA III, Kuchel GA. Detrusor underactivity: clinical features and pathogenesis of an underdiagnosed geriatric condition. J Am Geriatr Soc 2006;54: 1920–32.

20. Ransmayr GN, Holliger S, Schletterer K, et al. Lower urinary tract symptoms in dementia with Lewy bodies, Parkinson disease, and Alzheimer disease. Neurology 2008;70:299–303.

21. Sugaya K, Nishijima S, Oda M, et al. Biochemical and body composition analysis of nocturia in the elderly. Neurourol Urodyn 2008;27:205–11.

22. Kujubu DA, Aboseif SR. An overview of nocturia and the syndrome of nocturnal polyuria in the elderly. Nat Clin Pract Nephrol 2008;4:426–35.

23. Subak LL, Whitcomb E, Shen H, et al. Weight loss: a novel and effective treatment for urinary incontinence. J Urol 2005;174:190–5.

24. Ostaszkiewicz J, Johnston L, Roe B. Timed voiding for the management of urinary incontinence in adults. Cochrane Database Syst Rev 2004;1:CD002802.

25. van Houten P, Achterberg W, Ribbe M. Urinary incontinence in disabled elderly women: a randomized clinical trial of the effect of training mobility and toileting skills to achieve independent toileting. Gerontology 2007;53:205–10.

26. Kegel AH. Physiologic therapy for urinary incontinence. JAMA 1951;146:915–7.

27. Burgio KL, Goode PS, Locher JL, et al. Behavioral training with and without biofeedback in the treatment of urge incontinence in older women: a randomized controlled trial. JAMA 2002;288:2293–9.

28. Perrin L, Dauphinée SW, Corcos J, et al. Pelvic floor muscle training with biofeedback and bladder training in elderly women: a feasibility study. J Wound Ostomy Continence Nurs 2005;32:186–99.

29. Goode PS. Behavioral and drug therapy for urinary incontinence. Urology 2004; 63:58–64.

30. Burgio KL, Locher JL, Goode PS. Combined behavioral and drug therapy for urge incontinence in older women. J Am Geriatr Soc 2000;48:370–4.

31. Komesu YM, Ketai LH, Rogers RG, et al. Restoration of continence by pessaries: magnetic resonance imaging assessment of mechanism of action. Am J Obstet Gynecol 2008;198:563. e1–6.
32. Staskin DR. Overactive bladder in the elderly: a guide to pharmacological management. Drugs Aging 2005;22:1013–28.
33. Feinberg M. The problems of anticholinergic adverse effects in older patients. Drugs Aging 1993;3:335–48.
34. Johnell K, Fastborn J. Concurrent use of anticholinergic drugs and cholinesterase inhibitors: register-based study of over 700,000 elderly patients. Drugs Aging 2008;25:871–7.
35. Sink KM, Thomas J III, Xu H, et al. Dual use of bladder anticholinergics and cholinesterase inhibitors: long-term functional and cognitive outcomes. J Am Geriatr Soc 2008;56:847–53.
36. Dalpiaz O, Primus G, Schips L. SPARC sling system for treatment of female stress urinary incontinence in the elderly. Eur Urol 2006;50:826–31.
37. Campeau L, Tu LM, Lemieux MC, et al. A multicenter, prospective, randomized clinical trial comparing tension-free vaginal tape surgery and no treatment for the management of stress urinary incontinence in elderly women. Neurourol Urodyn 2007;26:990–4.
38. Anger JT, Litwin MS, Wang Q, et al. Complications of sling surgery among female Medicare beneficiaries. Obstet Gynecol 2007;109:707–14.
39. Isom-Batz G, Zimmern PE. Collagen injection for female urinary incontinence after urethral or periurethral surgery. J Urol 2009;181:701–4.
40. Aboseif SR, Kim DH, Rieder JM, et al. Sacral neuromodulation: cost considerations and clinical benefits. Urology 2007;70:1069–73.
41. Edlund C, Dijkema HE, Hassouna MM, et al. Sacral nerve stimulation for refractory urge symptoms in elderly patients. Scand J Urol Nephrol 2004;38:131–5.
42. Landefeld CS, Bowers BJ, Feld AD, et al. National Institutes of Health State-of-the-Science Conference Statement: prevention of fecal and urinary incontinence in adults. Ann Intern Med 2008;148:449–58.
43. Newman DK, Ee CH, Gordon D, et al. Continence promotion, education, and primary prevention. Chapter 21. In: Abrams P, Cardozo L, Khoury S, et al, editors. 4th International Consultation on Incontinence. Paris: Health Publication Ltd; 2009. p. 1643–84.

Drug Dosing in the Elderly Patients with Chronic Kidney Disease

Ali J. Olyaei, PharmD[a],*, William M. Bennett, MD[b]

KEYWORDS

- Kidney disease • Drug dosing • Toxicity
- Therapeutic drug monitoring

Chronic kidney disease is a common disorder that affects many patients with a prevalence approaching 19 million people in the United States. Kidney failure and renal impairment is a common occurrence in the geriatric population.[1,2] Most types of kidney diseases are chronic conditions and frequently manifest at the late stages of life. Aging effects the biologic, psychological, and cognitive function of individuals.[3] Age-related changes in the kidney and renal function have been well documented.[4] Epidemiologic studies suggest that older patients are at a greater risk for renal failure if the kidney experiences insults from ischemia or exposure to pharmacologic and diagnostic nephrotoxins.[5,6] Geriatric patients often take medications for several indications to treat or prevent common conditions. In one study, patients aged 65 years on renal replacement therapy (hemodialysis) were taking an average of 12.5 ± 4.2 medications, and 15.7 ± 7.2 doses per day.[7]

In the early 1970s and 1980s, dialysis was not routinely offered to patients aged more than 65 years. It was assumed that older patients did not benefit from any form of renal replacement therapy. Today, however, 10% of renal transplant recipients are more than 65 years of age.[8]

Pharmacologic management of most common diseases in elderly individuals is a difficult task, particularly in older individuals with chronic kidney disease. Aging and renal dysfunction may influence the pharmacokinetics and pharmacodynamics of many drugs.[9,10] Thus, primary care providers must proceed with caution when prescribing drugs for elderly patients with kidney disease. Geriatric patients are at greater risk for adverse drug reactions and medication errors. The expenditure of the United States health care system is approaching $85 billion for the management of adverse drug complications.[11] This disproportionate spending is related to adverse

[a] Division of Nephrology & Hypertension, Oregon Health and Science University, 3314 SW US Veterans Hospital Road, Portland, OR 97201, USA
[b] Northwest Renal Clinic, Legacy Good Samaritan Hospital Transplant Services, 1130 NW 22nd Avenue, Suite 640, Portland, OR 97210, USA
* Corresponding author.
E-mail address: olyaeia@ohsu.edu (A.J. Olyaei).

Clin Geriatr Med 25 (2009) 459–527
doi:10.1016/j.cger.2009.04.004
0749-0690/09/$ – see front matter © 2009 Elsevier Inc. All rights reserved.

geriatric.theclinics.com

drug reactions in elderly patients. Although the elderly only constitute 15% of the population, they use 30% of all prescription drugs prescribed in the United States and account for 60% of all admissions to intensive care units in the United States. In addition, the elderly most often self-diagnose or obtain wrong information about their health from Web sites. Self-medication is a common problem in this population; they consume more than 40% to 50% of all over-the-counter medications.[12,13]

Limited data exist regarding drug use in elderly patients with chronic kidney disease. National prescribing guidelines for management of common conditions are deficient or mostly formulated by opinion without any solid clinical evidence in the geriatric population. McLean and colleagues have documented that only 3.45% of subjects were more than 65 years old in 8945 randomized controlled studies. In addition, only 1.2% of the meta-analysis (n = 706) included the geriatric population.[14] National guidelines do not reflect comorbid conditions, drug-drug interactions, and the immune or the functional status of older patients. In addition, proven therapies are often underutilized in the geriatric population. To a certain extent, limiting pharmacologic treatment is due to the lack of data or resources. For example, recent data indicate that aggressive management of hypertension may be beneficial in older patients.[15] However, most physicians hesitate to treat older patients more aggressively.[15,16] This is due, in part, to a high risk of drug-drug interactions, adverse drug reactions, and lack of clinical data in this population. Monitoring the medications used in older adults and identifying drug interactions and adverse events are crucial.

Drug therapy management in older adults is challenging and many factors related to normal aging, disease states, and lifestyle should be considered before initiation of pharmacotherapy. Most drugs and dosage recommendation are driven from studies in younger individuals with normal renal function.[17] Understanding of aging and renal function on drug disposition is the important factor in the pharmacologic management of common conditions. For most drugs, in particular drugs with a narrow therapeutic index, the margin of safety is much smaller in older patients with chronic kidney disease.[17–19] Primary care providers must understand the basic concept of pharmacokinetics and pharmacodynamics to provide effective treatment when exposing older patients to adverse drug interactions.

PHARMACOKINETICS

Pharmacokinetics defines and analyzes the time course of the drug in the body. Pharmacokinetic properties are altered in chronic kidney disease and in the natural aging process. These include bioavailability, volume of distribution (V_d), protein binding, and biotransformation.

Drug Absorption

Following oral administration, the drug must be absorbed before reaching its site of action. Absorption is the first stage of pharmacokinetics. Bioavailability is a better pharmacokinetic phrase compared with drug absorption. Bioavailability defines the percentage of the drug that reaches the systemic circulation.[11] In older patients with kidney disease, especially patients on continuous ambulatory peritoneal dialysis (CAPD), gastritis, gastroesophageal reflux, and vomiting are common problems. For the most part, drug absorption is variable and incomplete. Bioavailability is primarily calculated by considering the rate of drug absorption and route of administration. For example, drugs administered intravenously are generally 100% bioavailable, because the entire dosage reaches the systemic circulation. If given orally, subcutaneously, or intramuscularly, bioavailability decreases for most drugs compared with intravenous administration. Uremia also alters drug absorption or bioavailability. Most drugs require an acidic environment to be absorbed. Poor absorption may occur because of edema at the site of absorption. Older patients or patients with chronic kidney disease have higher gastric pH because of uremia or they are taking proton pump inhibitors. For many drugs, an acidic environment is needed for complete absorption.[20,21] For example, phenytoin and phenobarbital require an acidic atmosphere to be absorbed completely.[22]

Drugs that increase gastric pH, such as phosphate binders and H2-receptor blockers, may impair absorption of concomitantly administered drugs. Most pharmacologic agents are absorbed by passive diffusion and changing ionization states may change drug diffusion through the gastrointestinal wall. Concomitant administration of some phosphate binders for the treatment of hyperphosphatemia (aluminum- or calcium-containing) with antibiotics or iron-containing supplements may result in the formation of insoluble complexes that limit absorption and slow gastrointestinal motility.[23] Parenteral drug administration might provide a more reliable route of administration but may be more painful and should be avoided as much as possible. In addition, because of a low muscle mass and poor blood flow to the muscle, drug bioavailability is unpredictable following intramuscular administration. Finally, some intramuscular preparations are oil-based formulations and have a prolonged absorption period.

Drug Distribution

The volume of distribution is inversely correlated to plasma concentration. The hydrophilicity or lipophilicity of drugs affect their distribution through the body. Following absorption, most drugs reach the systemic circulation and are then distributed throughout different body compartments in several phases. Initially, drugs are distributed to highly perfused organs such as the heart, liver, kidney, and brain. Next, drugs are distributed to other areas with less or slower blood flow such as fat, bone, and skin. The rate of distribution and extent of drug concentration at the site of action determines the onset of drug action. Geriatric patients have significantly lower total body water and a smaller volume of distribution (V_d). The volume of distribution can be calculated by dividing the total amount of drug in the body by the concentration of the drug in the blood. It is important to mention that the volume of distribution does not refer to a specific anatomic compartment. It is only a mathematical model, which is useful for calculating the appropriate dosage regimen needed to achieve a desired systemic plasma concentration. An inverse correlation exists between the serum concentration and the volume of distribution.[24–26] With hydrophilic drugs such as aminoglycosides, renal failure and total body water may affect the volume of distribution. This increase in extracellular fluid volume from renal failure results in a lower serum concentration of aminoglycosides. However, older patients and patients with chronic kidney disease (stages II–IV) are at greater risk for nephrotoxicity from aminoglycosides.[27,28] Drug distribution could be affected by protein binding and lipid solubility. Pharmacologically, only unbound drugs are active and able to bind to specific receptors. The affinity of pharmacologic agents to receptors and the degree of protein binding determines the pharmacodynamic properties of any drug. Drugs that are highly bound to protein have a large volume distribution. Any changes to protein binding due to decreased protein synthesis or proteinuria may alter the therapeutic plasma concentration and desired outcomes.[29,30] In addition, drugs with high affinity to protein mostly distribute in the vascular compartment. Older patients with renal impairment and proteinuria have decreased protein synthesis and increased protein elimination. For drugs such as phenytoin, mycophenolate, and warfarin, which are highly protein bound, the free fraction concentration is elevated and total plasma levels are subtherapeutic. For phenytoin, only free, unbound phenytoin should be measured to avoid toxicities.[31,32] For other drugs, other biomarkers such as the international normalized ratio (INR) or white blood cell count should be monitored closely. For example, about 97% of mycophenolate in the plasma is bound to albumin and 2% to 3% is free. Hypoalbuminemia may cause an increase in the free fraction of mycophenolate.[33] Although small increases in free fractions seem trivial, the amount of free mycophenolate available to exert immunosuppressive or adverse drug reactions is doubled, with possible serious consequences. Hypoalbuminemia (albumin less than 2.5 g/dL) causes increased risk of toxicities due to an increased concentration of free mycophenolate in the plasma. In patients with hepatorenal syndrome and high bilirubin, most of the sites for drug binding are occupied with endogenous bilirubin or uremic molecules, resulting in increased plasma concentrations of drugs that are highly protein bound.[32,34]

DRUG METABOLISM

Most drugs are metabolized to more soluble compounds, which are then removed from the circulation. Drug metabolites are pharmacologically inactive; however, several drugs have active metabolites that are excreted through the kidney. Patients with chronic kidney disease are at a higher risk of drug accumulation and toxicities in this setting. For example, procainamide has an active metabolite, N-acetyl procainamide (NAPA). NAPA has pro-arrhythmic properties and is excreted by the kidneys.[35]

There are two major metabolic pathways. In phase 1, reaction drugs are metabolized through oxidation, reduction, and hydrolysis. In oxidation reactions, oxygen atoms cause a lipophilic pharmacologic agent to become more water soluble. Oxidative reactions typically involve the cytochrome P450 enzymatic system.[36] Age-dependent changes in hepatic function and the size of liver have been documented. A 25% to 35% reduction of drugs that are eliminated, predominantly through hepatic metabolism, can be expected. The activity of cytochrome P450 enzyme systems is reduced significantly during adulthood or renal failure.[37] The second important pathway for drug metabolism is called synthetic or conjugation reactions. Phase 2 reactions involve the attachment of another chemical group to the drug resulting in greater water solubility and renal elimination.[38] Most drugs undergo one or both of the phase 1 and 2 reactions to be eliminated from the systemic circulation and the body. There is increasing evidence to suggest that the phase 2 pathway does not significantly alter during age-related changes, but the pathway is subject to a significant amount of polymorphism.[39] Most patients with kidney disease take several drugs and the enzyme systems can be induced or inhibited by other pharmacotherapeutic agents. Drugs that stimulate this enzymatic system are considered inducers and may decrease the therapeutic benefit of other agents. For example, phenytoin may increase the metabolism of warfarin and result in risk of thrombotic events. Some drugs may inhibit the metabolism of another drug and increase the risk of toxicity. Metronidiazole may decrease the metabolism of warfarin and cause warfarin toxicity and bleeding.[40,41]

APPROACH TO DOSAGE ADJUSTMENT IN OLDER ADULTS

Most guidelines recommend a small drug dose and dosing adjustments in older adults with or without chronic kidney disease. Age-related changes in organ function may alter the renal elimination rate of the drugs. The following recommendations provide a simple approach for health care providers, and attempt to reduce the risk of drug toxicity and improve pharmacotherapeutic efficacy.[42] At any point of care, patient-specific risk factors such as comorbidity, drug interactions and health care insurance coverage should be considered and monitored during therapy. The cause and duration of renal dysfunction should be determined and defined as acute or chronic whenever possible. A review of current medications, prescription and nonprescription, should be obtained to identify potential nephrotoxins or interacting medications. In elderly patients, the use of nephrotoxins should be limited only in circumstances whereby the benefits clearly outweigh the risks of nephrotoxicty.[43,44] Age-related nephrotoxicity has not been researched well and most reported cases are documented in a general population. **Table 1** in the Appendix lists common nephrotoxins and the management of nephrotoxicity. Body mass index (BMI) and ideal body weight (IBW) should be calculated using the following formula:

BMI: (weight in kilograms)/(height in meters)^2
IBW (men): 50.0 kg + 2.3 kg for every 2.5 cm over 152 cm
IBW (women): 45.5 kg + 2.3 kg for every 2.5 cm over 152 cm

The Cockcroft-Gault formula is a simple and widely used method to approximate creatinine clearance or glomerular filtration rate (GFR) in patients with stable chronic kidney disease.[45–47] The formula is practical and well accepted for dosage modification in patients with stable renal dysfunction. The Cockcroft-Gault is not a valuable tool in patients with acute kidney injury, or patients with increasing levels of serum creatinine (SCr). For anuric patients, creatinine clearance should be assumed to be generally less than 10 mL/min. The Cockcroft-Gault formula includes the variables of age (years), IBW (kg), and SCr (mg/dL) and calculates the CrCl (mL/min):

CrCl = (140 − age) × IBW/72 × SCr
Multiply result by 0.85 in women

The Modification of Diet in Renal Disease (MDRD) study recently reported a new formula to estimate renal function. This method provides a more accurate estimation of renal function in the geriatric population and in patients with low muscle mass or who have a low protein intake. The MDRD formula gives a predictive sensitivity in patients with GFR <60 mL/min/1.73 m^2. Normal or near normal renal function is often underestimated by this equation. In addition, the MDRD formula is subject to less artifact interference. However, the method has not been studied for dosage adjustment or drug dosing in chronic kidney disease. Therefore both methods lack precision.[42] The maintenance dose of drugs that are primarily eliminated unchanged through the kidneys should be modified in patients with chronic kidney disease.[48] Dosage modification in older adults with kidney disease can be accomplished by dose reduction, prolonging the dosing interval or both methods. The dosing interval should be adjusted for drugs with a clinical efficacy that correlates with adequate peak concentrations (aminoglycosides, cephalosporines). The dosage interval should be prolonged for agents with efficacy that correlates with the area under of the curve, or a rapid increase in plasma concentration correlated with toxicity. In general, for most drugs, a combined approach using dose reduction and interval prolongation should be used. This combined method provides a constant plasma drug concentration without increasing the risk of toxicity from high peak or trough levels. Commonly used drugs and dosage adjustment in the geriatric population with chronic kidney disease are listed in each therapeutic category in **Table 3** in the Appendix.

Despite dosage adjustments and prolonged dosage intervals, drug toxicity is a common problem in older adults with chronic kidney disease. Because of inter- and intra-individual pharmacokinetic variabilities, comorbid conditions, and drug interactions, therapeutic drug monitoring is important in older patients with renal impairment. The diagnostic value of therapeutic drug monitoring relies on correct interpretation of plasma drug concentrations. It is important to know the exact dose given, the route of administration, time of administration and time since the last dose. Peak levels are meaningful for only a few drugs. Peak drug levels represent the highest drug concentration achieved after initial rapid distribution. For most drugs, trough levels, obtained immediately before the next dose, represent the lowest serum concentration and predict drug toxicity. Therapeutic drug monitoring is not available and could be costly. This type of drug monitoring should be used only for drugs in which plasma concentrations are correlated to toxicity or efficacy. Even with therapeutic drug monitoring, drug toxicities cannot always be avoided. For example, aminoglycoside antibiotics can accumulate in tissues such as the inner ear and renal tubules. Aminoglycoside toxicity can occur after a single dose or in some cases without associated high plasma concentrations. Clinical practitioners must incorporate ongoing clinical assessment and therapeutic drug monitoring simultaneously. Assessment of adverse drug reactions is important even when drug levels are within the established therapeutic range. Finally, in older adults with kidney disease, protein binding is altered significantly. For highly protein-bound drugs, the free fraction can be elevated significantly while the total plasma concentration is within therapeutic range. Most assays do not distinguish between free and protein-bound drug in the plasma. An increase in unbound drug is common in patients with renal failure. For example, a dialysis patient with albumin of less than 2 g/dL and phenytoin level of 6 mg/L could experience phenytoin toxicities although phenytoin levels are within therapeutic range (therapeutic level 10–20 mg/L). Free phenytoin levels provide better therapeutic drug monitoring in older patients with renal impairment.[34] **Table 1** in the Appendix summarizes the therapeutic drug monitoring parameters in renal insufficiency for those drugs for which monitoring of levels is routinely recommended.

DIALYSIS AND DRUG DOSING

In 2005, 1 in 1000 people received renal replacement therapy in the United States. Today it is estimated that more than 350,000 patients are on dialysis. There are a limited number of published studies on drug pharmacokinetics and clearance in the geriatric population that who undergoes various dialytic modalities. Therefore, most of the data are extrapolated from the general population on dialysis. Hemodynamically unstable patients also require continuous arteriovenous hemofiltration (CAVH), continuous venovenous hemofiltration (CVVH), continuous arteriovenous hemodialysis (CAVHD), and continuous venovenous hemodialysis (CVVHD).[49,50] Several dialysis methods are employed for the management of solute and solvents in patients with end-stage kidney disease. Drugs that are eliminated primarily by the renal system are significantly affected by different modes of dialysis. Drug removal during hemodialysis is a function of the dialysis dose (Kt/V), where K is the dialyzer clearance, t is the time on dialysis, and V is the urea volume of distribution, which is practically equivalent to total body water (approximately 60% of body weight). The dialyzability of a drug is dependent on several factors: type of dialysis, drug characteristics, and duration and rate of dialysis. The drug characteristics that affect drug removal are molecular weight and size, protein binding, volume of distribution, and electrostatic charge. If low-flux dialysis membranes are used, drugs of small molecular size or volume (<500 Da) are more readily dialyzable compared with drugs of larger molecular size. However, when high-flux dialysis membranes are used, the molecular weight becomes less relevant. In high-flux membrane dialysis, drugs with a molecular weight of more than 30,000 to 40,000 Da can pass freely through the dialysis membrane. For example, vancomycin with a molecular weight 1450 Da can be eliminated readily with high-flux membranes, whereas an insignificant amount is cleared by low-flux membranes.[51] Any changes to the rate of blood flow or dialysis flow rate may alter the clearance of many drugs. A change in blood flow rate may play a more important role in drug clearance. For example, an increase in rate of blood flow from 100 to 300 mL/min could increase the clearance of tobramycin by 100%.

Drugs that are highly protein bound are not dialyzable. Only unbound drugs are removed during dialysis. However, in patients with chronic kidney disease, the concentration of the unbound fraction for most drugs is altered due to changes in the metabolic stage or a reduction in plasma proteins and albuminuria.[52]

The volume of distribution of drugs also affects drug removal by dialysis. Drugs with a low volume of distribution (eg, hydrophilic drugs, such as β-lactam antibiotics, aminoglycosides, and glycopeptides), are usually confined to the intravascular and extracellular spaces, and therefore, are effectively removed by dialysis. Drugs with a large volume of distribution are usually highly tissue bound and distributed throughout the extravascular and intracellular compartments such as adipose tissue (eg, lipophilic drugs, such as the macrolides, tetracyclines, fluoroquinolones, and linezolid), and are not removed effectively by dialysis even if the extraction across the dialysis membrane is 100%. In general, drugs with a volume of distribution less than 0.7 L/kg are well dialyzed, whereas drugs with a volume of distribution greater than 2 L/kg are not. Drugs with a volume of distribution between 0.7 and 2 L/kg have variable but low dialyzability.[53]

Drug molecular charge may also affect dialytic clearance. The anionic drug, clavulinic acid, is cleared rapidly by high-flux membranes compared with cationic drugs. Cationic drugs may be retained by anionic protein charges in the blood, and therefore may not cross the dialysis membrane to the dialysate compartment, even if the molecular weight and other drug properties favor its dialyzability.[54]

DOSING TABLES

Tables 2–16 in the Appendix present key information required for prescribing drugs in patients with chronic kidney disease. These tables should be used with caution and the overall situation of each patient should be fully considered. For some drugs, adjustment is an interval extension (I), whereby the dosage stays the same as an adult without kidney disease. On the other hand, if the dose reduction method (D) is recommended, the adjustment refers to the percentage of the dose given to a patient with normal renal function. This dose should be given at the usual dosing interval. Finally, it is vital to incorporate patient-specific factors such as age, disease state, nutrition, and body fluid when considering a dosage adjustment.[48]

APPENDIX

Table 1
Common nephrotoxins and management of nephrotoxicity

	Therapeutic Range	When to Draw a Sample	How Often to Draw Levels
Aminoglycosides (conventional dosing) gentamicin, tobramycin, amikacin	Gentamicin and tobramycin: Trough: 0.5–2 mg/L Peak: 5–8 mg/L Amikacin: Peak: 20–30 mg/L Trough: <10 mg/L	Obtain drug level 30 min before and after dose	Check peak and trough with third dose For therapy less than 72 h, levels not necessary. Repeat drug levels weekly or if renal function changes
Aminoglycosides (24-h dosing), gentamicin, tobramycin, amikacin	0.5–3 mg/L	Obtain random drug level 12 h after dose	After initial dose. Repeat drug level in 1 week or if renal function changes
Carbamazepine	4–12 µg/mL	Trough: immediately before dosing	Check 2–4 d after first dose or change in dose
Cyclosporin	150–400 ng/mL	Trough: immediately before dosing	Daily for first week, then weekly
Digoxin	0.8–2.0 ng/mL	23 h after maintenance dose	5–7 d after first dose for patients with normal renal and hepatic function, 15–20 d in anephric patients
Lidocaine	1–5 µg/mL	8 h after intravenous infusion started or changed	—
Lithium	Acute: 0.8–1.2 mmol/L Chronic: 0.6–0.8 mmol/L	Trough: before morning dose at least 12 h since last dose	—
Phenobarbital	15–40 µg/mL	Trough: immediately before dosing	Check 2 weeks after first dose or change in dose. Follow-up level in 1–2 months

Phenytoin Free phenytoin	10–20 µg/mL 1–2 µg/mL	Trough: immediately before dosing	5–7 d after first dose or after change in dose
Procainamide NAPA (*N*-acetyl procainamide) a procainamide metabolite	4–10 µg/mL Trough: 4 µg/mL Peak: 8 µg/mL 10–30 µg/mL	Trough: immediately before next dose or 12–18 h after starting or changing an infusion draw with procainamide sample	–
Quinidine	1–5 µg/mL	Trough: immediately before next dose	–
Sirolimus	10–20 ng/dL	Trough: immediately before next dose	–
Tacrolimus (FK-506)	10–15 ng/mL	Trough: immediately before next dose	Daily for first week, then weekly
Theophylline by mouth or aminophylline intravenously	15–20 µg/mL	Trough: immediately before next dose	–
Valproic acid (divalproex sodium)	40–100 µg/mL	Trough: immediately before next dose	Check 2–4 d after first dose or change in dose
Vancomycin	Trough: 5–15 mg/L Peak: 25–40 mg/L	Trough: Immediately before dose Peak: 60 min after a 60-min infusion	With third dose (when initially starting therapy, or after each dosage adjustment). For therapy less than 72 h, levels not necessary. Repeat drug levels if renal function changes

Table 2
Drug-induced kidney injury

Drug	Risk Factor	Pathophysiology	Prevention	Management
NSAIDS	Volume and Na depletion, diuretic used Large dose and long therapy Severe liver disease	Hemodynamically induced acute renal failure due to vasoconstriction by decreased PG production, decreased GFR → acute renal failure, Na retention, and edema Increased recruitment and activation of lymphocyte → acute and chronic tubulointerstitial nephropathy, with or without nephrotic syndrome Direct toxicity → chronic interstitial nephritis and papillary necrosis	Avoid diuretic used at the same time. Avoid large doses	DC medication Consider opiate
Aminoglycoside (neomycin, gentamicin, tobramicin, amikacin, streptomycin)	Dose, duration and frequency of administration, concurrent renal ischemia or administration of nephrotoxin, liver disease plasma concentration >10 mg/dL for peak and >2–3 for trough	In PCT, AG bound to anionic phospholipid, then delivered to megalin and undergoes endocytic uptake into the cell. Within the cell, AG accumulates within → acute tubular necrosis Acute renal failure, decreased GFR	Maintain therapeutic range Give once-daily dose if necessary	Reduce the dose, decrease frequency and duration of therapy Oral Mg supplement in Mg wasting

Acyclovir	High dose, intravenous bolus dose	Deposition of acyclovir crystals in the tubules, resulting in intratubular obstruction and foci of interstitial inflammation → acute interstitial nephritis and obstruction → ARF Chronic renal disease Crystal nephropathy Proximal tubulopathy	Avoid bolus dose Prior hydration (with the urine output maintained above 75 mL/h) and slow drug infusion over 1–2 h	DC hydration and loop diuretic
Adefovir dipivoxil	≥30 mg/d renal impairment Preexisting tubular dysfunction Duration of therapy	Depletion of mitochondrial DNA (mtDNA) from proximal tubular cells through inhibition of mtDNA replication → enlargement and dysmorphia of mitochondria of PCT → acute tubular degeneration	–	–
Cidofovir	–	Induced apoptosis in PCT, PCT dysfunction, diabetes insipidus, renal failure	–	Probenecid (human organic anion transporter inhibitor) → reduce uptake of cidofovir in PCT
Tenofovir	Dose and duration	Tubular cell karyomegaly, degeneration, and necrosis → interstitial nephritis, diabetes insipidus, ARF Fanconi syndrome	–	–
Indinavir	Bolus dose	Crystal neuropathy, nephrolithiasis → obstructive ARF	Hydration, establish high urine flow Avoid bolus dose	DC

(continued on next page)

Table 2
(continued)

Drug	Risk Factor	Pathophysiology	Prevention	Management
Foscarnet	–	Direct tubular toxicity → acute tubular necrosis, nephrogenic diabetes insipidus Crystal in glomerular capillary lumen and PCT	0.5–1 L NS infusion	Dose reduction
Interferon	–	Prerenal acute renal failure, tubulointerstitial nephritis, throbotic microangiopathy, membranoproliferative glomerular sclerosis	–	Discontinuation
Cimetidine	Men >50 y	Cellular hypersensitivity → acute interstitial nephritis characterized by heavy infiltrate of lymph, macrophage, eosinophil and PMN ↓ renal blood flow by inhibition of H2 receptor	Early recognition	Discontinuation
IVIG	Sucrose-containing product Dehydration	Accumulation of sucrose in PCT forms vesicle, ↑ osmolarity → cell swelling, vacuolization, and tubular luminal occlusion	Infusion rate: <3 mg sucrose/kg/min Avoid radiocontrast concomitantly Avoid sucrose-containing product	Hydration DC sucrose-containing product

Lithium	Renal impairment Dehydration from fever, N/V, sun exposure Hyponatremia Diuretic, especially thiazide used	Impairment of collecting duct conc. ability → diabetes insipidus Chronic tubulointerstitial nephropathy (tubular atrophy and interstitial fibrosis) Glomerulosclerosis	Therapeutic range (0.6–1.2 mEq/L) Prevent dehydration Avoid low Na diet Avoid thiazide and nephrotoxic drug	Amiloride for nephrogenic diabetes insipidus Fluid restoration Furosemide up to 40 mg/h Acetazolamide + $NaHCO_3Na$, K supplement Hemodialysis (rebound can occur if stopped too early)
CSA/ tacrolimus	Dose, age, lower pretransplant GFR, female, postoperative ARF, diabetes, HTN, and hepatitis C infection	↓ PG and ↑ 20-HETE acid production → vasoconstriction Generation of H_2O_2 resulting in depleted glutathione → ↓ GFR, ischemic collapse or scarring of the glomeruli, vacuolization of the tubules, and focal areas of tubular atrophy and interstitial fibrosis (striped fibrosis), ↑ apoptosis → calcineurin inhibitor nephrotoxicity (CIN)	Maintain in therapeutic range Avoid drugs that raise levels (CYP 3A4 inhibitor) Calcium channel blocker	Dose reduction
ACE-I	–	Vasoconstriction → prerenal ARF	Avoid in bilateral renal artery stenosis	–

(continued on next page)

Table 2
(continued)

Drug	Risk Factor	Pathophysiology	Prevention	Management
Methotrexate	Acidic urine High dose	Precipitate in the urine and induce tubular injury	Prior hydration, alkalize urine to pH >7.0 (3 L of dextrose in water + 44–66 mEq of $NaHCO_3$/d)	Loop diuretic Leucovorin rescue with or without thymidine for systemic toxicities [a]Dialysis use not effective because MTX is protein bound
Ifosfamide	Use cisplatin at the same time	Direct tubular injury and mitochondrial damage → renal tubular acidosis, ↓ PCT phosphate, glucose, amino acid reabsorption, marked ↑ b2-microglobulin excretion (Fanconi-like syndrome), nephrogenic diabetes insipidus, hypokalemia	Mesna	Discontinuation
Cisplatin	Low chloride High dose used for bone marrow ablation	The Cl in *cis* position replaced by H_2O → highly reactive hydoxyl radical by cytochrome P450 → DNA injury and cell death in renal tubule, especially PCT, also DCT, CT and loop of Henle Nephrogenic diabetes insipidus	Vigorous hydration with forced diuresis: 2500 mL NS/h before and several hours after administration Mannitol or furosemide used Amifostine (thiophosphate) thiosulfate	Discontinue Mg supplementation
Sulfonamide (sulfadiazine and sulfa-methoxazole)	High dose during the treatment of toxoplasmosis in patients with AIDS Urine pH <5.5	Intrarenal precipitation → kidney stone formation	Fluid intake >3 L/d, monitor urine for crystals, if crystals are seen, alkalinization of urine to pH >7.15	–

Radiocontrast	Dose and frequency, osmolarity of contrast medium	High osmolarity, medullary vasoconstriction, ↑ active transport in thick ascending loop of Henle → ↑ O$_2$ needs	Hydration before and after the administration Acetylcysteine (600 mg by mouth), or NaHCO$_3$ before and after administration	Hydration
Aristolochia acid (Chinese herbal neuropathy and endemic Balkan nephropathy)	Use vasoconstrictor such as fenfluramine/diethylpropion at the same time Batch to batch variability in toxin content Female gender Dose Genetic predisposition	Chronic tubulointerstitial nephritis, thickening of the walls of interlobular and afferent arterioles → ischemia → extensive interstitial fibrosis and loss of tubules → proteinuria Overexpress protein p53 → cellular atypia and urothelial carcinoma and genitourinary tract	—	Discontinue Corticosteroid
Amphotericin B	High dose and long duration of therapy	Afferent vasoconstriction by TGF system and direct action → decreased GFR Distal tubular injury by creation of pores that increase membrane permeability → hypokalemia, hypomagnesemia, metabolic acidosis due to tubular acidosis, polyuria due to nephrogenic diabetes insipidus	Use liposomal formulation (does not contain deoxycholate) Sodium loading (500–1000 mL of NS 30 min before administration Regularly monitor K, Mg, Na serum concentration	Hydration Dose reduction

The dose of all of the medications listed should be based on renal function. Avoid concomitant use of nephrotoxic medications and diuretics. Patient-related risk factors for all the drugs listed are age, previous renal insufficiency, dehydration and volume depletion, concurrent use of nephrotoxic drugs, CRF, diabetic neuropathy, severe CHF, and so forth. Adequate hydration is necessary before therapy and during the treatment of acute renal failure because volume depletion is one of the most important risk factors. Obtain baseline BUN, SCr, and electrolytes and closely monitor renal function during the treatments.

Abbreviations: ACE-I, angiotensin-converting enzyme inhibitors; AG, aminoglycoside; ARF, acute renal failure; BUN, blood urea nitrogen; HF, heart failure; CKD, chronic kidney disease; CSA, cyclosporine; DC, discontinue; GFR, glomerular filtration rate; HETE, 20-hydroxyeicosatetraenoic acid; HTN, hypertension; IVIG, immunoglobulin; MTX, methotrexate; N/V, nausea and vomiting; NS, normal saline; PCT, proximal convoluted tubule; PG, prostaglandin; PMN, Polymorphonuclear; Scr, serum creatinine; TGF, Transforming growth factor.

Table 3
Antimicrobial dosing in renal failure

| Drugs | Normal Dosage | % of Renal Excretion | Dosage Adjustment in Renal Failure | | | Comments | HD | CAPD | CVVH |
			GFR >50	GFR 10–50	GFR <10				
Aminoglycoside antibiotics	–	–	–	–	–	Nephrotoxic. Ototoxic. Toxicity worse when hyperbilirubinemic. Measure serum levels for efficacy and toxicity. Peritoneal absorption increases with presence of inflammation. V_d increases with edema, obesity, and ascites	–	–	–
Streptomycin	7.5 mg/kg every 12 h (1.0 g every 24 h for tuberculosis)	60	Every 24 h	Every 24–72 h	Every 72–96 h	For the treatment of tuberculosis. May be less nephrotoxic than other members of class	1/2 normal dose after dialysis	20–40 mg/L/d	Dose for GFR 10–50 and measure levels

Drug	Dose						Toxicity / Comments	After dialysis		
Kanamycin	7.5 mg/kg every 8 h	50–90	60%–90% every 12 h or 100% every 12–24 h	30%–70% every 12–18 h or 100% every 24–48 h	20%–30% every 24–48 h or 100% every 48–72 h		Nephrotoxic. Ototoxic. Toxicity worse when hyperbilirubinemic. V_d increases with edema, obesity, and ascites. Do not use once-daily dosing in patients with creatinine clearance less than 30–40 mL/min or in patients with acute renal failure or uncertain level of kidney function	1/2 full does after dialysis	15–20 mg/L/d	Dose for GFR 10–50 and measure levels
Gentamicin	1.7 mg/kg every 8 h	95	60%–90% every 8–12 h or 100% every 12–24 h	30%–70% every 12 h or 100% every 24–48 h	20%–30% every 24–48 h or 100% every 48–72 h		Concurrent penicillins may result in subtherapeutic aminoglycoside levels. Peak 6–8, trough <2	1/2 full dose after dialysis	3–4 mg/L/d	Dose for GFR 10–50 and measure levels
Tobramicin	1.7 mg/kg every 8 h	95	60%–90% every 8–12 h or 100% every 12–24 h	30%–70% every 12 h or 100% every 24–48 h	20%–30% every 24–48 h or 100% every 48–72 h		Concurrent penicillins may result in subtherapeutic aminoglycoside levels. Peak 6–8, trough <2	1/2 full dose after dialysis	3–4 mg/L/d	Dose for GFR 10–50 and measure levels
Netilmicin	2 mg/kg every 8 h	95	50%–90% every 8–12 h or 100% every 12–24 h	20%–60% every 12 h or 100% every 24–48 h	10%–20% every 24–48 h or 100% every 48–72 h		May be less ototoxic than other members of class. Peak 6–8, trough <2	1/2 full dose after dialysis	3–4 mg/L/d	Dose for GFR 10–50 and measure levels

(continued on next page)

Table 3
(continued)

Drugs	Normal Dosage	% of Renal Excretion	Dosage Adjustment in Renal Failure			Comments	HD	CAPD	CVVH
			GFR >50	GFR 10–50	GFR <10				
Amikacin	7.5 mg/kg every 12 h	95	60%–90% every 12 h or 100% every 12–24 h	30%–70% every 12–18 h or 100% every 24–48 h	20%–30% every 24–48 h or 100% every 48–72 h	Monitor levels. Peak 20–30, trough <5	1/2 full does after dialysis	15–20 mg/L/d	Dose for GFR 10–50 and measure levels
Cephalosporin –	–	–	–	–	–	Coagulation abnormalities, transitory elevation of BUN, rash and serum sickness-like syndrome	–	–	–
Oral cephalosporin									
Cefaclor	250–500 mg three times a day	70	100%	100%	50%	–	250 mg twice a day after dialysis	250 mg every 8–12 h	N/A
Cefadroxil	500 mg to 1 g twice a day	80	100%	100%	50%	–	0.5–1.0 g after dialysis	0.5 g/d	N/A
Cefixime	200 to 400 mg every 12 h	85	100%	100%	50%	–	300 mg after dialysis	200 mg/d	Not recommended
Cefpodoxime	200 mg every 12 h	30	100%	100%	100%	–	200 mg after dialysis	Dose for GFR <10	N/A
Ceftibuten	400 mg every 24 h	70	100%	100%	50%	–	300 mg after dialysis	No data: dose for GFR <10	Dose for GFR 10–50

Drug		Dose				Comments			
Cefuroxime axetil	90	250–500 mg three times a day	100%	100%	100%	Malabsorbed in presence of H2 blockers. Absorbed better with food	Dose after dialysis	Dose for GFR <10	N/A
Cephalexin	95	250–500 mg three times a day	100%	100%	100%	Rare allergic interstitial nephritis. Absorbed well when given intraperitoneally. May cause bleeding from impaired prothrombin biosynthesis	Dose after dialysis	Dose for GFR <10	N/A
Cephradine	100	250–500 mg three times a day	100%	100%	50%	Rare allergic interstitial nephritis. Absorbed well when given intraperitoneally. May cause bleeding from impaired prothrombin biosynthesis	Dose after dialysis	Dose for GFR <10	N/A
Intravenous cephalosporin									
Cefamandole	100	1–2 g intravenously every 6–8 h	Every 6 h	Every 8 h	Every 12 h	—	0.5–1.0 g after dialysis	0.5–1.0 g every 12 h	Dose for GFR 10–50
Cefazolin	80	1–2 g intravenously every 8 h	Every 8 h	Every 12 h	Every 12–24 h	—	0.5–1.0 g after dialysis	0.5 g every 12 h	Dose for GFR 10–50
Cefepime	85	1–2 g intravenously every 8 h	Every 8–12 h	Every 12 h	Every 24 h	—	1 g after dialysis	Dose for GFR <10	Not recommended

(continued on next page)

Table 3
(continued)

Drugs	Normal Dosage	% of Renal Excretion	Dosage Adjustment in Renal Failure			Comments	HD	CAPD	CVVH
			GFR >50	GFR 10–50	GFR <10				
Cefmetazole	1–2 g intravenously every 8 h	85	Every 8 h	Every 12 h	Every 24 h	–	Dose after dialysis	Dose for GFR <10	Dose for GFR 10–50
Cefoperazone	1–2 g intravenously every 12 h	20	No renal adjustment is required			Displaced from protein by bilirubin. Reduce dose by 50% for jaundice. May prolong prothrombin time	1 g after dialysis	None	None
Cefotaxime	1–2 g intravenously every 6–8 h	60	Every 8 h	Every 12 h	Every 12–24 h	Active metabolite in ESRD. Reduce dose further for combined hepatic and renal failure	1 g after dialysis	1 g/d	1g every 12 h
Cefotetan	1–2 g intravenously every 12 h	75	Every 12 h	Every 12–24 h	Every 24 h	–	1 g after dialysis	1 g/d	750 mg every 12 h
Cefoxitin	1–2 g intravenously every 6 h	80	Every 6 h	Every 8–12 h	Every 12 h	May produce false increase in serum creatinine by interference with assay	1 g after dialysis	1 g/d	Dose for GFR 10–50
Ceftazidime	1–2 g intravenously every 8 h	70	Every 8 h	Every 12 h	Every 24 h	–	1 g after dialysis	0.5 g/d	Dose for GFR 10–50

Drug	Dose		Dose for GFR >50	Dose for GFR 10–50	Dose for GFR <10	Toxicity	Dose after dialysis	Dose for GFR 10–50
Ceftriaxone	1–2 g intravenously every 24 h	50	No renal adjustment is required	—	—	—	—	—
Cefuroxime sodium	0.75–1.5 g intravenously every 8 h	90	Every 8 h	Every 8–12 h	Every 12–24 h	Rare allergic interstitial nephritis. Absorbed well when given intraperitoneally. May cause bleeding from impaired prothrombin biosynthesis	750 mg every 12 h	1.0 g every 12 h
Penicillin	—	—	—	—	—	Bleeding abnormalities, hypersensitivity. Seizures	—	—
Oral penicillin								
Amoxicillin	500 mg by mouth three times a day	60	100%	100%	50%–75%	—	250 mg every 12 h	N/A
Ampicillin	500 mg by mouth every 6 h	60	100%	100%	50%–75%	—	250 mg every 12 h	N/A
Dicloxacillin	250–500 mg by mouth every 6 h	50	100%	100%	50%–75%	—	None	N/A
Penicillin V	250–500 mg by mouth every 6 h	70	100%	100%	50%–75%	—	None	N/A

(continued on next page)

Table 3
(continued)

Drugs	Normal Dosage	% of Renal Excretion	Dosage Adjustment in Renal Failure			Comments	HD	CAPD	CVVH
			GFR >50	GFR 10–50	GFR <10				
Intravenous penicillin									
Ampicillin	1–2 g intravenously every 6 h	60	Every 6 h	Every 8 h	Every 12 h	—	Dose after dialysis	250 mg every 12 h	Dose for GFR 10–50
Nafcillin	1–2 g intravenously every 4 h	35	No renal adjustment is required			—	None	None	Dose for GFR 10–50
Penicillin G	2–3 million units intravenously every 4 h	70	Every 4–6 h	Every 6 h	Every 8 h	Seizures. False-positive urine protein reactions. Six million units/d upper limit dose in ESRD	Dose after dialysis	Dose for GFR <10	Dose for GFR 10–50
Piperacillin	3–4 g intravenously every 4–6 h	—	No renal adjustment is required			Specific toxicity: sodium, 1.9 mEq/g	Dose after dialysis	Dose for GFR <10	Dose for GFR 10–50
Ticarcillin/ clavulanate	3.1 g intravenously every 4–6 h	85	1–2 g every 4 h	1–2 g every 8 h	1–2 g every 12 h	Specific toxicity: sodium, 5.2 mEq/g	3.0 g after dialysis	Dose for GFR <10	Dose for GFR 10–50
Piperacillin/ tazobactam	3.375 g intravenously every 6–8 h	75–90	Every 4–6 h	Every 6–8 h	Every 8 h	Specific toxicity: sodium, 1.9 mEq/g	Dose after dialysis	Dose for GFR <10	Dose for GFR 10–50

Quinolones	–	–	–	–	Photosensitivity, food, dairy products, tube feeding and Al(OH)$_3$ may decrease the absorption of quinolones	–	–	–
Cinoxacin	500 mg every 12 h	55	100%	50%	Avoid	—	Avoid	Avoid	Avoid
Fleroxacin	400 mg every 12 h	70	100%	50%–75%	50%	—	Dose for GFR <10	400 mg/d	N/A
Ciprofloxacin	200–400 mg intravenously every 24 h	60	Every 12 h	Every 12–24 h	Every 24 h	Poorly absorbed with antacids, sucralfate, and phosphate binders. Intravenous dose one third of oral dose. Decreases phenytoin levels	250 mg every 12 h (200 mg if intravenously)	250 mg every 8 h (200 mg if intravenously)	200 mg intravenously every 12 h

(continued on next page)

Table 3
(continued)

Drugs	Normal Dosage	% of Renal Excretion	Dosage Adjustment in Renal Failure			Comments	HD	CAPD	CVVH
			GFR >50	GFR 10–50	GFR <10				
Lomefloxacin	400 mg every 24 h	76	100%	200–400 mg every 48 h	50%	Agents in this group are malabsorbed in the presence of magnesium, calcium, aluminum, and iron. Theophylline metabolism is impaired. Higher oral doses may be needed to treat CAPD peritonitis	Dose for GFR <10	Dose for GFR <10	N/A
Levofloxacin	500 mg by mouth every day	70	Every 12 h	250 every 12 h	250 every 12 h	L-isomer of ofloxacin: seems to have similar pharmacokinetics and toxicities	Dose for GFR <10	Dose for GFR <10	Dose for GFR 10–50
Moxifloxacin	400 mg every day	20	No renal adjustment is required			—	No data	No data	No data
Nalidixic acid	1.0 g every 6 h	High	100%	Avoid	Avoid	Agents in this group are malabsorbed in the presence of magnesium, calcium, aluminum, and iron. Theophylline metabolism is impaired. Higher oral doses may be needed to treat CAPD peritonitis	Avoid	Avoid	N/A
Norfloxacin	400 mg by mouth every 12 h	30	Every 12 h	Every 12–24 h	Every 24 h	See earlier	Dose for GFR <10	Dose for GFR <10	N/A

Drug / Dosing	t½ (h)	Every 12 h	Every 12–24 h	Every 24 h	Comments	Supplement after dialysis	Dose GFR <10	Dose for GFR 10–50
Ofloxacin 200–400 mg by mouth every 12 h	70				See earlier	100–200 mg after dialysis	Dose for GFR <10	300 mg/d
Pefloxacin 400 mg every 24 h	11	100%	100%	100%	Excellent bidirectional transperitoneal movement	None	None	Dose for GFR 10–50
Sparfloxacin 400 mg every 24 h	10	100%	50%–75%	50% every 48 h	—	No data: dose for GFR <10	No data	Dose for GFR 10–50
Trovafloxacin 200–300 mg by mouth every 12 h	10	No renal adjustment is required				No data	No data	No data
Miscellaneous agents								
Azithromycin 250–500 mg by mouth every day	6	No renal adjustment is required			No drug–drug interaction with CSA/FK	None	None	None
Clarithromycin 500 mg by mouth twice a day	—	—	—		20%	No renal adjustment is required	None	None
Clindamycin 150–450 mg by mouth three times a day	10	No renal adjustment is required			Increase CSA/FK level	None	None	None
Dirithromycin 500 mg by mouth every day	—	No renal adjustment is required			Nonenzymatically hydrolyzed to active compound erythomycylamine	None	No data: none	Dose for GFR 10–50

(continued on next page)

Table 3
(continued)

Drugs	Normal Dosage	% of Renal Excretion	Dosage Adjustment in Renal Failure			Comments	HD	CAPD	CVVH
			GFR >50	GFR 10–50	GFR <10				
Erythromycin	250–500 mg by mouth 4 times a day	15	No renal adjustment is required			Increase CSA/FK level, avoid in transplant patients	None	None	None
Imipenem/ cilastatin	250–500 mg intravenously every 6 h	50	500 mg every 8 h	250–500 mg every 8–12 h	250 mg every 12 h	Seizures in ESRD. Nonrenal clearance in acute renal failure is less than in chronic renal failure. Administered with cilastin to prevent nephrotoxicity of renal metabolite	Dose after dialysis	Dose for GFR <10	Dose for GFR 10–50
Meropenem	1 g intravenously every 8 h	65	1 g every 8 h	0.5–1g every 12 h	0.5–1 g every 24 h		Dose after dialysis	Dose for GFR <10	Dose for GFR 10–50
Metronidazole	500 mg intravenously every 6 h	20	No renal adjustment is required			Peripheral neuropathy, increase LFTs, disulfiram reaction with alcoholic beverages	Dose after dialysis	Dose for GFR <10	Dose for GFR 10–50
Pentamidine	4 mg/kg/d	5	Every 24 h	Every 24 h	Every 48 h	Inhalation may cause bronchospasm, intravenously administration may cause hypotension, hypoglycemia and nephrotoxicity	None	None	None

Drug	Dose	%	GFR >50	GFR 10–50	GFR <10	Toxicity/comments	Dose after dialysis		
Trimethoprim/ sulfamethoxazole	800/160 mg by mouth twice a day	70	Every 12 h	Every 18 h	Every 24 h	Increase serum creatinine. Can cause hyperkalemia		Every 24 h	Every 18 h
Vancomycin	1 g intravenously every 12 h	90	Every 12 h	Every 24–36 h	Every 48–72 h	Nephrotoxic, ototoxic, may prolong the neuromuscular blockade effect of muscle relaxants. Peak 30, trough 5–10	500 mg every 12–24 h (high FLX)	1.0 g every 24–96 h	500 mg every 12 h
Vancomycin	125–250 mg by mouth 4 times a day	0	100%	100%	100%	Oral vancomycin is indicated only for the treatment of *Clostridium difficile*	100%	100%	100%
Antituberculosis antibiotics									
Rifampin	300–600 mg by mouth every day	20	No renal adjustment is required			Decrease CSA/FK level. Many drug interactions	None	Dose for GFR <10	Dose for GFR <10
Antifungal agents									
Amphotericin B	0.5 mg–1.5 mg/kg/d	<1	No renal adjustment is required			Nephrotoxic, infusion-related reactions, give 250 cm³ NS before each dose	every 24 h	Every 24 h	Every 24–36 h
Amphotec	4–6 mg/kg/d	<1	No renal adjustment is required			—	—	—	—
Abelcet	5 mg/kg/d	<1	No renal adjustment is required			—	—	—	—
AmBisome	3–5 mg/kg/d	<1	No renal adjustment is required			—	—	—	—
Azoles and other antifungals	—	—	—	—	—	Increase CSA/FK level	—	—	—

(continued on next page)

Table 3
(continued)

Drugs	Normal Dosage	% of Renal Excretion	Dosage Adjustment in Renal Failure			Comments	HD	CAPD	CVVH
			GFR >50	GFR 10–50	GFR <10				
Fluconazole	200–800 mg intravenously every day, twice a day	70	100%	100%	50%	–	200 mg after dialysis	Dose for GFR <10	Dose for GFR 10–50
Flucytosine	37.5 mg/kg	90	Every 12 h	Every 16 h	Every 24 h	Hepatic dysfunction. Marrow suppression more common in azotemic patients	Dose after dialysis	0.5–1.0 g/d	Dose for GFR 10–50
Griseofulvin	125–250 mg every 6 h	1	100%	100%	100%	–	None	None	None
Itraconazole	200 mg every 12 h	35	100%	100%	50%	Poor oral absorption	100 mg every 12–24 h	100 mg every 12–24 h	100 mg every 12–24 h
Ketoconazole	200–400 mg by mouth every day	15	100%	100%	100%	Hepatotoxic	None	None	None
Miconazole	1200–3600 mg/d	1	100%	100%	100%	–	None	None	None
Terbinafine	250 mg by mouth every day	>1	100%	100%	100%	–	–	–	–
Voriconazole	4 mg/kg every 12 h	>1	100%	100%	100%	Intravenous use should be limited to only a few doses in patients with CrCl less than 30 mL/min	–	–	–

Antiviral agents

Drug	Dose	% renal	GFR >50	GFR 10–50	GFR <10	Toxicity	Dose after dialysis	Dose for GFR <10	
Acyclovir	200–800 mg by mouth 5 times day	50	100%	100%	50%	Poor absorption. Neurotoxicity in ESRD. Intravenous preparation can cause renal failure if injected rapidly	Dose after dialysis	Dose for GFR <10	3.5 mg/kg/d
Adefovir	10 mg	45	100%	10 mg every 48 h	10 mg every 72 h	Nephrotoxic	Dose for GFR <10	Dose for GFR <10	Dose for GFR <10
Amantadine	100–200 mg every 12 h	90	100%	50%	25%	—	None	None	Dose for GFR 10–50
Cidofovir	5 mg/kg weekly × 2 (induction), 5 mg/kg every 2 weeks	90	No data: avoid	No data: avoid	No data: avoid	Dose-limiting nephrotoxicity with proteinuria, glycosuria, renal insufficiency, nephrotoxicity and renal clearance reduced with coadministration of probenecid	No data	No data	Avoid
Delavirdine	400 mg every 8 h	5	No data: 100%	No data: 100%	No data: 100%	—	No data: none	No data	No data: dose for GFR 10–50
Didanosine	200 mg every 12 h (125 mg if <60 kg)	40–69	Every 12 h	Every 24 h	50% every 24 h	Pancreatitis	Dose after dialysis	Dose for GFR <10	Dose for GFR <10
Famciclovir	250–500 mg by mouth twice a day to three times a day	60	Every 8 h	Every 12 h	Every 24 h	VZV: 500 mg by mouth three times a day. HSV: 250 by mouth twice a day. Metabolized to active compound penciclovir	Dose after dialysis	No data	No data: dose for GFR 10–50

(continued on next page)

Table 3
(continued)

Drugs	Normal Dosage	% of Renal Excretion	Dosage Adjustment in Renal Failure			Comments	HD	CAPD	CVVH
			GFR >50	GFR 10–50	GFR <10				
Foscarnet	40–80 mg intravenously every 8 h	85	40–20 mg every 8–24 h according to ClCr			Nephrotoxic, neurotoxic, hypocalcemia, hypophosphatemia, hypomagnesemia and hypokalemia	Dose after dialysis	Dose for GFR <10	Dose for GFR 10–50
Ganciclovir intravenously	5 mg/kg every 12 h	95	Every 12 h	Every 24 h	2,5 mg/kg every day	Granulocytopenia and thrombocytopenia	Dose after dialysis	Dose for GFR <10	2.5 mg/kg every 24 h
Ganciclovir by mouth	1000 mg by mouth three times a day	95	1000 mg three times a day	1000 mg twice a day	1000 mg every day	Oral ganciclovir should be used ONLY for prevention of CMV infection. Always use intravenous ganciclovir for the treatment of CMV infection	No data: dose after dialysis	No data: dose for GFR <10	N/A
Indinavir	800 mg every 8 h	10	No data: 100%	No data: 100%	No data: 100%	Nephrolithiasis, acute renal failure due to crystalluria, tubulointerstitial nephritis	No data: none	No data: dose for GFR <10	No data
Lamivudine	150 mg by mouth twice a day	80	Every 12 h	Every 24 h	50 mg every 24 h	For hepatitis B	Dose after dialysis	No data: dose for GFR <10	Dose for GFR 10–50
Nelfinavir	750 mg every 8 h	No data	No data	No data	No data	—	No data	No data	No data
Nevirapine	200 mg every 24 h for 14 d	<3	No data: 100%	No data: 100%	No data: 100%	May be partially cleared by hemodialysis and peritoneal dialysis	Dose after dialysis	No data: dose for GFR <10	No data: dose for GFR 10–50
Ribavirin	500–600 mg	30	100%	100%	50%	Hemolytic uremic	Dose after	Dose for	Dose for

Drug	Dose								
Rifabutin	300 mg every 24 h	5–10	100%	100%	100%	–	None	None	No data: dose for GFR 10–50
Rimantadine	100 mg by mouth twice a day	25	100%	100%	50%	–	–	–	–
Ritonavir	600 mg every 12 h	3.50	No data: 100%	No data: 100%	No data: 100%	Many drug interactions	No data: none	No data: dose for GFR <10	No data: dose for GFR 10–50
Saquinavir	600 mg every 8 h	<4	No data: 100%	No data: 100%	No data: 100%	—	No data: none	No data: dose for GFR <10	No data: dose for GFR 10–50
Stavudine	30–40 mg every 12 h	35–40	100%	50% every 12–24 h	50% every 24 h	—	Dose for GFR <10 after dialysis	No data	No data: dose for GFR 10–50
Valacyclovir	500–1000 mg every 8 h	50	100%	50%	25%	Thrombotic thrombocytopenic purpura/hemolytic uremic syndrome	Dose after dialysis	Dose for GFR <10	No data: dose for GFR 10–50
Vidarabine	15 mg/kg infusion every 24 h	50	100%	100%	75%	–	Infuse after dialysis	Dose for GFR <10	Dose for GFR 10–50
Zanamivir	2 puffs twice a day for 5 d	1	100%	100%	100%	Bioavailability from inhalation and systemic exposure to drug is low	None	None	No data
Zalcitabine	0.75 mg every 8 h	75	100%	Every 12 h	Every 24 h	–	No data: dose after dialysis	No data: dose No data	No data: dose for GFR 10–50
Zidovudine	200 mg every 8 h, 300 mg every 12 h	8–25	100%	100%	100 mg every 8 h	Enormous interpatient variation. Metabolite renally excreted	Dose for GFR <10	Dose for GFR	100 mg every 8 h

Table 4
Analgesic drug dosing in renal failure

Analgesics	Normal Dosage	% of Renal Excretion	Dosage Adjustment in Renal Failure			Comments	HD	CAPD	CVVH
			GFR >50	GFR 10–50	GFR <10				
Narcotics and narcotic antagonists									
Alfentanil	Anesthetic induction 8–40 µg/kg	Hepatic	100%	100%	100%	Titrate the dose regimen	N/A	N/A	N/A
Butorphanol	2 mg every 3–4 h	Hepatic	100%	75%	50%	–	No data	No data	N/A
Codeine	30–60 mg every 4–6 h	Hepatic	100%	75%	50%	–	No data	No data	Dose for GFR 10–50
Fentanyl	Anesthetic induction (individualized)	Hepatic	100%	75%	50%	CRRT, titrate	N/A	N/A	N/A
Meperidine	50–100 mg every 3–4 h	Hepatic	100%	Avoid	Avoid	Normeperidine, an active metabolite, accumulates in ESRD and may cause seizures. Protein binding is reduced in ESRD. 20%–25% excreted unchanged in acidic urine	Avoid	Avoid	Avoid
Methadone	2.5–5 mg every 6–8 h	Hepatic	100%	100%	50%–75%	Should not be used for acute pain	None	None	N/A
Morphine	20–25 mg every 4 h	Hepatic	100%	75%	50%	Increased sensitivity to drug effect in ESRD. Active metabolites	None	No data	Dose for GFR 10–50

Naloxone	2 mg intravenously	Hepatic	100%	100%	100%	–	N/A	N/A	Dose for GFR 10–50
Pentazocine	50 mg every 4 h	Hepatic	100%	75%	75%	–	None	No data	Dose for GFR 10–50
Propoxyphene	65 mg by mouth every 6–8 h	Hepatic	100%	100%	Avoid	Active metabolite norpropoxyphene accumulates in ESRD. Cardiotoxic	Avoid	Avoid	N/A
Sufentanil	Anesthetic induction	Hepatic	100%	100%	100%	CRRT, titrate	N/A	N/A	N/A
Non-narcotics									
Acetaminophen	650 mg every 4 h	Hepatic	Every 4 h	Every 6 h	Every 8 h	Overdose may be nephrotoxic. Drug is major metabolite of phenacetin	None	None	Dose for GFR 10–50
Acetylsalicylic acid	650 mg every 4 h	Hepatic (renal)	Every 4 h	Every 4–6 h	Avoid	Nephrotoxic in high doses. May decrease GFR when renal blood flow is prostaglandin dependent. May add to uremic GI and hematologic symptoms. Protein binding reduced in ESRD	Dose after dialysis	None	Dose for GFR 10–50

Table 5
Antihypertensive and cardiovascular agent dosing in renal failure

Antihypertensive and Cardiovascular Agents	Normal Dosage	% of Renal Excretion	Dosage Adjustment in Renal Failure			Comments	HD	CAPD	VVH
			GFR >50	GFR 10–50	GFR <10				
ACE inhibitors	—	—	—	—	—	Hyperkalemia, acute renal failure, angioedema, rash, cough, anemia and liver toxicity	—	—	—
Benazepril	10 mg every day, 80 mg every day	20	100%	75%	25%–50%	—	None	None	Dose for GFR 10–50
Captopril	6.25–25 mg by mouth three times a day, 100 mg three times a day	35	100%	75%	50%	Rare proteinuria, nephrotic syndrome, dysgeusia, granulocytopenia. Increases serum digoxin levels	25%–30%	None	Dose for GFR 10–50
Enalapril	5 mg every day, 20 mg twice a day	45	100%	75%	50%	Enalaprilat, the active moiety formed in liver	20%–25%	None	Dose for GFR 10–50
Fosinopril	10 mg by mouth every day, 40 mg twice a day	20	100%	100%	75%	Fosinoprilat, the active moiety formed in liver. Drug less likely than other angiotensin-converting enzyme inhibitors to accumulate in renal failure	None	None	Dose for GFR 10–50
Lisinopril	2.5 mg every day, 20 mg twice a day	80	100%	50%–75%	25%–50%	Lysine analog of a pharmacologically active enalapril metabolite	20%	None	Dose for GFR 10–50
Pentopril	125 mg every 24 h	80–90	100%	50%–75%	50%	—	No data	No data	Dose for GFR 10–50

Drug	Dose					Comments			
Perindopril	2 mg every 24 h		<10	100%	75%	50%	Active metabolite is perindoprilat. The clearance of perindoprilat and its metabolites is almost exclusively renal. Approximately 60% of circulating perindopril is bound to plasma proteins, and only 10%–20% of perindoprilat is bound	25%–50%	No data	Dose for GFR 10–50
Quinapril	10 mg every day	20 mg every day	30	100%	75%–100%	75%	Active metabolite is quinaprilat. 96% of quinaprilat is excreted renally	25%	None	Dose for GFR 10–50
Ramipril	2.5 mg every day	10 twice a day	15	100%	50%–75%	25%–50%	Active metabolite is ramiprilat. Data are for ramipril	20%	None	Dose for GFR 10–50
Trandolapril	1–2 mg every day	4 mg every day	33	100%	50%–100%	50%	–	None	None	Dose for GFR 10–50
Angiotensin-II receptor antagonists	–	–	–	–	–	–	Hyperkalemia, angioedema (less common than ACE inhibitors	–	–	–
Candesartan	16 mg every day	32 mg every day	33	100%	100%	50%	Candesartan cilexetil is rapidly and completely bioactivated by ester hydrolysis during absorption from the gastrointestinal tract to candesartan	None	None	None

(continued on next page)

Table 5 (continued)

Antihypertensive and Cardiovascular Agents	Normal Dosage	% of Renal Excretion	Dosage Adjustment in Renal Failure			Comments	HD	CAPD	VVH
			GFR >50	GFR 10–50	GFR <10				
Eprosartan	600 mg every day; 400–800 mg every day	25	100%	100%	100%	Eprosartan pharmacokinetics more variable ESRD. Decreased protein binding in uremia	None	None	None
Irbesartan	150 mg every day; 300 mg every day	20	100%	100%	100%	–	None	None	None
Losartan	50 mg every day; 100 mg every day	13	100%	100%	100%	–	No data	No data	Dose for GFR 10–50
Valsartan	80 mg every day; 160 mg twice a day	7	100%	100%	100%	–	None	None	None
Telmisartan	20–80 mg every day	<5	100%	100%	100%	–	None	None	None
Beta blockers	–	–	–	–	–	Decrease HDL, mask symptoms of hypoglycemia, bronchospasm, fatigue, insomnia, depression and sexual dysfunction	–	–	–
Acebutolol	400 mg every 24 h or twice a day; 600 mg every 24 h or twice a day	55	100%	50%	30%–50%	Active metabolites with long half-life	None	None	Dose for GFR 10–50
Atenolol	25 mg every day; 100 mg every day	90	100%	75%	50%	Accumulates in ESRD	25–50 mg	None	Dose for GFR 10–50
Betaxolol	20 mg every 24 h; 80%–90%	100	100%	50%	50%	–	None	Dose for GFR 10–50	Dose for GFR 10–50

Bopindolol	1 mg every 24 h	4 mg every 24 h	<10	100%	100%	100%	–	None	None	Dose for GFR 10–50
Carteolol	0.5 mg every 24 h	10 mg every 24 h	<50	100%	50%	25%	–	No data	None	Dose for GFR 10–50
Carvedilol	3.125 mg by mouth three times a day	25 mg three times a day	2	100%	100%	100%	Kinetics are dose dependent. Plasma concentrations of carvedilol have been reported to be increased in patients with renal impairment	None	None	Dose for GFR 10–50
Celiprolol	200 mg every 24 h		10	100%	100%	75%	–	No data	None	Dose for GFR 10–50
Dilevalol	200 mg twice a day	400 mg twice a day	<5	100%	100%	100%	–	None	None	No data
Esmolol (intravenously only)	50 µg/kg/min	300 µg/kg/min	10	100%	100%	100%	Active metabolite retained in renal failure	None	None	No data

(continued on next page)

Table 5
(continued)

Antihypertensive and Cardiovascular Agents	Normal Dosage	% of Renal Excretion	GFR >50	GFR 10–50	GFR <10	Comments	HD	CAPD	VVH
				Dosage Adjustment in Renal Failure					
Labetalol	50 mg by mouth twice a day	5	100%	100%	100%	For intravenous use: 20 mg slow intravenous injection over a 2-min period. Additional injections of 40 mg or 80 mg can be given at 10-min intervals until a total of 300 mg or continuous infusion of 2 mg/min	None	None	Dose for GFR 10–50
Metoprolol	50 mg twice a day	100 mg twice a day	< 5%	100%	100%	–	None	None	None
Nadolol	80 mg every day	90	100%	50%	25%	Start with prolonged interval and titrate	40 mg	None	Dose for GFR 10–50
Penbutolol	10 mg every 24 h	<10	100%	100%	100%	–	None	None	Dose for GFR 10–50
Pindolol	10 mg twice a day	40	100%	100%	100%	–	None	None	Dose for GFR 10–50
Propranolol	40–160 mg three times a day	<5	100%	100%	100%	Bioavailability may increase in ESRD. Metabolites may cause increased bilirubin by assay interference in ESRD. Hypoglycemia reported in ESRD	None	None	Dose for GFR 10–50

Normal Dosage for Nadolol: 160 mg twice a day. Normal Dosage for Penbutolol: 40 mg every 24 h. Normal Dosage for Pindolol: 40 mg twice a day. Normal Dosage for Propranolol: 320 mg/d.

Drug				GFR >50	GFR 10–50	GFR <10	Comments			Dose for GFR 10–50
Sotalol	80 twice a day	160 mg twice a day	70	100%	50%	25%–50%	Extreme caution should be exercised in the use of sotalol in patients with renal failure undergoing hemodialysis. To minimize the risk of induced arrhythmia, patients initiated or re-initiated on BETAPACE should be placed for a minimum of 3 d (on their maintenance dose) in a facility that can provide cardiac resuscitation and continuous electrocardiographic monitoring	80 mg	None	Dose for GFR 10–50
Timolol	10 mg twice a day	20 mg twice a day	15	100%	100%	100%	—	None	None	Dose for GFR 10–50
Calcium channel blockers	—	—	—	—	—	—	Dihydropyridine: headache, ankle edema, gingival hyperplasia and flushing Nondihydropyridine: bradycardia, constipation, gingival hyperplasia and AV block	—	—	—

(continued on next page)

Table 5
(continued)

Antihypertensive and Cardiovascular Agents	Normal Dosage	% of Renal Excretion	Dosage Adjustment in Renal Failure			Comments	HD	CAPD	VVH
			GFR >50	GFR 10–50	GFR <10				
Amlodipine	2.5 by mouth every day / 10 mg every day	10	100%	100%	100%	May increase digoxin and cyclosporine levels	None	None	Dose for GFR 10–50
Bepridil	No data	<1%	No data	No data	Weak vasodilator and antihypertensive	—	None	No data	No data
Diltiazem	30 mg three times a day / 90 mg three times a day	10	100%	100%	100%	Acute renal dysfunction. May exacerbate hyperkalemia. May increase digoxin and cyclosporine levels	None	None	Dose for GFR 10–50
Felodipine	5 mg by mouth twice a day / 20 mg every day	1	100%	100%	100%	May increase digoxin levels	None	None	Dose for GFR 10–50
Isradipine	5 mg by mouth twice a day / 10 mg twice a day	<5	100%	100%	100%	May increase digoxin levels	None	None	Dose for GFR 10–50
Nicardipine	20 mg by mouth three times a day / 30 mg by mouth three times a day	<1%	100%	100%	Uremia inhibits hepatic metabolism. May increase digoxin levels	None	None	None	
Nifedipine XL	30 every day / 90 mg twice a day	10	100%	100%	100%	Avoid short-acting nifedipine formulation	None	None	None
Nimodipine	30mg every 8 h	100%	100%	100%	May lower blood pressure	None	None	Dose for GFR 10–50	None
Nisoldipine	20 mg every day / 30 mg twice a day	10	100%	100%	100%	May increase digoxin levels	None	None	Dose for GFR 10–50

Drug										Dose for GFR 10–50
Verapamil	40 mg three times a day	240 mg/d	10	100%	100%	100%	Acute renal dysfunction. Active metabolites accumulate particularly with sustained-release forms	None	None	None
Diuretics	—	—	—	—	—	—	Hypokalemia/hyperkalemia (potassium sparing agents), hyperuricemia, hyperglycemia, hypomagnesemia, increase serum cholesterol	—	—	—
Acetazolamide	125 mg by mouth three times a day	500 mg by mouth three times a day	90	100%	50%	Avoid	May potentiate acidosis. Ineffective as diuretic in ESRD. May cause neurologic side effects in dialysis patients	No data	No data	Avoid
Amiloride	5 mg by mouth every day	10 mg by mouth every day	50	100%	100%	Avoid	Hyperkalemia with GFR <30 mL/min, especially in diabetics. Hyperchloremic metabolic acidosis	N/A	N/A	N/A
Bumetanide	1–2 mg by mouth every day	2–4 mg by mouth every day	35	100%	100%	100%	Ototoxicity increased in ESRD in combination with aminoglycosides. High doses effective in ESRD. Muscle pain, gynecomastia	None	None	N/A
Chlorthalidone	25 mg every 24 h	50%	Every 24 h	Every 24 h	Avoid	Ineffective with low GFR	—	N/A	N/A	N/A
Ethacrynic acid	50 mg by mouth every day	100 mg by mouth twice a day	20	100%	100%	100%	Ototoxicity increased in ESRD in combination with aminoglycosides	None	None	N/A

(continued on next page)

Table 5
(continued)

Antihypertensive and Cardiovascular Agents	Normal Dosage	% of Renal Excretion	Dosage Adjustment in Renal Failure GFR >50	GFR 10–50	GFR <10	Comments	HD	CAPD	VVH
Furosemide	40–80 mg by mouth every day; 120 mg by mouth three times a day	70	100%	100%	100%	Ototoxicity increased in ESRD, especially in combination with aminoglycosides. High doses effective in ESRD	None	None	N/A
Indapamide	2.5 mg every 24 h	<5%	100%	Avoid	Ineffective in ESRD	–	None	N/A	None
Metolazone	2.5 mg by mouth every day; 10 mg by mouth twice a day	70%	100%	100%	100%	High doses effective in ESRD. Gynecomastia, impotence	None	None	None
Piretanide	6 mg every 24 h; 12 mg every 24 h	40%–60%	100%	100%	100%	High doses effective in ESRD. Ototoxicity.	None	None	N/A
Spironolactone	100 mg by mouth every day; 300 mg by mouth every day	25	100%	100%	Avoid	Active metabolites with long half-life. Hyperkalemia common when GFR <30, especially in diabetics. Gynecomastia, hyperchloremic acidosis. Increases serum by immunoassay interference	N/A	N/A	Avoid

	Dose			GFR >50	GFR 10–50	GFR <10		Comments		
Thiazides	25 mg twice a day	50 mg twice a day		>95%	100%	100%	Avoid	Usually ineffective with GFR <30 mL/min. Effective at low GFR in combination with loop diuretic. Hyperuricemia	N/A	N/A
Torasemide	5 mg by mouth twice a day	20 mg every day	25	100%	100%	100%	None	High doses effective in ESRD. Ototoxicity	None	N/A
Triamterene	25 mg twice a day	50 mg twice a day	5–10	every 12 h	Every 12 h	Avoid	Avoid	Hyperkalemia common when GFR <30, especially in diabetics. Active metabolite with long half-life in ESRD. Folic acid antagonist. Urolithiasis. Crystalluria in acid urine. May cause acute renal failure	Avoid	Avoid
Miscellaneous agents										
Amrinone	5 mg/kg/min daily dose <10 mg/kg	10 mg/kg/min daily does <10 mg/kg	10–40	100%	100%	100%	No data	Thrombocytopenia. Nausea, vomiting in ESRD	No data	Dose for GFR 10–50
Clonidine	0.1 by mouth twice a day/ three times a day	1.2 mg/d	45	100%	100%	100%	None	Sexual dysfunction, dizziness, postal hypotension	None	Dose for GFR 10–50

(continued on next page)

Table 5
(continued)

Antihypertensive and Cardiovascular Agents	Normal Dosage	% of Renal Excretion	Dosage Adjustment in Renal Failure				Comments	HD	CAPD	VVH
			GFR >50	GFR 10–50	GFR <10					
Digoxin	0.125 mg every other day/every day	0.25 mg by mouth every day	25	100%	100%	100%	Decrease loading dose by 50% in ESRD. Radioimmunoassay may overestimate serum levels in uremia. Clearance decreased by amiodarone, spironolactone, quinidine, verapamil. Hypokalemia, hypomagnesemia enhance toxicity. V_d and total body clearance decreased in ESRD. Serum level 12 h after dose is best guide in ESRD. Digoxin immune antibodies can treat severe toxicity in ESRD	None	None	Dose for GFR 10–50
Hydralazine	10 mg by mouth four times a day	100 mg by mouth four times a day	25	100%	100%	100%	Lupus-like reaction	None	None	Dose for GFR 10–50

Drug							Toxicity			
Midodrine	No data	No data	75–80	5–10 mg every 8 h	5–10 mg every 8 h	No data	Increased blood pressure	5 mg every 8 h	No data	Dose for GFR 10–50
Minoxidil	2.5 mg by mouth twice a day	10 mg by mouth twice a day	20	100%	100%	100%	Pericardial effusion, fluid retention, hypertrichosis and tachycardia	None	None	Dose for GFR 10–50
Nitroprusside	1 µg/kg/min	10 µg/kg/min	<10	100%	100%	100%	Cyanide toxicity	None	None	Dose for GFR 10–50
Amrinone	5 µg/kg/min	10 µg/kg/min	25	100%	100%	100%	Thrombocytopenia. Nausea, vomiting in ESRD	No data	No data	Dose for GFR 10–50
Dobutamine	2.5 µg/kg/min	15 µg/kg/min	10	100%	100%	100%	–	No data	No data	Dose for GFR 10–50
Milrinone	0.375 µg/kg/min	0.75 µg/kg/min	–	100%	100%	100%	–	No data	No data	Dose for GFR 10–50

Table 6
Endocrine and metabolic agent dosing in renal failure

Hypoglycemic Agents	Normal Dosage	% of Renal Excretion	Dosage Adjustment in Renal Failure				Comments	HD	CAPD	CVVH
			GFR >50	GFR 10–50	GFR <10					
–	–	–	–	–	–		Avoid all oral hypoglycemic agents on CRRT	–	–	–
Acarbose	25 mg three times a day	35	100%	50%	Avoid		Abdominal pain, N/V and flatulence	No data	No data	Avoid
Acetohexamide	250 mg every 24 h	None	Avoid	Avoid	Avoid		Diuretic effect. May falsely elevate serum creatinine. Active metabolite has $T_{1/2}$ of 5–8 h in healthy subjects and is eliminated by the kidney. Prolonged hypoglycemia in azotemic patients	No data	None	Avoid
Chlorpropamide	100 mg every 24 h	47	50%	Avoid	Avoid		Impairs water excretion. Prolonged hypoglycemia in azotemic patients	No data	None	Avoid

Glibornuride	12.5 mg every 24 h	100 mg every 14 h	No data	No data	No data	No data	–	No data	No data	Avoid
Gliclazide	80 mg every 24 h	320 mg every 24 h	<20	50%–100%	Avoid	Avoid	–	No data	No data	Avoid
Glipizide	5 mg every day	20 mg twice a day	5	100%	50%	50%	–	No data	No data	Avoid
Glyburide	2.5 mg every day	10 mg twice a day	50	100%	50%	Avoid	–	None	None	Avoid
Metformin	500 mg twice a day	2550 mg/d (twice a day or three times a day)	95	100%	Avoid	Avoid	Lactic acidosis	No data	No data	Avoid
Repaglinide	0.5–1 mg	4 mg three times a day	–	–	–	–	–	–	–	–
Tolazamide	100 mg every 24 h	250 mg every 24 h	7	100%	100%	No data	Diuretic effects	No data	No data	Avoid
Tolbutamide	1 g every 24 h	2 g every 24 h	None	100%	100%	100%	May impair water excretion	None	None	Avoid
Troglitazone	200 mg every day	600 mg every day	3	100%	Avoid	Avoid	Decrease CSA level, hepatotoxic	–	–	–
Parenteral agents	–	–	–	–	–	–	Dosage guided by blood glucose levels	–	–	–
Insulin	Variable		None	100%	75%	50%	Renal metabolism of insulin decreases with azotemia	None	None	Dose for GFR 10–50
Lispro insulin	Variable	No data	No data	100%	75%	50%	Avoid all oral hypoglycemic agents on CRRT	None	None	None

Table 7
Endocrine and metabolic agent dosing in renal failure

Hyperlipidemic Agents	Normal Dosage	% of Renal Excretion	Dosage Adjustment in Renal Failure				Comments	HD	CAPD	CVVH
			GFR >50	GFR 10–50	GFR <10					
Atorvastatin	10 mg/d	<2	100%	100%	100%	Liver dysfunction, myalgia and rhabdomyolysis with CSA/FK	No data	No data	No data
Bezafibrate	200 mg 2–4 times a day 400 mg SR every 24 h	50	50%–100%	25%–50%	Avoid	–	No data	No data	No data
Cholestyramine	4 g twice a day	24 g/d	None	100%	100%	100%	–	No data	No data	No data
Clofibrate	500 mg twice a day	1000 mg twice a day	40–70	Every 6–12 h	Every 12–18 h	Avoid	–	No data	No data	No data
Colestipol	5 g twice a day	30 g/d	None	100%	100%	100%	–	No data	No data	No data
Fluvastatin	20 mg daily	80 mg/d	<1	100%	100%	100%	–	No data	No data	No data
Gemfibrozil	600 twice a day	600 twice a day	None	100%	100%	100%	–	No data	No data	No data
Lovastatin	5 mg daily	20 mg/d	None	100%	100%	100%	–	No data	No data	No data
Nicotinic acid	1 g three times a day	2 g three times a day	None	100%	50%	25%	–	No data	No data	No data
Pravastatin	10–40 mg daily	80 mg/d	<10%	100%	100%	100%	–	No data	No data	No data
Probucol	500 mg twice a day		<2	100%	100%	100%	–	No data	No data	No data
Crestor	5–20 mg/d	40 mg/d	–	100%	100%	100%	–	No data	No data	No data
Simvastatin	5–20 mg daily	20 mg/d	13	100%	100%	100%	–	No data	No data	No data

Table 8
Antithyroid dosing in renal failure

Antithyroid Drugs	Normal Dosage	% of Renal Excretion	Dosage Adjustment in Renal Failure			Comments	HD	CAPD	CVVH
			GFR > 50	GFR 10–50	GFR <10				
Methimazole	5–20 mg three times a day	7	100%	100%	100%	–	No data	No data	Dose for GFR 10–50
Propylthiouracil	100 mg three times a day	<10	100%	100%	100%	–	No data	No data	Dose for GFR 10–50

Table 9
Gastrointestinal agents

Gastrointestinal Agents	Normal Doses		% of Renal Excretion	Dosage Adjustment in Renal Failure			Comments
	Starting Dose	Maximum Dose		GFR >50	GFR 10–50	GFR <10	
Cimetidine	300 mg by mouth three times a day	800 mg by mouth twice a day	60	100%	75%	25%	Multiple drug–drug interactions, beta blockers, sulfonylurea, theophylline, warfarin, and so forth
Famotidine	20 mg by mouth twice a day	40 mg by mouth twice a day	70	100%	75%	25%	Headache, fatigue, thrombocytopenia, alopecia
Lansoprazole	15 mg by mouth every day	30 mg twice a day	None	100%	100%	100%	Headache, diarrhea
Nizatidine	150 mg by mouth twice a day	300 mg by mouth twice a day	20	100%	75%	25%	Headache, fatigue, thrombocytopenia, alopecia
Omeprazole	20 mg by mouth every day	40 mg by mouth twice a day	None	100%	100%	100%	Headache, diarrhea
Rabeprazole	20 mg by mouth every day	40 mg by mouth twice a day	None	100%	100%	100%	Headache, diarrhea
Pantoprazole	40 mg by mouth every day	80 mg by mouth twice a day	None	100%	100%	100%	Headache, diarrhea
Ranitidine	150 mg by mouth twice a day	300 mg by mouth twice a day	80	100%	75%	25%	Headache, fatigue, thrombocytopenia, alopecia
Cisapride	10 mg by mouth three times a day	20 mg four times a day	5	100%	100%	50%–75%	Avoid with azole antifungal, macrolide antibiotics and other P450 IIIA-4 inhibitors
Metoclopramide	10 mg by mouth three times a day	30 mg by mouth four times a day	15	100%	100%	50%–75%	Increase cyclosporine/tacrolimus level. Neurotoxic
Misoprostol	100 µg by mouth twice a day	200 µg by mouth four times a day	–	100%	100%	100%	Diarrhea, N/V. Abortifacient agent
Sucralfate	1 g by mouth four times a day	1 g by mouth four times a day	None	100%	100%	100%	Constipation, decrease absorption of MMF

Table 10
Neurologic/anticonvulsant dosing in renal failure

Anticonvulsants	Normal Dosage	% of renal Excretion	Dosage Adjustment in Renal Failure				Comments	HD	CAPD	CVVH
			GFR >50	GFR 10–50	GFR <10					
Carbamazepine	2–8 mg/kg/d, adjust for side effect and TDM	2	100%	100%	100%	Plasma concentration: 4–12, double vision, fluid retention, myelosuppression	None	None	None
Clonazepam	0.5 mg 2 mg three three times times a day a day	1	100%	100%	100%	Although no dose reduction is recommended, the drug has not been studied in patients with renal impairment. Recommendations are based on known drug characteristics not clinical trials data	None	No data	N/A
Ethosuximide	5 mg/kg/d, adjust for side effect and TDM	20	100%	100%	100%	Plasma concentration: 40–100, headache	None	No data	No data
Felbamate	400 mg/ 1200 three mg/ times three a day times a day	90	100%	50%	25%	Anorexia, vomiting, insomnia, nausea	Dose after dialysis	Dose for GFR <10	Dose for GFR 10–50
Gabapentin	150 mg 900 mg three three times times a day a day	77	100%	50%	25%	Less CNS side effects compared with other agents	300 mg load, then 200–300 after hemodialysis	300 mg four times a day	Dose for GFR 10–50

(continued on next page)

Table 10
(continued)

Anticonvulsants	Normal Dosage	% of renal Excretion	Dosage Adjustment in Renal Failure			Comments	HD	CAPD	CVVH
			GFR >50	GFR 10–50	GFR <10				
Lamotrigine	25–50 150 mg/d mg/d	1	100%	100%	100%	Auto-induction, major drug–drug interaction with valproate	No data	No data	Dose for GFR 10–50
Levetiracetam	500 mg 1500 twice mg a day twice a day	66	100%	50%	50%	—	250–500 mg after dialysis	Dose for GFR <10	Dose for GFR 10–50
Oxcarbazepine	300 mg 600 mg twice twice a day a day	1	100%	100%	100%	Less effect on P450 compared with carbamazepine	No data	No data	No data
Phenobarbital	20 mg/kg/d, adjust for side effect and TDM	1	100%	100%	100%	Plasma concentration: 15–40, insomnia	—	—	—
Phenytoin	20 mg/kg/d, adjust for side effect and TDM	1	Adjust for renal failure and low albumin			Plasma concentration: 10–20, nystagmus, check free phenytoin level	None	None	None
Primidone	50 mg 100 mg	1	100%	100%	100%	Plasma concentration: 5–20	One third dose	No data	No data
Sodium valproate	7.5 to 15 mg/kg/d, adjust for side effect and TDM	1	100%	100%	100%	Plasma concentration: 50–150, weight gain, hepatitis, check free valproate level	None	None	None
Tiagabine	4 mg every day, Increase 4 mg/d, titrate weekly	2	100%	100%	100%	Total daily dose may be increased by 4–8 mg at weekly intervals until clinical response is achieved or up to 32 mg/d. The total daily dose should be given in divided doses	None	None	Dose for GFR 10–50

Drug										
Topiramate	50 mg/d	200 mg twice a day	70	100%	50%	Avoid	Kidney stone	No data	No data	Dose for GFR 10-50
Trimethadione	300 mg 3–4 times a day	600 mg 3–4 times a day	None	Every 8 h	Every 8–12 h	Every 12–24 h	Active metabolites with long half-life in ESRD. Nephrotic syndrome	No data	No data	Dose for GFR 10-50
Vigabatrin	1 g twice a day	2 g twice a day	70	100%	50%	25%	Encephalopathy with drug accumulation	No data	No data	Dose for GFR 10-50
Zonisamide	100 mg every day	100–300 mg every day-twice a day	30	100%	75%	50%	Manufacturer recommends that Zonisamide should not be used in patients with renal failure (estimated GFR <50 mL/min) as there has been insufficient experience concerning drug dosing and toxicity. Zonisamide doses of 100–600 mg/d are effective for normal renal function. Dose recommendations for renal impairment based on clearance ratios	Dose for GFR <10	Dose for GFR <10	Dose for GFR <10 – 50

Table 11
Rheumatologic dosing in renal failure

Arthritis and Gout Agents	Normal Dosage	% of Renal Excretion	Dosage Adjustment in Renal Failure			Comments	HD	CAPD	CVVH
			GFR >50	GFR 10–50	GFR <10				
Allopurinol	300 mg every 24 h	30	75%	50%	25%	Interstitial nephritis. Rare xanthine stones. Renal excretion of active metabolite with $T_{1/2}$ of 25 h in normal renal function, $T_{1/2}$ 1 week in patients with ESRD. Exfoliative dermatitis	Half dose	No data	Dose for GFR 10–50
Auranofin	6 mg every 24 h	50	50%	Avoid	Avoid	Proteinuria and Nephritic syndrome	None	None	None
Colchicine	Acute: 2 mg then 0.5 mg every 6 h Chronic: 0.5–1.0 mg every 24 h	5–17	100%	50%–100%	25%	Avoid prolonged use if GFR <50 mL/min	None	No data	Dose for GFR 10–50
Gold sodium	25–50 mg	60–90	50%	Avoid	Avoid	Thiomalate, proteinuria, nephritic syndrome, membranous nephritis	None	None	Avoid
Penicillamine	250–1000 mg every 24 h	40	100%	Avoid	Avoid	Nephrotic syndrome	One third dose	No data	Dose for GFR 10–50
Probenecid	500 mg twice a day	<2	100%	Avoid	Avoid	Ineffective at decreased GFR	Avoid	No data	Avoid
Nonsteroidal antiinflammatory drugs	–	–	–	–	–	May decrease renal function. Decrease platelet aggregation. Nephrotic syndrome. Interstitial nephritis. Hyperkalemia. Sodium retention	–	–	–

Drug	Dose								
Diclofenac	25–75 mg twice a day	<1	50%–100%	25%–50%	25%	–	None	None	Dose for GFR 10–50
Diflunisal	250–500 mg twice a day	<3	100%	50%	50%	–	None	None	Dose for GFR 10–50
Etodolac	200 mg twice a day	Negligible	100%	100%	100%	–	None	None	Dose for GFR 10–50
Fenoprofen	300–600 mg four times a day	30	100%	100%	100%	–	None	None	Dose for GFR 10–50
Flurbiprofen	100 mg twice a day to three times a day	20	100%	100%	100%	–	None	None	Dose for GFR 10–50
Ibuprofen	800 mg three times a day	1	100%	100%	100%	–	None	None	Dose for GFR 10–50
Indomethacin	25–50 mg three times a day	30	100%	100%	100%	–	None	None	Dose for GFR 10–50
Ketoprofen	25–75 mg three times a day	<1	100%	100%	100%	–	None	None	Dose for GFR 10–50
Ketorolac	30–60 mg load then 15–30 mg every 6 h	30–60	100%	50%	25%–50%	Acute hearing loss in ESRD	None	None	Dose for GFR 10–50
Meclofenamic acid	50–100 3–4 times a day	2–4	100%	100%	100%	–	None	None	Dose for GFR 10–50
Mefanamic acid	250 mg four times a day	<6	100%	100%	100%	–	None	None	Dose for GFR 10–50
Nabumetone	1.0–2.0 g every 24 h	<1	100%	50%–100%	50%–100%	–	None	None	Dose for GFR 10–50

(continued on next page)

Table 11
(continued)

Arthritis and Gout Agents	Normal Dosage	% of Renal Excretion	Dosage Adjustment in Renal Failure				Comments	HD	CAPD	CVVH
			GFR >50	GFR 10–50	GFR <10					
Naproxen	500 mg twice a day	<1	100%	100%	100%	–	None	None	Dose for GFR 10–50
Oxaproxin	1200 mg every 24 h	<1	100%	100%	100%	–	None	None	Dose for GFR 10–50
Phenylbutazone	100 mg 3–4 times a day	1	100%	100%	100%	–	None	None	Dose for GFR 10–50
Piroxicam	20 mg every 24 h	10	100%	100%	100%	–	None	None	Dose for GFR 10–50
Sulindac	200 mg twice a day	7	100%	100%	100%	Active sulfide metabolite in ESRD	None	None	Dose for GFR 10–50
Tolmetin	400 mg three times a day	15	100%	100%	100%	–	None	None	Dose for GFR 10–50

Table 12
Sedative dosing in renal failure

Sedatives	Normal Dosage	% of Renal Excretion	Dosage Adjustment in Renal Failure			Comments	HD	CAPD	CVVH
			GFR >50	GFR 10–50	GFR <10				
Barbiturates	–	–	–	–	–	May cause excessive sedation, increase osteomalacia in ESRD. Charcoal hemoperfusion and hemodialysis more effective than peritoneal dialysis for poisoning	–	–	–
Pentobarbital	30 mg every 6–8 h	Hepatic	100%	100%	100%	–	None	No data	Dose for GFR 10–50
Phenobarbital	50–100 mg every 8–12 h	Hepatic (renal)	Every 8–12 h	Every 8–12 h	Every 12–16 h	Up to 50% unchanged drug excreted with urine with alkaline diuresis	Dose after dialysis	Half normal dose	Dose for GFR 10–50
Secobarbital	30–50 mg every 6–8 h	Hepatic	100%	100%	100%	–	None	None	N/A
Thiopental	Anesthesia induction (individualized)	Hepatic	100%	100%	100%	–	N/A	N/A	N/A
Benzodiazepines	–	–	–	–	–	May cause excessive sedation and encephalopathy in ESRD	–	–	–
Alprazolam	0.25–5.0 mg every 8 h	Hepatic	100%	100%	100%	–	None	No data	N/A
Clorazepate	15–60 mg every 24 h	Hepatic (renal)	100%	100%	100%	–	No data	No data	N/A
Chlordiazepoxide	15–100 mg every 24 h	Hepatic	100%	100%	50%	–	None	No data	Dose for GFR 10–50

(continued on next page)

Table 12
(continued)

Sedatives	Normal Dosage	% of Renal Excretion	GFR >50	GFR 10–50	GFR <10	Comments	HD	CAPD	CVVH
			Dosage Adjustment in Renal Failure						
Clonazepam	1.5 mg every 24 h	Hepatic	100%	100%	100%	Although no dose reduction is recommended, the drug has not been studied in patients with renal impairment. Recommendations are based on known drug characteristics not clinical trials data	None	No data	N/A
Diazepam	5–40 mg every 24 h	Hepatic	100%	100%	100%	Active metabolites, desmethyldiazepam and oxazepam may accumulate in renal failure. Dose should be reduced if given longer than a few days. Protein binding decreases in uremia	None	No data	None
Estazolam	1 mg every hour of sleep	Hepatic	100%	100%	100%	–	No data	No data	N/A
Flurazepam	15–30 mg every hour of sleep	Hepatic	100%	100%	100%	–	None	No data	N/A
Lorazepam	1–2 mg every 8–12 h	Hepatic	100%	100%	100%	–	None	No data	Dose for GFR 10–50
Midazolam	Individualized	Hepatic	100%	100%	50%	–	N/A	N/A	N/A
Oxazepam	30–120 mg every 24 h	Hepatic	100%	100%	100%	–	None	No data	Dose for GFR 10–50

Drug	Dose	Route	GFR >50	GFR 10–50	GFR <10	Comments	Supplement for hemodialysis	Supplement for peritoneal dialysis	Supplement for CAVH
Quazepam	15 mg every hour of sleep	Unknown	No data	No data	No data	–	None	No data	N/A
Temazepam	30 mg every hour of sleep	Hepatic	100%	100%	100%	–	None	None	N/A
Triazolam	0.25–0.50 mg every h	Hepatic	100%	100%	100%	Protein binding correlates with alpha-1 acid glycoprotein concentration	None	None	N/A
Benzodiazepines: benzodiazepine antagonist	–	–	–	–	–	May cause excessive sedation and encephalopathy in ESRD	–	–	–
Flumazenil	0.2 mg intravenously over 15 s	Hepatic	100%	100%	100%	–	None	No data	N/A
Miscellaneous sedative agents									
Buspirone	5 mg every 8 h	Hepatic	100%	100%	100%	–	None	No data	N/A
Ethchlorvynol	500 mg every hour of sleep	Hepatic	100%	Avoid	Avoid	Removed by hemoperfusion. Excessive sedation	Avoid	Avoid	N/A
Haloperidol	1–2 mg every 8–12 h	Hepatic	100%	100%	100%	Hypertension, excessive sedation	None	None	Dose for GFR 10–50

(continued on next page)

Table 12
(continued)

Sedatives	Normal Dosage	% of Renal Excretion	Dosage Adjustment in Renal Failure				Comments	HD	CAPD	CVVH
			GFR >50	GFR 10–50	GFR <10					
			100%	50%–75%	25%–50%					
Lithium carbonate	0.9–1.2 g every 24 h	Renal	100%	50%–75%	25%–50%	Nephrotoxic. Nephrogenic diabetes insipidus. Nephrotic syndrome. Renal tubular acidosis. Interstitial fibrosis. Acute toxicity when serum levels > 1.2 mEq/L. Serum levels should be measure periodically 12 h after dose. $T_{1/2}$ does not reflect extensive tissue accumulation. Plasma levels rebound after dialysis. Toxicity enhanced by volume depletion, NSAIDs, and diuretics	Dose after dialysis	None	Dose for GFR 10–50
Meprobamate	1.2–1.6 g every 24 h	Hepatic (renal)	Every 6 h	Every 9–12 h	Every 12–18 h	Excessive sedation. Excretion enhanced by forced diuresis	None	No data	N/A

Table 13
Antiparkinson dosing in renal failure

Antiparkinson Agents	Normal Dosage	% of Renal Excretion	Dosage Adjustment in Renal Failure			Comments	HD	CAPD	CVVH
			GFR >50	GFR 10–50	GFR <10				
Carbidopa	1 tablet three times a day to 6 tablets daily	30	100%	100%	100%	Require careful titration of dose according to clinical response	No data	No data	No data
Levodopa	25–500 mg twice a day to 8 g every 24 h	None	100%	50%–100%	50%–100%	Active and inactive metabolites excreted in urine. Active metabolites with long $T_{1/2}$ in ESRD	No data	No data	Dose for GFR 10–50

Table 14
Antipsychotic dosing in renal failure

Antipsychotics	Normal Dosage	% of Renal Excretion	Dosage Adjustment in Renal Failure			Comments	HD	CAPD	CVVH
			GFR >50	GFR 10-50	GFR <10				
Phenothiazines	–	–	–	–	–	Orthostatic hypotension, extrapyramidal symptoms, and confusion can occur	No data	No data	No data
Chlorpromazine	300–800 mg every 24 h	Hepatic	100%	100%	100%	No comments	None	None	Dose for GFR 10–50
Promethazine	20–100 mg every 24 h	Hepatic	100%	100%	100%	Excessive sedation may occur in ESRD	No data	No data	Dose for GFR 10–50
Thioridazine	50–100 mg by mouth three times a day. Increase gradually. Maximum of 800 mg/d	Hepatic	100%	100%	100%	–	No data	No data	No data
Trifluoperazine	1–2 mg twice a day. Increase to no more than 6 mg	Hepatic	100%	100%	100%	–	No data	No data	No data
Perphenazine	8–16 mg by mouth twice a day, three times a day, or four times a day. Increase to 64 mg daily	Hepatic	100%	100%	100%	–	No data	No data	No data
Thiothixene	2 mg by mouth three times a day. Increase gradually to 15 mg daily	Hepatic	100%	100%	100%	–	No data	No data	No data

Drug	Dose	Metabolism	GFR >50	GFR 10–50	GFR <10	Comments	Hemodialysis	Peritoneal dialysis	CRRT
Haloperidol	1–2 mg every 8–12 h	Hepatic	100%	100%	100%	Hypotension, excessive sedation	None	None	Dose for GFR 10–50
Loxapine	12.5–50 mg intramuscularly every 4–6 h	—	—	—	—	Do not administer drug intravenously	No data	No data	No data
Clozapine	12.5 mg by mouth, 25–50 mg daily to 300–450 mg by end of 2 weeks. Maximum: 900 mg daily	Metabolism nearly complete	100%	100%	100%	—	No data	No data	No data
Risperidone	1 mg by mouth twice a day. Increase to 3 mg twice a day	—	100%	100%	100%	—	No data	No data	No data
Olanzapine	5–10 mg	Hepatic	100%	100%	100%	Potential hypotensive effects	No data	No data	No data
Quetiapine	25 mg by mouth twice a day. Increase in increments of 25–50 mg twice a day or three times a day. 300–400 mg daily by day 4	Hepatic	100%	100%	100%	—	No data	No data	No data
Ziprasideone	20–100 mg every 12 h	Hepatic	100%	100%	100%	—	No data	No data	No data

Table 15
Miscellaneous dosing in renal failure

Corticosteroids	Normal Dosage	% of Renal Excretion	Dosage Adjustment in Renal Failure			Comments	HD	CAPD	CVVH
			GFR >50	GFR 10-50	GFR <10				
—	—	—	—	—	—	May aggravate azotemia, Na$^+$ retention, glucose intolerance, and hypertension	—	—	—
Betamethasone	0.5–9.0 mg every 24 h	5	100%	100%	100%	—	No data	No data	Dose for GFR 10–50
Budesonide	No data	None	100%	100%	100%	—	No data	No data	Dose for GFR 10–50
Cortisone	25–500 mg every 24 h	None	100%	100%	100%	—	None	No data	Dose for GFR 10–50
Dexamethasone	0.75–9.0 mg every 24 h	8	100%	100%	100%	—	No data	No data	Dose for GFR 10–50
Hydrocortisone	20–500 mg every 24 h	None	100%	100%	100%	—	No data	No data	Dose for GFR 10–50
Methylprednisolone	4–48 mg every 24 h	<10	100%	100%	100%	—	Yes	No data	Dose for GFR 10–50
Prednisolone	5–60 mg every 24 h	34	100%	100%	100%	—	Yes	No data	Dose for GFR 10–50
Prednisone	5–60 mg every 24 h	34	100%	100%	100%	—	None	No data	Dose for GFR 10–50
Triamcinolone	4–48 mg every 24 h	No data	100%	100%	100%	—	No data	No data	Dose for GFR 10–50

Table 16
Anticoagulant dosing in renal failure

Anticoagulants	Normal Dosage		% of Renal Excretion	Dosage Adjustment in Renal Failure			Comments	HD	CAPD	CVVH
				GFR >50	GFR 10–50	GFR <10				
Alteplase	60 mg over 1 h then 20 mg/h for 2 h		No data	100%	100%	100%	Tissue-type plasminogen activator (tPa)	No data	No data	Dose for GFR 10–50
Aspirin	81 mg/d	325 mg/d	10%	100%	100%	100%	GI irritation and bleeding tendency	No data	No data	Dose for GFR 10–50
Clopidogrel	75 mg/d	75 mg/d	50%	100%	100%	100%	GI irritation and bleeding tendency	No data	No data	Dose for GFR 10–50
Dalteparin	2500 units Sq/d	5000 units Sq/d	Unknown	100%	100%	50%	—	No data	No data	Dose for GFR 10–50
Dipyridamole	50 mg three times a day		No data	100%	100%	100%	—	No data	No data	N/A
Enoxaparin	20 mg/d	30 mg twice a day	8%	100%	75%–50%	50%	1 mg/kg every 12 h for treatment of DVT. Check antifactor Xa activity 4 h after second dose in patients with renal dysfunction. Some evidence of drug accumulation in renal failure	No data	No data	N/A

(continued on next page)

Table 16
(continued)

Anticoagulants	Normal Dosage	% of Renal Excretion	Dosage Adjustment in Renal Failure			Comments	HD	CAPD	CVVH
			GFR >50	GFR 10–50	GFR <10				
Heparin	75 U/kg load then 15 U/kg/h	None	100%	100%	100%	Half-life increases with dose	None	None	Dose for GFR 10–50
Iloprost	0.5–2.0 ng/kg/min for 5–12 h	No data	100%	100%	50%	–	No data	No data	Dose for GFR 10–50
Indobufen	100 mg twice a day / 200 mg twice a day	<15%	100%	50%	25%	–	No data	No data	N/A
Streptokinase	250,000 U load then 100,000 U/h	None	100%	100%	100%	–	N/A	N/A	Dose for GFR 10–50
Sulfinpyrazone	200 mg twice a day	25%–50%	100%	100%	Avoid	Acute renal failure. Uricosuric effect at low GFR	None	None	Dose for GFR 10–50
Ticlopidine	250 mg twice a day	2%	100%	100%	100%	Decrease CSA level, may cause severe neutropenia and thrombocytopenia	No data	No data	Dose for GFR 10–50
Tranexamic acid	25 mg/kg 3–4 times a day	90%	50%	25%	10%	–	No data	No data	No data
Urokinase	4400 U/kg load then 4400 U/kg every hour	No data	No data	No data	No data	–	No data	No data	Dose for GFR 10–50
Warfarin	2.5–5 mg/d / Adjust per INR	<1%	100%	100%	100%	Monitor INR closely. Start at 5 mg/d. 1 mg vitamin K intravenously over 30 min or 2.5–5 mg by mouth can be used to normalize INR	None	None	None

REFERENCES

1. Hossain MP, Goyder EC, Rigby JE, et al. CKD and poverty: a growing global challenge. Am J Kidney Dis 2009;53(1):166–74.
2. Abdelhafiz AH, Tan E, El Nahas M. The epidemic challenge of chronic kidney disease in older patients. Postgrad Med 2008;120(4):87–94.
3. Culberson JW, Ziska M. Prescription drug misuse/abuse in the elderly. Geriatrics 2008;63(9):22–31.
4. Le Couteur DG, Kendig H. Pharmaco-epistemology for the prescribing geriatrician. Aust J Ageing 2008;27(1):3–7.
5. Pannu N, Nadim MK. An overview of drug-induced acute kidney injury. Crit Care Med 2008;36(4 Suppl):S216–23.
6. Venkataraman R. Can we prevent acute kidney injury? Crit Care Med 2008;36(4 Suppl):S166–71.
7. Manley HJ, Drayer DK, Muther RS. Medication-related problem type and appearance rate in ambulatory hemodialysis patients. BMC Nephrol 2003;4:10–6.
8. Ladriere M. [What is the best immunosuppression for the elderly kidney transplantation patient?]. Nephrol Ther 2008;3(4 Suppl):S179–83 [in French].
9. Molony SL. Monitoring medication use in older adults. Am J Nurs 2009;109(1):68–78.
10. Pollock B, Forsyth C, Bies R. The critical role of clinical pharmacology in geriatric psychopharmacology. Clin Pharmacol Ther 2009;85(1):89–93.
11. Bond CA, Raehl CL. Adverse drug reactions in United States hospitals. Pharmacotherapy 2006;26(5):601–8.
12. Miller SW. Evaluating medication regimens in the elderly. Consult Pharm 2008;23(7):538–47.
13. Messinger-Rapport BJ, Thomas DR, Gammack JK, et al. Clinical update on nursing home medicine: 2008. J Am Med Dir Assoc 2008;9(7):460–75.
14. McLean AJ, Le Couteur DG. Aging biology and geriatric clinical pharmacology. Pharmacol Rev 2004;56(2):163–84.
15. Aronow WS. Treatment of hypertension in the elderly. Compr Ther 2008;34(3–4):171–6.
16. Divakaran VG, Murugan AT. Polypharmacy: an undervalued component of complexity in the care of elderly patients. Eur J Intern Med 2008;19(3):225–6.
17. Ferrario CG. Geropharmacology: a primer for advanced practice acute care and critical care nurses, part I. AACN Adv Crit Care 2008;19(1):23–35.
18. Cantu TG, Ellerbeck EF, Yun SW, et al. Drug prescribing for patients with changing renal function. Am J Hosp Pharm 1992;49(12):2944–8.
19. Ferrario CG. Geropharmacology: a primer for advanced practice. Acute care and critical care nurses, part II. AACN Adv Crit Care 2008;19(2):134–49.
20. Jain V, Pitchumoni CS. Gastrointestinal side effects of prescription medications in the older adult. J Clin Gastroenterol 2009;43:103–10.
21. Sitar DS. Aging issues in drug disposition and efficacy. Proc West Pharmacol Soc 2007;50:16–20.
22. Diamond AM, Blum AS. Epilepsy in the elderly. Med Health R I 2008;91(5):138–9.
23. Bushardt RL, Massey EB, Simpson TW, et al. Polypharmacy: misleading, but manageable. Clin Interv Aging 2008;3(2):383–9.
24. Turnheim K. Pharmacokinetic dosage guidelines for elderly subjects. Expert Opin Drug Metab Toxicol 2005;1(1):33–48.
25. Turnheim K. Drug therapy in the elderly. Exp Gerontol 2004;39(11–12):1731–8.

26. Turnheim K. When drug therapy gets old: pharmacokinetics and pharmacodynamics in the elderly. Exp Gerontol 2003;38(8):843–53.
27. Thatte L, Vaamonde CA. Drug-induced nephrotoxicity: the crucial role of risk factors. Postgrad Med 1996;100(6):83–8, 91.
28. Appel GB. Aminoglycoside nephrotoxicity. Am J Med 1990;88(3C):16S–20S.
29. Vanholder R, De Smet R, Ringoir S. Factors influencing drug protein binding in patients with end stage renal failure. Eur J Clin Pharmacol 1993;1(Suppl 44): S17–21.
30. Cherry KE, Morton MR. Drug sensitivity in older adults: the role of physiologic and pharmacokinetic factors. Int J Aging Hum Dev 1989;28(3):159–74.
31. von Winckelmann SL, Spriet I, Willems L. Therapeutic drug monitoring of phenytoin in critically ill patients. Pharmacotherapy 2008;28(11):1391–400.
32. Richens A. Clinical pharmacokinetics of phenytoin. Clin Pharmacokinet 1979; 4(3):153–69.
33. Barraclough KA, Staatz CE, Isbel NM, et al. Therapeutic monitoring of mycophenolate in transplantation: is it justified? Curr Drug Metab 2009;10(2):179–87.
34. Perucca E. Plasma protein binding of phenytoin in health and disease: relevance to therapeutic drug monitoring. Ther Drug Monit 1980;2(4):331–44.
35. Raehl CL, Patel AK, LeRoy M. Drug-induced torsade de pointes. Clin Pharm 1985;4(6):675–90.
36. Wynne H. Drug metabolism and ageing. J Br Menopause Soc 2005;11(2):51–6.
37. Nolin TD. Altered nonrenal drug clearance in ESRD. Curr Opin Nephrol Hypertens 2008;17(6):555–9.
38. Dreisbach AW, Lertora JJ. The effect of chronic renal failure on drug metabolism and transport. Expert Opin Drug Metab Toxicol 2008;4(8):1065–74.
39. Nivoix Y, Leveque D, Herbrecht R, et al. The enzymatic basis of drug-drug interactions with systemic triazole antifungals. Clin Pharmacokinet 2008;47(12): 779–92.
40. Li YD, Davis G, Lewis D. General principles of warfarin interactions in orthopedic patients. Orthopedics 2008;31(10):pii.
41. Freeman WD, Aguilar MI. Management of warfarin-related intracerebral hemorrhage. Expert Rev Neurother 2008;8(2):271–90.
42. Prigent A. Monitoring renal function and limitations of renal function tests. Semin Nucl Med 2008;38(1):32–46.
43. Schmitt R, Coca S, Kanbay M, et al. Recovery of kidney function after acute kidney injury in the elderly: a systematic review and meta-analysis. Am J Kidney Dis 2008;52(2):262–71.
44. Tedla FM, Friedman EA. The trend toward geriatric nephrology. Prim Care 2008; 35(3):515–30, vii.
45. Cholongitas E, Shusang V, Marelli L, et al. Review article: renal function assessment in cirrhosis – difficulties and alternative measurements. Aliment Pharmacol Ther 2007;26(7):969–78.
46. Winston JA. Assessing kidney function in HIV infection. AIDS Read 2007;17(5): 257–61, 264.
47. Coresh J, Stevens LA. Kidney function estimating equations: where do we stand? Curr Opin Nephrol Hypertens 2006;15(3):276–84.
48. Olyaei A, deMattos AM, Bennett WM. Drug usage in dialysis patients in Clinical Dialysis. NY: McGraw-Hill; 2005. p. 891–926.
49. Bouman CS. Antimicrobial dosing strategies in critically ill patients with acute kidney injury and high-dose continuous veno-venous hemofiltration. Curr Opin Crit Care 2008;14(6):654–9.

50. Pittrow L, Penk A. Dosage adjustment of fluconazole during continuous renal replacement therapy (CAVH, CVVH, CAVHD, CVVHD). Mycoses 1999;42(1–2): 17–9.

51. Foote EF, Dreitlein WB, Steward CA, et al. Pharmacokinetics of vancomycin when administered during high flux hemodialysis. Clin Nephrol 1998;50(1):51–5.

52. Joy MS, Matzke GR, Armstrong DK, et al. A primer on continuous renal replacement therapy for critically ill patients. Ann Pharmacother 1998;32(3):362–75.

53. Matzke GR, Frye RF. Drug administration in patients with renal insufficiency. Minimising renal and extrarenal toxicity. Drug Saf 1997;16(3):205–31.

54. Matzke GR. Pharmacotherapeutic consequences of recent advances in hemodialysis therapy. Ann Pharmacother 1994;28(4):512–4.

Renal Replacement Therapy in the Elderly

Xiaoyi Ye, MD[a,*], Anjay Rastogi, MD[a], Allen R. Nissenson, MD[a,b]

KEYWORDS

- Dialysis • Geriatric • Elderly • Renal replacement therapy
- End-stage renal disease

With the aging of the United States population, the number of patients with chronic kidney disease (CKD) and end-stage renal disease (ESRD) is increasing dramatically. CKD is a widespread condition in the elderly population. Among Medicare patients aged 65 years or greater, the prevalence of CKD has increased from 1.8% in 1995 to 6.4% in 2006, representing a 3.6-fold increase.[1] The adjusted incident rate of ESRD reached 360 per million population in 2006, with the median age stable since the late 1990s at about 64 years.[1]

As more clinical laboratories are reporting estimated glomerular filtration rates, more cases of CKD are being recognized by physicians, whereas in the past, serum creatinine alone often resulted in under-recognition of this disorder. Aside from diabetes and hypertension, age is a risk factor for CKD and elderly individuals comprise a substantial proportion of the population with renal impairment. Diabetes remains the primary cause of ESRD, with rates continuing to increase annually. In contrast, the incident rate of ESRD due to glomerulonephritis is decreasing (**Fig. 1**).

For the elderly who do progress to ESRD, renal replacement therapy (RRT) is often employed as treatment. Unlike several decades ago when there was often an age limit for who would be eligible for RRT, current practice does not simply exclude individuals on the basis of age alone. However, with more and more elderly patients needing dialysis, the complexities of managing those with renal failure are ever growing. Ethical, socioeconomic, and psychosocial concerns are involved, in addition to medical issues. The elderly in general have a high prevalence of comorbid conditions such as heart disease, vascular disease, dementia, and disability, issues that must be considered by physicians when deciding on how to care for those with ESRD. This article discusses issues specific to the geriatric dialysis population. Although the specific age of "elderly" is not strictly defined in the literature, for purposes of this presentation "elderly" is defined as those aged 65 years or older.

This work was supported in part by National Institutes of Health Training Grant T32-DK-07789.
[a] Division of Nephrology, Department of Medicine, David Geffen School of Medicine at UCLA, 10833 Le Conte Avenue, Room 7-155 Factor Building, Los Angeles, CA 90095, USA
[b] DaVita Inc., 611 Hawaii Street, El Segundo, CA 90245, USA
* Corresponding author.
E-mail address: xye@mednet.ucla.edu (X. Ye).

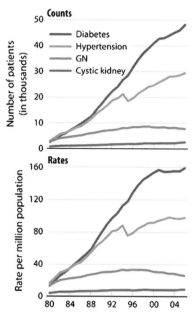

Fig. 1. Incident counts and adjusted rates, by primary diagnosis (incident ESRD patients). (*From* US Renal Data System, USRDS 2008 annual data report: atlas of end-stage renal disease in the United States. Bethesda (MD): National Institutes of Health, National Institute of Diabetes and Digestive and Kidney Diseases; 2008 (figure II 2.8).)

RRT MODALITY

Dialysis (hemodialysis and peritoneal dialysis) and transplantation may be successfully used in appropriate elderly patients with ESRD. Based on United States Renal Data System (USRDS) data, as of December 31, 2006, nearly 328,000 patients were on hemodialysis compared with more than 26,000 on peritoneal dialysis (representing 8.2% of the dialysis population), and more than 150,000 patients were living with a functioning kidney transplant.[1] **Table 1** shows the prevalent counts of ESRD patients separated by age, gender, race, ethnicity, and primary diagnosis for 2006. The largest portion of the prevalent ESRD population by age is the 45–64-year-old group. Over time, there has been a general decline in the use of peritoneal dialysis (decreased from more than 10% of the dialysis population in the mid-1990s), although there are certain states where use has increased such as in the Dakotas and Nebraska. In terms of home therapy, peritoneal dialysis is much more common than home hemodialysis. Home hemodialysis peaked in the 1980s and steadily declined thereafter, but there seems to be a resurgence of this modality as the prevalent population is currently on the increase.

Several studies have compared hemodialysis and peritoneal dialysis in the elderly, examining factors such as survival, quality of life, and morbidity. A meta-analysis performed by Selgas and colleagues (2001)[2] of eight studies comparing these two techniques suggests that the mortality and hospitalization rate of elderly people treated by peritoneal dialysis is similar to that of elderly people treated by hemodialysis. Most studies confirm that the survival of elderly patients on peritoneal dialysis is no different than for hemodialysis. However, subgroup analyses have shown that the presence of diabetes does modify the effect of treatment modality on mortality. In the United

Table 1
Prevalent counts and rates per million population, 2006, by age, gender, race, ethnicity, and primary diagnosis

		Number of Patients				Rate Per Million Population			
		HD	PD	Tx	Unknown	HD	PD	Tx	Unknown
Age (years)	0–19	1201	815	5001	57	13.4	9.6	59.4	0.6
	20–44	44,656	5633	43,043	269	415.7	52.7	403.8	2.5
	45–64	130,134	11,229	75,877	391	2012.8	163.2	1,054.8	5.6
	65–74	72,921	4667	19,515	89	4361.2	259.5	1,074.8	4.9
	75+	71,050	3094	3953	29	4569.5	179.2	212.8	1.7
Gender	Male	174,899	13,311	87,353	488	1288.5	94.6	597.1	3.4
	Female	145,063	12,127	60,036	347	867.2	75.9	385.4	2.2
Race	White	176,940	16,787	110,267	542	684.6	66.1	440.6	2.2
	African American	124,184	6743	28,213	236	3978.9	195.9	822.4	6.6
	Native American	4809	330	1537	11	2000.1	124.7	562.6	3.9
	Asian	14,029	1578	7372	46	1184.0	119.6	524.5	3.3
Ethnicity	Hispanic	44,578	2903	16,917	119	1717.8	93.5	511.6	3.4
	Non-Hispanic	275,384	22,535	130,472	716	1001.6	83.3	488.5	2.7
Primary diagnosis	Diabetes	140,630	8568	34,323	185	462.1	28.2	113.1	0.6
	Hypertension	91,440	6173	22,563	127	300.9	20.4	74.2	0.4
	Glomerulonephritis	33,241	4615	40,067	204	109.7	15.3	132.4	0.7
	Cystic kidney	7969	1340	13,947	56	26.2	4.4	45.8	0.2
	Other urologic	6896	634	5508	29	22.8	2.7	18.3	0.1
	Other cause	27,622	3062	21,301	159	91.3	10.2	70.7	0.5
	Unknown/missing	12,164	1046	9680	75	20.1	1.7	16.0	0.1
All		319,962	25,438	147,389	835	1053.1	83.9	486.6	2.8

Abbreviations: HD, hemodialysis; PD, peritoneal dialysis; Tx, transplant.
From US Renal Data System, USRDS 2008 annual data report: atlas of end-stage renal disease in the United States. Bethesda (MD): National Institutes of Health, National Institute of Diabetes and Digestive and Kidney Diseases; 2008 (table II 4.b).

States, peritoneal dialysis compared with hemodialysis is associated with poorer survival among diabetic patients more than 45 years of age.[3] Thus, although overall patient survival is similar for peritoneal dialysis and hemodialysis, there are differences within select subgroups of patients. The final decision on modality should be made after the patient is fully informed about the advantages and disadvantages of both options, taking into account the specific circumstances, comorbidities, and wishes of the individual.

The advantages of peritoneal dialysis include the fact that it is performed at home, thus avoiding the need for frequent transport to the dialysis center. For the elderly on peritoneal dialysis who remain active, travel may be easier to arrange without the burden of scheduling visits to other hemodialysis units. Many older individuals can be trained to carry out their own peritoneal dialysis, or have family members assist in the procedure. There is the simplicity of dialysis access, and decreased risk of hypotension on peritoneal dialysis as it avoids the large fluid shifts seen with hemodialysis. Peritoneal dialysis may also maintain residual renal function to a greater extent than hemodialysis, and diet can be less restricted. Disadvantages of peritoneal dialysis include difficulty in learning the procedure by some patients, risk of peritonitis and possible social isolation because it is a home-based therapy. The advantages of in-center hemodialysis include a source of social support for many elderly patients and the technique is independent of the individual's ability for self-care. However, vascular access problems are a common occurrence and there is a higher risk of hypotension on hemodialysis.[2]

Compared with a younger cohort, there are fewer elderly patients who are initiated on peritoneal dialysis. Living alone has been shown to be a barrier to home-based therapy. Late nephrology referral and therefore lack of predialysis care and lack of education regarding peritoneal dialysis often predispose patients to be initiated on in-center hemodialysis instead of home-based peritoneal dialysis.[4] Oftentimes, once hemodialysis is initiated, there is no consideration of switching modality. However, based on studies such as the North Thames Dialysis Study[5] showing that mortality is not influenced by dialysis modality, peritoneal dialysis is a suitable alternative and should be offered to elderly patients if it suits their lifestyle and there are no contraindications.

Elderly patients value their independence, which can be a factor in which modality they choose. With home dialysis treatment, most patients are treated with peritoneal dialysis. Home hemodialysis was more common a few decades ago, but decreased in popularity as for-profit hemodialysis centers grew in number along with the increased use of renal transplantation and peritoneal dialysis.[6] Self-care home-based therapy, whether hemodialysis (usually performed 5–7 times per week) or peritoneal dialysis, is more cost-effective than in-center dialysis. Self-care dialysis is an underutilized modality, with less than 10% of all dialysis-dependent patients using this form of treatment in the United States. Ledebo[7] reports on the results of a questionnaire distributed to participants at five major international dialysis conferences in 2006 to identify the barriers limiting self-care dialysis at home. Of 7000 responses collected, nephrology professionals felt that patient motivation is the strongest driver of self-care dialysis, and the reason patients decline this option is due to a knowledge barrier regarding home dialysis modalities. There is a need for dedicated resources to work with the patients to promote and teach home dialysis, to convert patients who are accustomed to full-care in-center dialysis to managing their own treatments at home. Studies show that longer and more frequent dialysis results in better patient outcomes compared with the standard three times per week regimen, and thus home hemodialysis is now increasing in popularity again.

Renal transplantation is the renal replacement modality of choice in ESRD for whom there are no medical contradictions to the surgery or the potential complications of immunosuppression. With the large and increasing number of patients on the waiting list for a renal transplant in the United States, the supply of available kidneys is not keeping up with the demand. Due to the aging population, there is an increasing need for kidney transplants among older individuals. In 2006, 57% of the wait-listed population was aged 50 years or older, increased from 29% in 1991.[1] In the past, elderly age was considered to be a contraindication to renal transplantation. However, the growing number of elderly patients with ESRD in conjunction with improvements in transplant care has resulted in an increase in the number of elderly patients receiving kidney transplants.[8]

Due to the shortage of organs, the concept of expanded criteria donor (ECD) kidneys has developed. ECD refers to a kidney from a donor 60 years of age or older, or a donor 50 to 59 years of age with two comorbidities (hypertension, death from cerebrovascular accident, or a terminal creatinine level ≥ 1.5 mg/dL). To optimize the use of ECD kidneys, appropriate donor and recipient selection is necessary, with the concept of age-matching becoming more accepted. For example, the kidney from an older donor is transplanted into an older recipient, so as not to "waste" a kidney from a younger donor to somebody with a limited post-transplant life span. Older recipients can achieve excellent renal outcomes with transplantation and studies have shown that compared with dialysis, kidney transplantation considerably prolongs the life expectancy of the elderly recipient.[8] Thus, renal transplantation in the elderly is not a waste of a scarce resource.

Regardless of age, living donor transplantation results in better recipient prognosis than deceased donor transplantation. Gill and colleagues (2008),[9] in a review of more than 23,000 kidney transplants from 1996 to 2005 in recipients aged 60 years or older, showed that the recipients of transplants from older living donors (>55 years of age) had superior allograft and patient survival compared with those who received ECD or standard criteria deceased donor kidneys. Thus, for elderly transplantation candidates, an older living donor is a suitable alternative to a deceased donor if a willing donor is available.

At the University of California, Los Angeles Ronald Reagan Medical Center, where more than 300 deceased and living renal transplants are performed annually, there is no absolute chronologic age limit to be a recipient for transplantation. What matters more is the general health, associated surgical risk, and projected life span of the recipient. In general, the likelihood of being removed from the transplant waiting list is higher as one ages, due to an age-related decline in health. However, for the elderly who receive a kidney transplant, there is a survival benefit compared with dialysis (**Table 2**), and thus age itself should not be a barrier to receiving a kidney transplant.

COST OF DIALYSIS

Although medical suitability is often the main reason in selecting a dialysis modality, the economic cost of RRT can be a factor in deciding which modality is chosen for a patient. A review of articles comparing cost evaluations of hemodialysis and peritoneal dialysis was conducted by Just and colleagues (2007).[10] In the United States, there is a cost saving for peritoneal dialysis compared with hemodialysis of roughly $10,000 to $20,000 annually; this has been confirmed in several studies. In other developed countries such as Canada, Denmark, France and Sweden, in-center hemodialysis is more expensive for the payer than peritoneal dialysis, particularly continuous ambulatory peritoneal dialysis, which is cost saving. However, for developing

Table 2
Expected remaining lifetimes (years) of the United States population and of dialysis and transplant patients, by age, gender, and race

Age (Years)	General United States Population, 2004									ESRD Patients, 2006					
	All Races			White			African American			Dialysis			Transplant		
	All	M	F	All	M	F	All	M	F	All	M	F	All	M	F
0–14	71.4	68.8	73.9	71.8	69.2	74.3	67.2	63.7	70.3	19.8	20.2	19.4	53.3	52.8	54.1
15–19	61.6	59.1	64.1	62.0	59.5	64.4	57.5	54.0	60.6	16.8	17.7	15.9	41.5	41.0	42.3
20–24	56.9	54.4	59.2	57.2	54.8	59.5	52.7	49.4	55.7	14.5	15.3	13.6	37.8	37.3	38.6
25–29	52.1	49.7	54.4	52.5	50.1	54.7	48.1	44.9	50.9	12.8	13.4	12.1	34.5	34.0	35.3
30–34	47.4	45.1	49.5	47.7	45.4	49.8	43.5	40.5	46.2	11.1	11.5	10.7	30.7	30.2	31.7
35–39	42.7	40.4	44.7	42.9	40.7	45.0	39.0	36.0	41.5	9.6	9.9	9.3	27.1	26.5	28.2
40–44	38.0	35.8	40.0	38.3	36.1	40.2	34.5	31.6	37.0	8.3	8.4	8.1	23.7	23.1	24.8
45–49	33.5	31.4	35.4	33.7	31.7	35.6	30.3	27.5	32.6	7.2	7.2	7.1	20.5	19.9	21.7
50–54	29.2	27.2	30.9	29.3	27.4	31.1	26.3	23.7	28.5	6.3	6.3	6.2	17.6	17.0	18.8
55–59	25.0	23.1	26.5	25.1	23.3	26.6	22.6	20.1	24.5	5.4	5.4	5.4	15.1	14.4	16.2
60–64	21.0	19.3	22.4	21.0	19.4	22.4	19.1	16.9	20.7	4.6	4.6	4.7	12.7	12.1	13.8
65–69	17.2	15.7	18.5	17.3	15.8	18.5	15.9	14.0	17.2	3.9	3.9	4.0	10.6	10.0	11.7
70–74	13.8	12.5	14.8	13.8	12.5	14.8	13.0	11.4	14.0	3.3	3.2	3.4	8.9	8.3	9.9
75–79	10.8	9.7	11.5	10.7	9.6	11.5	10.4	9.1	11.2	2.8	2.7	2.8	7.4	6.8	8.4
80–84	8.2	7.3	8.7	8.1	7.2	8.6	8.3	7.3	8.7	2.3	2.3	2.4			
85+	4.4	3.9	4.6	4.3	3.8	4.5	5.0	4.4	5.1	1.9	1.8	2.0			
Overall	25.3	23.6	26.7	25.4	23.7	26.8	23.2	21.0	24.9	5.8	5.8	5.7	16.1	15.5	17.2

Abbreviations: M, males; F, females.
From US Renal Data System, USRDS 2008 annual data report: atlas of end-stage renal disease in the United States. Bethesda (MD): National Institutes of Health, National Institute of Diabetes and Digestive and Kidney Diseases; 2008 (table II 6.b).

nations such as Mexico and the Philippines, the economics of dialysis seem different from developed nations. In the developing countries, where labor is inexpensive and imported equipment and solutions are costly, peritoneal dialysis is often perceived to be more expensive than hemodialysis. However, there is a lack of well-conducted economic evaluations for those countries to make a definitive conclusion. Nonetheless, the economics of dialysis including funding and reimbursement vary by region, and can be another factor in determining the modality for a patient.

Renal transplantation has long been recognized as the best option for quality of life and cost effectiveness.[11] However, many elderly patients are not suitable transplant candidates given multiple comorbidities, and thus another modality has to be offered. Several studies have shown that average treatment costs for elderly dialysis patients are not higher than estimates for dialysis patients in general.[12] Thus, the cost of dialysis should not be a limiting factor in providing dialysis to the elderly. Frequently, nonmedical reasons are the determining factors for dialysis modality selection, including financial reimbursement, lack of trained nephrologists/nurses, as well as poor education of patients about dialysis options, resource availability, social mores, and cultural habits.[13] This may explain why choice of dialysis modality varies from country to country. The most important of these factors is financial reimbursement, which can influence a physician's decision on what modality to prescribe for a patient.

IMPACT OF LATE REFERRAL

As the number of individuals suffering from CKD is increasing, it is important for patients to be referred to a nephrologist early in the course of their disease, so treatment can be initiated earlier to prevent progression to ESRD, and to have adequate time to prepare patients for RRT if need be. Unfortunately, a substantial percentage of patients are referred to nephrologists late in the course of disease. Based on USRDS data, in 2006, 42% of new ESRD patients had no nephrology care before initiation of treatment of ESRD. Only 23% of patients had greater than 1 year of nephrology care before being initiated on RRT. This has profound consequences, such as the type of vascular access the patient has when starting dialysis. For the patients with no pre-ESRD nephrology care, 90% have a catheter as initial access, compared with 55% in those with at least a year of nephrology care.[1] There are other consequences of late referral, including increased morbidity and mortality, and missed opportunity for preemptive transplantation.

Some of the reasons for late referral include nonrecognition of abnormal renal function, the attitudes of nonnephrologists toward the usefulness of dialysis or the role of nephrologists, and in some cases, physician concerns about loss of income.[14] Consequently, late referral results in lost opportunities for early intervention. If long-term patient outcomes are to be improved, then early identification of renal disease with early intervention is necessary. In some cases, such as the elderly with multiple comorbidities, it is unclear how many are never referred to a nephrologist at all due to the perception by the physician or patient that dialysis would be futile. Ultimately, this results in death for the patient. However, even if RRT is not undertaken, a nephrologist can be of value in managing the complications of ESRD including anemia, hyperparathyroidism, malnutrition and hypertension, among others.

VASCULAR ACCESS FOR HEMODIALYSIS

For permanent vascular access in hemodialysis, the options include arteriovenous fistulas (AVF), arteriovenous grafts (AVG), and central venous catheters. AVF are the preferred type of vascular access compared with AVG or catheters secondary to lower complication rates and greater survival. AVF are recommended worldwide as the first choice of hemodialysis access.[15] For elderly patients requiring hemodialysis, consideration of vascular access is paramount. The 2006 National Kidney Foundation Kidney Disease Outcome Quality Initiative (K/DOQI) Vascular Access Guidelines recommend that the prevalence rate of AVF should be greater than 65% by June 2009 and catheter prevalence rate to be less than 10%.[16] The Fistula First Breakthrough Initiative is a collaborative effort between ESRD Networks, Centers for Medicare and Medicaid Services, and the Institute for Healthcare Improvement to increase the proportion of patients undergoing dialysis through AVF. Although the campaign has achieved some success, the use of catheters remains high. USRDS data show that for incident hemodialysis patients in 2006, more than 60% had a catheter as access at their first outpatient dialysis, compared with less than 20% using an AVF or AVG (**Fig. 2**). The chances of having a fistula at the initiation of dialysis are greater for patients who had nephrology care before starting RRT, thus reiterating the need for early referral. Because the median age of those who initiate dialysis is now in the mid-60s, the K/DOQI goal will not be achievable unless more AVF are constructed in the elderly.

The elderly are less likely to have AVF placed as initial vascular access compared with a younger cohort. They often do not have suitable vessels for successful creation of AVF, especially if they suffer from peripheral vascular disease or diabetes. Conflicting results of the success rates of AVF in the elderly have been reported in the literature. Studies have suggested that the elderly have decreased AVF patency rates and higher failure to mature rates secondary to vascular anatomy, given the higher incidence of atherosclerosis, systolic hypertension, and arterial stiffness.[17] In contrast, Lok and colleagues (2004),[15] in a retrospective analysis of 444 patients with first-time AVF, demonstrated that patency outcomes were similar in young and old alike, and thus they promote AVF as the permanent access of choice regardless of age. More research is needed to elucidate which risk factors play a role in access failure, especially in the elderly.

In a retrospective study of patients aged 70 years or older, Ekbal and colleagues (2008)[18] showed that access survival was significantly longer in the AVF group

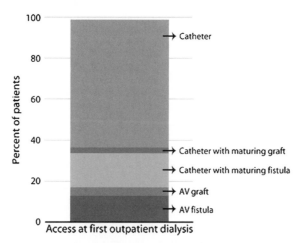

Fig. 2. Vascular access use at initiation (incident hemodialysis patients, 2006). (*From* US Renal Data System, USRDS 2008 annual data report: atlas of end-stage renal disease in the United States. Bethesda (MD): National Institutes of Health, National Institute of Diabetes and Digestive and Kidney Diseases; 2008 (figure II 3.1).)

compared with the catheter group. In addition, there was a significantly greater loss of vascular access due to infection in the catheter group. Sepsis is a common source of morbidity and mortality in hemodialysis patients, particularly with central venous catheters. Studies consistently show that catheter use is associated with the greatest risk of infection-related mortality compared with AVF or AVG. AVF have the lowest risk of infection, greater quality of life and lower all-cause mortality compared with AVG or catheters.[19] However, despite the recommendations of the National Kidney Foundation, most new dialysis patients start treatment with a catheter. The reasons for high rates of catheter use include limited access to medical care for many patients, limited patient education regarding access choices, failure of AVF to mature, inadequate surgical training of local surgeons in AVF construction, and late referral to a nephrologist.[19] The benefits of catheter use include immediate use, relative ease of placement and pain-free dialysis. For some patients with difficult vasculature, a catheter may be the only viable alternative. However, the high rates of central venous catheter dysfunction and associated morbidity preclude it from being an access of choice.

COMORBIDITIES

The elderly face various issues, such as cognitive decline, depression, frailty and disability, that are more common compared with a younger population. These issues are especially magnified in the elderly ESRD patient. Those with cognitive impairment are at greater risk of becoming dependent and requiring help with activities of daily living. In addition, depression can often be under detected, resulting in under treatment. The usual ESRD patient is prescribed approximately 12 different medications for their five to six chronic medical conditions. This places the elderly ESRD patient at especially high risk of medication-related problems, including adverse drug reactions, drug interactions, risk of noncompliance, subtherapeutic dose, or overdose.[20] To provide effective care to the elderly ESRD patient is to realize that they are frail, and thus require extra vigilance to ensure their well-being.

Aging is a complex process that does not start at a fixed age, varies in pace among individuals, and may last many decades. Genetic makeup and environmental factors modify the aging process, and so the elderly comprise a heterogeneous population. Thus, there are octogenarians who have much better functional status and less comorbidity than some 60-year-old individuals. Elderly patients are subject to the same complications seen with all patients on maintenance hemodialysis, but these complications occur more frequently in the elderly. In general, the elderly have more comorbidities such as coronary disease that produce more complications on RRT and affect patient survival. The mortality rate of a prevalent dialysis patient aged 65 years or older is 6 times greater than the general population.[1] Age is a predictor of death later in the first year of dialysis (**Fig. 3**).

CKD is a significant risk factor for cardiovascular disease, with a 10- to 30-fold higher risk relative to those with normal renal function.[21] Several studies have demonstrated that the risk of progression to ESRD in those with CKD declines with age,[22] and ESRD is a less common outcome than death or cardiovascular events in those with CKD. In other words, most CKD patients will die from a cardiovascular event before progressing to ESRD or requiring RRT. Cardiovascular disease is the main cause of death in all ESRD patients regardless of age.

Older patients, by their nature, have been subjected to numerous cardiovascular risk factors such as hypertension for many years, and thus, cardiomyopathies, left ventricular hypertrophy, and valvular heart disease are common among the elderly.[23] This increases the chance of a common complication seen in elderly hemodialysis

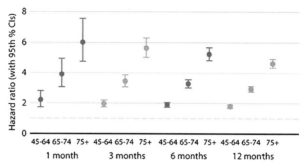

Fig. 3. Age as a predictor of mortality in the first months of ESRD (incident dialysis patients, 2005). (*From* US Renal Data System, USRDS 2008 annual data report: atlas of end-stage renal disease in the United States. Bethesda (MD): National Institutes of Health, National Institute of Diabetes and Digestive and Kidney Diseases; 2008 (figure II 1.13).)

patients: intradialytic hypotension. Hypotension is the most frequently noted complication during dialysis, and can occur in up to 30% of dialysis treatments.[24] Mechanisms leading to hypotension include removal of fluid from the intravascular space that exceeds the plasma refilling rate, aggressive fluid removal in an attempt to reach dry weight, autonomic dysfunction, which is more common in the elderly diabetic patient, intake of antihypertensive medications, and poor cardiac reserve. Various strategies are implemented to avoid intradialytic hypotension, including frequent assessment of dry weight, avoiding rapid fluid removal, aiming for a hematocrit >30%, using dialysate sodium ≥140 mEq/L, avoiding heavy meals before dialysis, and improving nutritional status and hypoalbuminemia.[24] Frequently, a dialysis session is stopped prematurely due to hypotension, resulting in decreased adequacy of dialysis, which is a factor in increased mortality.

Malnutrition is common among all dialysis patients, and is more prevalent in the elderly dialysis patient. Low serum albumin has been associated with increased mortality in dialysis patients.[25] Malnutrition may occur due to reduced protein-energy intake as a result of: inappropriate dietary restrictions, anorexia, and taste alterations; frequent hospitalizations and other comorbidities adding to dietary disturbances; and loss of nutrients such as glucose, amino acids and protein during the hemodialysis treatment.[26] For the elderly, factors such as low income, social isolation, malabsorption, and depression compound this problem. Glucose absorption in peritoneal dialysis can provide the necessary caloric intake, but can also suppress appetite, thus contributing to protein malnutrition. Once a diagnosis of malnutrition is made, therapeutic interventions are warranted, such as improving dialysis adequacy to remove the uremic toxins that are producing anorexia, encouraging oral nutritional supplements and even parental supplementation if necessary. K/DOQI recommends checking nutritional status every 3 months using markers such as body weight, albumin level, and protein consumption. A caloric intake of 30 to 35 kcal/kg/d is recommended for those patients who do not practice intense physical activity, including a protein intake of 0.8 g/kg/d.[27]

Infections are one of the major causes of morbidity and mortality in dialysis patients and contribute to the high rate of hospitalizations in this population. Sepsis is significantly greater than in the general population, and is frequently related to vascular access. As a result of hospitalizations, many patients become frail and develop a significant loss of personal independence, which negatively impacts on quality of life.[28] Elderly dialysis patients are especially prone to loss of functional status following hospitalizations, which contributes to permanent disability and admission to long-term care institutions. Thus, preventative measures and rehabilitative interventions following hospitalizations are necessary to avoid functional decline.

PSYCHOSOCIAL/ETHICAL ISSUES

When evaluating whether a patient should be initiated on long-term dialysis, important issues that have to be considered include the life expectancy of the patient, and the effect of dialysis on life expectancy and quality of life. One of the hardest dilemmas facing a general practitioner or nephrologist is deciding whether to even offer RRT to a patient with ESRD. This decision is especially difficult in the case of the elderly patient with multiple comorbidities for which dialysis may not prolong survival or improve quality of life. Thus, the risks and benefits of dialysis should be weighed in each specific case, factoring in prognosis, treatment burden, and patient wishes. Not initiating dialysis should be an option for all patients.

Conservative management is the other option for treatment if dialysis is decided against. Conservative management is not simply the absence of dialysis. Rather, it entails active disease management of the complications of ESRD, such as treatment of volume overload, anemia, electrolyte abnormalities, and other supportive care.[29] Ideally this involves care by a multidisciplinary team including physicians, nutritionists, and social workers, up until the end of life. In certain situations, such as severe dementia, terminal cancer, or multiple comorbidities, conservative treatment may be the best option. Borderline situations have to be dealt with on a case by case basis, and the decision should be made jointly between physician and patient. Geriatric consultation may be of help in these situations, especially in cases involving dementia.

Murtagh and colleagues (2007)[30] studied survival in elderly patients with CKD stage five treated with dialysis compared with conservative management. Patients greater than 75 years of age attending multidisciplinary predialysis care clinics in the South Thames region of the United Kingdom were included in this retrospective study. Analysis showed that survival rates were significantly improved for those in the dialysis group compared with the conservative group. The 1-year survival rate was 84% and 68% for those groups, respectively. The 2-year survival rate was 76% compared with 47%. However, in those with high comorbidity scores, the survival advantage of dialysis was lost, especially when ischemic heart disease was included. Thus, this study highlights the need to take into account the presence of comorbidities in elderly patients, in particular ischemic heart disease, when advising on dialysis treatment versus conservative treatment. Physicians need to consider if dialysis will offer survival advantage compared with conservative therapy without the burden of dialysis.

QUALITY OF LIFE

One of the goals of RRT is to maintain mental well-being in addition to physical well-being. Studies have shown that many elderly patients have a high quality of life on dialysis. An objective of the North Thames Dialysis Study,[5] a 12-month prospective cohort study from England, was to evaluate the quality of life in dialysis patients 70 years of age or more. This was assessed using the Short Form 36 and compared with general population norms of similar ages. The study showed that mental quality of life in elderly dialysis patients is preserved and is similar to those in the general population, in the initial period after starting dialysis and after having been on dialysis for several years. Although physical quality of life was lower in the dialysis population, this is expected and should not be a reason to withhold dialysis. With the expected increase in the number of elderly patients who will need RRT, age alone should not be used to ration who has access to dialysis.

An advantage of in-center hemodialysis includes the opportunity to socialize with other patients and staff members, a beneficial stimulus to those elderly patients who have limited access to outside activities. On the other hand, dialysis can take up more than 10 hours of time weekly, time that a patient could spend with his or her own family, which can contribute to depression and suicide. Suicide in the ESRD population is not a widely studied topic in the medical literature. Kurella and colleagues (2005)[31] examined the suicide rates of those with ESRD on RRT compared with the general population, and reported that those with ESRD are significantly more likely to commit suicide. Independent predictors of suicide included age 75 years or older, male gender, white or Asian race, geographic region, alcohol or drug dependence and recent hospitalization. The increased risk of suicide associated with ESRD should prompt physicians to seek help for those at high risk for suicide.

In addition to assessing who should be eligible for initiating dialysis, withdrawal of maintenance dialysis is another ethical issue that more and more physicians will have to confront. This is currently one of the leading causes of death in the ESRD population in the United States. The use of dialysis withdrawal and hospice care has increased substantially since the beginning of the decade, and has increased the most for patients aged 75 years or older.[1] This may be due to the establishment of the Renal Physicians Association/American Society of Nephrology (RPA/ASN) and their efforts to educate members of the health care community about quality care at the end of life. One of their educational efforts is to increase awareness among hospice providers that dialysis patients can continue to receive dialysis treatment while in the hospice. Based on USRDS data, the proportion of hospice patients who remain on dialysis has increased from approximately 20.3% in 2000 to 2001 to 26.8% in 2005 to 2006. Overall, the use of dialysis withdrawal has also increased, from 23.9% of deceased ESRD patients in 2005 to 2006, compared with 20.8% in 2000 to 2001.[1]

The ethical principles that support the right of an individual to withdraw from dialysis include the principles of autonomy and self-determination. This is further upheld by the Patient Self-Determination Act (PSDA), passed in 1991 by Congress, which gives patients the right to make decisions about medical care, including the right to refuse medical treatment such as dialysis. The PSDA also encouraged wider use of advance directives, which helps specify a patient's desires in the event they are unable to communicate their wishes or become incompetent. Studies have shown that in dialysis units, only a fraction of patients have completed advance directives. Despite a mortality rate that is higher than the general population, only 4% to 8% of the dialysis population has a completed advance directive.[32] This highlights the need for nephrologists and general practitioners to be more proactive in addressing these difficult decisions. Dialysis patients are not required to complete advanced directives, but it is encouraged.

There is a hesitancy by a large percentage of physicians to withhold or withdraw life-sustaining treatment such as dialysis in end of life cases when requested by the patient or surrogate, as demonstrated in a study by Farber and colleagues[33] in 2006. Of the 407 of the 1000 physicians who returned the survey about their views on withholding or withdrawing life-sustaining treatment, 49% were unwilling to withhold or withdraw treatment in at least 1 of 32 hypothetical situations. This may stem from the guilt that a physician can face knowing that the discontinuation of dialysis will lead directly to the patient's death, or due to the perception that the medical treatment is routine, or due to a lack of understanding of the legal or ethical issues involved in end-of-life care.[33] However, unwanted medical care may prolong the dying process and goes against patient wishes. Thus, it is important for advance directives to be in place to improve end-of-life care as specified by the individual. Physicians can facilitate the discussion to address end-of-life care by initiating the topic, providing information about the disease process and prognosis, and discussing the impact of treatment, using lay terms, listening empathetically, and affirming the self-worth of the patient.[34] Advance care planning should be part of the comprehensive care of dialysis patients, especially the elderly dialysis population.

SUMMARY

Elderly age no longer is a contraindication for initiation of RRT. If current epidemiologic trends persist, the typical patient who is started on dialysis will be greater than 65 years old. The elderly who are started on RRT can have hope for an enjoyable lifespan and thus should not be denied treatment on the basis of age alone. To provide optimal management and to personalize care, patient-specific factors such as comorbidities and patient preference should be taken into account when prescribing a treatment regimen. As the United States population ages, physicians will have to face the many challenges associated with aging, whether medical, psychosocial, or ethical. The decision to provide a life-sustaining treatment should be in the context of the goals of the patient, and thus advance directives will play an increasing role in the management of the elderly patient with ESRD.

REFERENCES

1. US Renal Data System, USRDS 2008 annual data report: atlas of end-stage renal disease in the United States. Bethesda (MD): National Institutes of Health, National Institute of Diabetes and Digestive and Kidney Diseases; 2008.
2. Selgas R, Cirugeda A, Fernandez-Perpén A, et al. Comparisons of hemodialysis and CAPD in patients over 65 years of age: a meta-analysis. Int Urol Nephrol 2001;33(2):259–64.
3. Vonesh EF, Snyder JJ, Foley RN, et al. Mortality studies comparing peritoneal dialysis and hemodialysis: what do they tell us? Kidney Int Suppl 2006;70(103): S3–11.
4. Brown EA. Peritoneal dialysis for older people: overcoming the barriers. Kidney Int Suppl 2008;73(108):S68–71.
5. Lamping DL, Constantinovici N, Roderick P, et al. Clinical outcomes, quality of life, and costs in the North Thames Dialysis Study of elderly people on dialysis: a prospective cohort study. Lancet 2000;356(9241):1543–50.
6. Kumar VA, Ledezma ML, Rasgon SA. Daily home hemodialysis at a health maintenance organization: three-year experience. Hemodial Int 2007;11(2):225–30.
7. Ledebo I. What limits the expansion of self-care dialysis at home? Hemodial Int 2008;12(Suppl 1):S55–60.
8. Saxena R, Yu X, Giraldo M, et al. Renal transplantation in the elderly. Int Urol Nephrol 2009;41(1):195–210.
9. Gill J, Bunnapradist S, Danovitch GM, et al. Outcomes of kidney transplantation from older living donors to older recipients. Am J Kidney Dis 2008;52(3):541–52.
10. Just PM, Riella MC, Tschosik EA, et al. Economic evaluations of dialysis treatment modalities. Health Policy 2008;86(2–3):163–80.
11. Peeters P, Rublee D, Just PM, et al. Analysis and interpretation of cost data in dialysis: review of Western European literature. Health Policy 2000;54(3):209–27.

12. Grun RP, Constantinovici N, Normand C, et al. Costs of dialysis for elderly people in the UK. Nephrol Dial Transplant 2003;18(10):2122–7.
13. Nissenson AR, Prichard SS, Cheng IK, et al. Non-medical factors that impact on ESRD modality selection. Kidney Int Suppl 1993;40:S120–7.
14. Levin A. Consequences of late referral on patient outcomes. Nephrol Dial Transplant 2000;15(Suppl 3):8–13.
15. Lok CE, Oliver MJ, Su J, et al. Arteriovenous fistula outcomes in the era of the elderly dialysis population. Kidney Int 2005;67(6):2462–9.
16. NKF KDOQI Guidelines. Available at: http://www.kidney.org/PROFESSIONALS/kdoqi/guideline_upHD_PD_VA/va_guide8.htm. Accessed December 12, 2008.
17. Chan MR, Sanchez RJ, Young HN, et al. Vascular access outcomes in the elderly hemodialysis population: a USRDS study. Semin Dial 2007;20(6):606–10.
18. Ekbal NJ, Swift PA, Chalisey A, et al. Hemodialysis access-related survival and morbidity in an elderly population in South West Thames, UK. Hemodial Int 2008;12(Suppl 2):S15–9.
19. Wasse H. Catheter-related mortality among ESRD patients. Semin Dial 2008; 21(6):547–9.
20. Katsikas JL, Nelson FV, Bacchus S, et al. Applying frail-elderly care principles. Semin Dial 2009;22(1):22–4.
21. Saran AM, DuBose TD Jr. Cardiovascular disease in chronic kidney disease. Ther Adv Cardiovasc Dis 2008;2(6):425–34.
22. Campbell KH, O'Hare AM. Kidney disease in the elderly: update on recent literature. Curr Opin Nephrol Hypertens 2008;17(3):298–303.
23. Latos DL. Chronic dialysis in patients over age 65. J Am Soc Nephrol 1996;7(5): 637–46.
24. Ismail N, Hakim RM, Oreopoulos DG, et al. Renal replacement therapies in the elderly: part 1. Hemodialysis and chronic peritoneal dialysis. Am J Kidney Dis 1993;22(6):759–82.
25. Chauveau P, Combe C, Laville M, et al. Factors influencing survival in hemodialysis patients aged older than 75 years: 2.5-year outcome study. Am J Kidney Dis 2001;37(5):997–1003.
26. Laville M, Fouque D. Nutritional aspects in hemodialysis. Kidney Int Suppl 2000; 76:S133–9.
27. Buemi M, Lacquaniti A, Bolignano D, et al. Dialysis and the elderly: an underestimated problem. Kidney Blood Press Res 2008;31(5):330–6.
28. Lo D, Chiu E, Jassal SV. A prospective pilot study to measure changes in functional status associated with hospitalization in elderly dialysis-dependent patients. Am J Kidney Dis 2008;52(5):956–61.
29. Brunori G, Viola BF, Maiorca P, et al. How to manage elderly patients with chronic renal failure: conservative management versus dialysis. Blood Purif 2008;26(1):36–40.
30. Murtagh FE, Marsh JE, Donohoe P, et al. Dialysis or not? A comparative survival study of patients over 75 years with chronic kidney disease stage 5. Nephrol Dial Transplant 2007;22(7):1955–62.
31. Kurella M, Kimmel PL, Young BS, et al. Suicide in the United States end-stage renal disease program. J Am Soc Nephrol 2005;16(3):774–81.
32. Bartlow B. In search of an advance directive that works for end-stage renal disease patients. Hemodial Int 2006;10(Suppl 2):S38–45.
33. Farber NJ, Simpson P, Salam T, et al. Physicians' decisions to withhold and withdraw life-sustaining treatment. Arch Intern Med 2006;166(5):560–4.
34. Davison SN. Facilitating advance care planning for patients with end-stage renal disease: the patient perspective. Clin J Am Soc Nephrol 2006;1(5):1023–8.

Ethical Issues in the Elderly with Renal Disease

Lucia Del Vecchio, MD, Francesco Locatelli, MD*

KEYWORDS

- Chronic kidney disease • Dialysis • Elderly
- Survival • Ethics • Dialysis withdrawal

Once seen as a temporary means of rescuing individuals from uremic coma, dialysis has allowed thousands of people with end-stage renal disease (ESRD) to survive for many years. As a consequence, the characteristics of the dialysis population have changed substantially over the last 40 years. This population now consists of considerably older patients with a greater number of coexisting diseases. Mortality and morbidity are high and quality of life is often poor.

This raises several ethical issues about the decision to start renal replacement therapy (RRT) in the elderly, particularly if life expectancy is poor or in the presence of dementia. It is often difficult to halt RRT even when medical conditions have became critical and quality of life has markedly decreased.

Clear behavior guidelines on these critical issues are still insufficient. The final decision is often the result of weighing beneficence (to maximize good) with nonmaleficence (to not cause harm).

The principle of justice plays an important role when considering financial resources. In Western countries, dialysis can be offered to everyone at the present time; however, the benefits of expensive treatments should be carefully considered in patients with a short life expectancy.

THE EXTENT OF THE PROBLEM: EPIDEMIOLOGIC DATA

There has been a striking increase in the incidence of ESRD over the last 30 years, with a 6% to 7% average annual increase in the number of new cases reported in the United States.[1] Despite some indications to the contrary, there is currently no conclusive evidence of any slowing down in this trend. Indeed, according to data from the United States Renal Data System (USRDS), in 2006 the incident population increased even more than predicted.[2]

Department of Nephrology, Dialysis, and Renal Transplant, Ospedale A. Manzoni, Via dell'Eremo 9, 23900 Lecco, Italy
* Corresponding author.
E-mail address: nefrologia@ospedale.lecco.it (F. Locatelli).

Clin Geriatr Med 25 (2009) 543–553
doi:10.1016/j.cger.2009.04.006
0749-0690/09/$ – see front matter © 2009 Published by Elsevier Inc.

The growing proportion of elderly patients mainly accounts for the total increase in the number of patients admitted to RRT. Since 2000, in the United States the adjusted incident rate for patients aged 45 to 64 years has increased by 2.4% reaching 625 per million population (pmp); in patients aged 75 years or older the increase is five times greater (11%) and has reached 1744 pmp.[2] The data are even more striking if only octogenarians and nonagenarians initiating dialysis are considered. In the United Stated this age group has nearly doubled in less than 10 years (from 7054 persons in 1996 to 13,577 persons in 2003), with an average annual increase of 9.8%.[3]

Similarly, less recent data from six national registries of the European Renal Association (ERA)-European Dialysis and Transplant Association (EDTA) showed a four- to five-fold increase over the period 1985 to 1999, with 48% of new patients older than 65 years in 1999.[4] However, in 2006 the adjusted incidence rate for patients aged 75 years or older was nearly the half that observed in the United States in the same period, suggesting important differences in acceptance criteria and patient characteristics between countries.[5]

Lombardy Registry data also indicate that the frequency of new patients aged 65 years or older more than doubled from 1983 to 1992 (from 19.7% to 41.6%) [6] and was still increasing in 1997 (nearly 54%).[7]

Several different factors probably account for this growth in the elderly RRT population. RRT has been found to lead to favorable results in elderly or diabetic patients, and other high-risk patients with malignancies, multi-organ failure, and so forth, who were previously excluded; this has been a major factor in the increase in RRT in the elderly. For the same reason, general practitioners now refer an increasing number of patients with chronic kidney disease (CKD) to renal units regardless of their age and clinical condition.

Concurrent with the increase in the number of patients admitted to RRT, which is only "the tip of the iceberg," CKD incidence and prevalence have also increased. In Europe, this has been well documented by an epidemiologic survey of the Ile de France, which showed a striking age-related increase in the annual incidence of CKD (ie, the first evidence of serum creatinine levels >2 mg/dL in the course of one year); the incidence rate among patients older than 75 years was almost seven times that of patients aged 20 to 39 years (619 versus 92 new cases per million population) and more than twice that of patients aged 40 to 59 years (619 versus 264 new cases per million population).[8] The increased incidence of CKD among the elderly translates into a similarly increased prevalence. An update to the Third National Health and Nutrition Examination Survey (NHANES III) program found an increase of 15.9% in the crude estimate of CKD prevalence in the adult United States population from 1988–1994 to 1999–2004 (14.5% and 16.8%, respectively).[9] By age group, CKD (all stages) was confirmed to be more prevalent among people aged 60 years and older (39.4%) than those aged 40 to 59 years (12.6%) or 20 to 39 years (8.5%).

The aging of the general population accounts for only a small fraction of the increase in the number of patients with CKD and ESRD. The observed decline in mortality due to stroke and coronary heart disease in the general population seems to be more important because of the consequent greater probability that those who survive longer are more likely to experience hypertensive or atherosclerotic kidney damage. However, improved survival after cardiovascular events, together with the population growth and increasing prevalence of diabetes explained less than 50% of the observed increase in new ESRD cases from 1978 to 1991.[10]

The high prevalence of diabetes and atherosclerotic kidney damage underlying renal disease in the ESRD population probably accounts for the other major change in today's dialytic population; that is, the high incidence of comorbidity factors.

Vascular disease and diabetes mellitus are the most common causes of ESRD in the elderly and, together with age, are the main determinants of morbidity and mortality in ESRD patients.

WHAT LIFE EXPECTANCY CAN BE OFFERED TO THE ELDERLY RECEIVING DIALYSIS?

As with many chronic medical conditions, the life expectancy of patients undergoing RRT is greatly reduced; however, overall survival has improved over the last few decades. The most consistent and greatest improvement has occurred in the younger adults and in those with diabetes. However, despite these improvements, which have been made possible by technical advances in medical care and dialysis delivery, several factors seem to contribute toward the high morbidity and mortality rates in patients on hemodialysis, and their poor quality of life. First-year mortality in the hemodialysis population has shown little changes over the last 9 years.[2]

Age is the most important demographic factor associated with increased mortality in patients with ESRD. The elderly are frailer and other medical conditions are more likely to occur with advancing age; furthermore, as vascular disease and diabetes are frequent causes of ESRD in the elderly, this further increases the risk of cardiovascular death. USRDS data for 2006 showed a progressive increase in all-cause mortality rates from the youngest to the older age groups in prevalent dialysis patients: 83 deaths per 1000 patient years at risk between 20 and 44 years, 174 between 45 and 64 years, more than 300 for patients aged 65 years or older.[2] Compared with the general population, mortality rates are six times higher in older prevalent dialysis patients.[2] A dialysis patient aged between 70 and 74 years is expected to survive nearly 3 years, but this prospective is markedly reduced by comorbidities.[2] Life expectancy is even shorter in octogenarians and nonagenarians starting dialysis in the United States.[3] In this age group, 1-year mortality after dialysis is 46%.[3] Median survival for octogenarians and nonagenarians ranges between 15 and 8 months, respectively.[3] This translates into a life expectancy nearly 14 times shorter than that of the age-matched general population.[3]

In European countries, the survival of geriatric patients, as well as that in the overall ESRD population, is slightly better than that reported in the United States. According to the data from the ERA-EDTA Registry,[4] the 1- and 2-year survival of patients aged 65 years or older was 69% and 51%, respectively. When the analysis was restricted to patients older than 75 years, median survival was 1.6 years (1995–1999 cohort). Nearly 40% of patients on hemodialysis died because of cardiovascular disease. Infections, cachexia, and social causes account for one third of the deaths.

An even older analysis of the outcomes of the 2447 ESRD patients aged 65 years or more who started RRT in Lombardy between 1983 and 1992 revealed that the mortality rate was 35.6% at 2 years[11]; only 13.1% of the elderly patients survived after 8 years of RRT. The main causes of death were again cardiovascular disease and cachexia.

HOW MUCH DO COMORBIDITIES IMPACT ON PATIENT OUTCOME AND QUALITY OF LIFE IN THE ELDERLY?

In addition to the basic factors of age, race, and underlying disease, comorbid conditions substantially modify the risk of mortality and impact on quality of life when receiving RRT. This is particularly true in the elderly.

Cardiovascular Disease

Cardiovascular diseases account for more than 50% of mortality in patients on hemo-dialysis, who have an incidence of cardiac death that is 5 to 10 times higher than that of the age-matched general population. The prevalence of ischemic heart disease, heart failure, and left ventricular disorders is high among patients beginning hemodi-alysis. According to the USRDS, of all patients who started dialysis in 2001, 32.3% had congestive heart failure, 33.8% had a history of coronary artery disease (including myocardial infarction), and peripheral vascular disease and other cardiovascular diseases were present in 14.1% and 9.5% of the patients, respectively.[12] Data obtained from the Registro Lombardo Dialisi e Trapianto (RLDT) on 4139 RRT patients showed that coronary artery disease, myocardial infarction, and congestive heart failure were present in 10.0%, 8.3% and 8.9% of the patients, respectively.[13] These abnormalities are all independent predictors of overall mortality and cardiac mortality.[13,14] More than two thirds of patients on dialysis with left ventricular hyper-trophy die from heart failure or sudden death, and the 5-year mortality rate increases from 23% to 52% when the left ventricular mass index is more than 125 g/m^2.[15] The survival rate in patients with recurrent or persistent congestive heart failure is also particularly low (2-year survival 33% versus 80% in patients without congestive heart failure).[16]

Underlying Renal Disease

The survival of patients with diabetes is generally shorter than that of their nondiabetic counterparts. Patients with diabetes have more comorbid conditions and higher levels of physical dysfunction, and are more dependent when it comes to daily activities. The higher prevalence of comorbid conditions is confirmed by the fact that dialysis with-drawal rates among patients with diabetes are 23 times those without diabetes.[17] It seems that the high mortality rate of patients with diabetes undergoing hemodialysis is largely related to factors connected to their predialysis life; the duration of diabetes typically exceeds 10 years, and its systemic complications are usually pronounced by the time end-stage renal disease (ESRD) is reached. A prospective study of 433 hemo-dialysis patients found that, at the beginning of dialysis, those with diabetes ($n = 116$) had more echocardiographic concentric left ventricular hypertrophy (50% versus 38%), ischemic heart disease (32% versus 18%), and cardiac failure (48% versus 24%) than those without diabetes.[18] After starting dialysis, the patients with diabetes had similar rates of progression of echocardiographic disorders and new cardiac failure to those observed in the patients without diabetes, but higher rates of new ischemic heart disease (RR 3.2, $P = .0002$), overall mortality (RR 2.6, $P < .0001$), and cardiovascular mortality (RR 2.6, $P < .0001$).[18] The difference in crude survival between age-matched patients with and without diabetes is greatest in younger patients (5-year survival of 56% versus 85% in patients aged 18 to 54 years, and 17% versus 28% in patients $\geq$65 years).[19]

Patients with renal vascular disease (which probably represents accompanying atherosclerotic disease in the coronary and cerebral beds) also fare poorly. The risk of mortality in these patients is double that of patients with other renal diseases (excluding diabetes), and the survival estimates at 5 and 10 years are only 16% and 5%, respectively.[20]

Malnutrition

Cachexia is an important cause of death in the elderly receiving RRT. However, the extent to which malnutrition reflects a cause–effect relationship is still not clear, because several comorbidity factors (which are more important causes of death) may have secondary effects on various parameters used to assess nutritional status. It has been suggested that malnutrition could be a uremic risk factor for cardiovascular disease, resulting in increased cardiovascular mortality in malnourished patients. In contrast, atherosclerosis is considered an inflammatory disease, and chronic inflammation may lead to a decline in appetite, increased rate of protein depletion, muscle and fat wasting, and hyper catabolism. The malnutrition, inflammation, and atherosclerosis (MIA) syndrome has been proposed to embrace these observations,[21] with the idea that chronic inflammation could be the missing link that casually ties malnutrition with poor outcome. In addition, malnutrition decreases the immune response, predisposing to latent or overt infections.

Walking Disability

The ability to walk is a robust measure of physical function and independence. In the United States, about 50% of incident dialysis patients older than 66 years have a walking disability; 10% are unable to walk.[2] The risk of mortality increases with the presence of walking disability and peaks in those unable to walk.[2] Obviously, the risk is further increased when the walking disability is associated with older age or other comorbidities; patients who are 85 years or older or those with dementia survive less than 1 year on average. Among prevalent patients, nearly 40% of patients aged 75 years or more have a walking disability or need an walking aid; dementia and stroke are the two comorbidities associated with any walking disability.[2] The mortality rates for these patients are alarming; after stratification by demographic factors and comorbidities, they are 50% higher than those of patients able to walk.

Cognitive Impairment

Dementia is a major cause of death and disability among elderly individuals in the general population; individuals with ESRD have a two- to seven-fold higher prevalence of cognitive impairment and dementia compared with the general population. This increased risk is explained by their older age, high prevalence of cardiovascular risk factors, previous stroke or transient ischemic attack, uremia-related factors and multiple metabolic abnormalities. According to a prospective study of 347 patients on hemodialysis aged 55 years and older, only a minority were classified with normal cognition; 37.3% had severe impairment, 36.1% had moderate deficit, and 13.9 had moderate impairment.[22] Factors independently associated with severe dementia were stroke, low education and, strangely enough, higher dialysis dose.[22] Cognitive impairment is often under evaluated; only 2.9% of these patients had a known history of dementia.

Similarly, data collected from a cohort of 16,694 patients in the Dialysis Outcomes and Practice Patterns Study (DOPPS) showed that only 4% of the patients had a recorded diagnosis of dementia,[23] suggesting that cognitive impairment is largely underestimated. After adjustment for several confounding factors, dementia was associated with an increased risk of death (RR 1.48, 95% confidence interval [CI], 1.32–1.66) and dialysis withdrawal (RR 2.01, 95% CI, 1.57–2.57).[23]

Moreover, severe cognitive impairment makes compliance with dialysis schedules, medications, and fluid and dietary restrictions difficult, and implies that such patients are mostly unable to properly judge whether to start or withdraw dialysis at a given time. Decisions regarding their care will then be in the hands of surrogates, proxies, family members, or close friends.

WHEN THE START OF DIALYSIS MAY BE CONSIDERED INAPPROPRIATE?

Given the high mortality rate and the high costs of RRT, ethical considerations are mandatory in relation to the potential benefits of treating ESRD in patients with a poor quality of life and long-term prognosis. The fact that elderly ESRD patients with multiple comorbidities can undergo dialysis successfully does not necessarily mean that they should do so without carefully evaluating each individual case. Like all physicians, nephrologists have the ethical need to offer all treatment options to their patients, but only if these are reasonable. However, bounds for defining the concept of "reasonable" are not so defined. Sometimes primary care physicians avoid nephrology referral of some patients with advanced CKD before dialysis evaluation.[24] However, this entails the risk that insufficient education of primary care physicians about outcomes and quality of life of the elderly receiving RRT might result in less referrals for patients who will benefit from dialysis.

Reasons for not starting dialysis include old age, neurologic impairment, end-stage organ failure other than the kidneys, metastatic cancer, multiple comorbidities, and patient or family refusal.

Providing dialysis to patients with severe dementia is considered by many people to be an unwise use of health resources. This view, although widespread, is not shared by everybody. Some people believe that brain and soul are different; others argue that it is difficult to discriminate the real perception of life and happiness of patients with moderate or severe dementia.[25] It would be advantageous if all patients with severe medical conditions discussed end-of-life care before they become mentally impaired.[25] For incapacitated patients who have not expressed a directive about their care in advance, hospitals should develop uniform policies and give adequate ethical education to all care providers.

In addition to the degree of mental impairment, the burden of comorbidities and life expectancy must also be considered in decision making. Recently, the French Renal Epidemiology and Information Network (REIN) registry proposed a clinical score to predict 6-month prognosis in elderly patients starting dialysis.[26] Nine risk factors were selected: body mass index less than 18.5 kg/m^2, diabetes, congestive heart failure stage III to IV, arrhythmia, active malignancy, severe behavioral disorder, total dependency on transfers, severe peripheral vascular disease, and unplanned dialysis. The prognostic score was then validated on a cohort of 1642 patients aged 75 years or older; at 6 months mortality ranged from 8% in the lowest risk group up to 70% in the highest risk group. However, prediction tools should not replace good clinical judgment.

To examine factors associated with the decision to propose RRT, Joly and colleagues[27] performed a single-center retrospective study of all consecutive octogenarian patients who reached ESRD from 1989 to 2000. During the observation period, the medical team recommended dialysis in two thirds of the patients. Among these, 6 refused dialysis. Those for whom conservative therapy was proposed were more likely to be socially isolated, referred late to nephrologists, have a lower Karnofsky performance status, and have diabetes.

In addition to medical judgment, cultural and educational differences may play a role. Surveys of nephrologists' opinions regarding the suitability of certain patients for dialysis have shown variations within and across countries. For instance, in a 1996 survey, nephrologists in the United Kingdom and Canada were significantly less likely than nephrologists in the United States to consider dialysis for patients with significant comorbidities, particularly dementia.[28] More recently, 242 hemodialysis units in six countries (France, Germany, Italy, Spain, United Kingdom, and the United States) were sent a questionnaire during the first phase of DOPPS asking opinions about access to dialysis.[29] Medical directors in France and the United Kingdom were least likely to start dialysis in patients with advanced renal failure and dementia, or in patients with multiple active and serious medical problems. Moreover, fewer medical directors in the United Kingdom than in the other countries were willing to start hemodialysis in patients who lived in nursing homes or were very old. Accordingly, the percentage of patients who were not self-sufficient was lower in the United Kingdom compared with other European countries.

In 2000 the Renal Physicians Association together with the American Society of Nephrology developed clinical practice guidelines aimed at helping physicians during decision making for appropriate initiation and withdrawal from dialysis.[30] According to these guidelines, dialysis should not be started when a patient or surrogate refuses it or, in the presence of profound neurologic impairment, a nonrenal terminal condition, a technical contraindication to the process of dialysis.

Another important issue that is related to the decision to start dialysis treatment is the right timing of surgical referral for creation of permanent access. Ideally, this referral should occur with enough time to allow for fistula maturation and repeated attempts at fistula creation if necessary. However, in the elderly, creation of vascular access is often a difficult task. Repeated surgical procedures and related hospitalizations may be the cause of further comorbidities or concurrent events in this frail population. Moreover, given the low life expectancy, many patients may die before starting dialysis without ever having used the vascular access.[31] In addition, older patients need longer times for fistula maturation and have a higher risk of infection when a vascular catheter has been placed.

ALTERNATIVES TO DIALYSIS IN THE ELDERLY WITH END-STAGE RENAL DISEASE

When dealing with the delicate decision of whether to start dialysis, it is important that attending physicians, and particularly nephrologists, provide the correct perspective and that the option of conservative management without dialysis is not simply the absence of treatment. According to medical conditions, patients are always offered active disease management and detailed supportive care. A few studies have examined the survival of patients with CKD on dialysis compared with those treated conservatively, and all suggest that elderly patients with CKD who start dialysis live longer. However, these studies are inevitably biased by the fact the patients who do not start RRT are more likely to have severe comorbidities, to be not self-sufficient, or socially isolated. Thus, it becomes difficult to discriminate whether the survival benefit of dialysis is due to the treatment modality itself or merely reflects important selection biases. Murtagh and colleagues[32] compared survival during dialysis and the conservative phase in 129 patients older than 75 years after the decision about access to RRT had already been taken. During the 12-month follow-up, 23% of the dialysis patients and 66% of those on conservative management died. However, for patients with a high comorbidity score (especially in the presence of ischemic heart disease) the survival advantage offered by dialysis was no longer evident. Similarly a retrospective study of 146 octogenarian patients with CKD in France found that those who began dialysis lived much longer than those who did not (median survival of 28.9 months versus 8.9 months, respectively).[27] Independent predictors of poor survival were malnourishment, late referral, and functional dependence; the burden of comorbidities was not significantly different in the two groups.

A small Italian study randomized 112 patients older than 70 years with a glomerular filtration rate (GFR) of 5 to 7 mL/min/1.73 m^2 to receive either a supplemented very-low-protein diet or dialysis.[33] During a median follow-up of nearly 2 years, the mortality rate in the two groups was comparable. However, nearly two thirds of the patients who were managed conservatively had to start dialysis after a median of 9.8 months because of either fluid overload or hyperkalemia. Even if this demanding diet could be an option for postponing dialysis for a while and does not seem to modify nutritional status, the applicability of these findings to everyday clinical practice is markedly reduced by the fact that patients with severe comorbidities, that is, those who are less likely to be started on RRT, were excluded from the trial.

Another option may be the use of an integrated diet and dialysis program, as proposed in the early 1990s.[34] This consisted of a low-protein diet (0.4 g/kg ideal body weight/d), supplemented with essential amino acids or a mixture of essential amino acids and keto analogs, and once-weekly hemodialysis, tailored to maintain predialytic blood urea nitrogen levels lower than 90 mg/dL. At 12-month follow-up, patient and technique survival were 89% and 56%, respectively. However, the success of this option is undermined by poor compliance to the diet and the risk of malnutrition in the long term. However, baseline GFR (2.54 ± 0.94 mL/min) was similar to that of patients starting dialysis in the study by Brunori and colleagues.[33]

DIALYSIS WITHDRAWAL: A DIFFICULT CHOICE

Dialysis withdrawal is a common occurrence, especially in the United States. According to the 2008 USRDS annual data report,[2] in the 2005 to 2006 cohort nearly one fourth of the patients withdrew dialysis before dying. Since 2000, this practice had increased considerably, mostly for patients aged 75 years or older. Failure to thrive is the most common cause of withdrawal, followed by the full comprehensive category of "medical complications." The diagnosis of failure to thrive is usually applied to patients with cachexia, to those who are unable to function independently, and sometimes to patients with dementia.

Withdrawal rates vary considerably throughout the world. Indeed, combined data from six European dialysis registries showed that mortality for social causes, also including dialysis withdrawal, accounted for 8% and 13% of dialysis deaths in patients aged 65 to 74 years or 75 years or more, respectively.[4] These dissimilarities likely reflect not only differences in the burden of comorbidities among the patients who receive RRT but also cultural and educational aspects. In addition, it is likely that the phenomenon is underreported in many countries. To better understand ESRD mortality, in the United States withdrawal from dialysis was removed as a cause of death from the Death Notification Form in 1990, and since then it has been asked if dialysis withdrawal occurred before death. Probably reflecting this change, the fraction of patients who withdrew from dialysis nearly doubled in the following 2 years (from 8.4% in 1998 to 1990 to 17.6% in 1991 to 1993).[35]

In 1996, the National Kidney Foundation started a huge educational effort concerning dialysis withholding or withdrawal.[36] Following this, the American Society of Nephrology and the Renal Physicians Association published a new set of practice guidelines in 2000.[30] According to them, dialysis withdrawal may be appropriate for patients with a limited life expectancy, or for those with poor quality of life, pain refractory to treatment, or progressive debilitation from an untreatable medical condition.

Other important points, such as shared decision making, informed consent or refusal, and conflict resolution are discussed. Even more significantly, these guidelines stress the importance of providing the most comfortable death possible for the patient once a decision to withdraw dialysis has been made. Unfortunately, despite the high mortality rate of older patients receiving RRT, education about end-of-life care is still insufficient among nephrologists.[37]

SUMMARY

Given the increasing gap between limited economic resources and the exponential increase in the dialysis population, there is the need to weigh operative choices to obtain the optimal use of human and technological resources. Furthermore, the high rates of morbidity and mortality and the high costs of RRT certainly require ethical considerations in relation to the potential benefits of treating ESRD patients with a poor quality of life and long-term prognosis.

Older age by itself is not a good reason for denying dialysis treatment; the survival and quality of life of many older patients on dialysis is reasonable and they often fare better than expected. However, dialysis withdrawal should be considered at least in the presence of severe dementia, permanent unconsciousness, or severe cachexia (which represent a prolongation of death rather than life).

Finally, it is important to take into account the social context in which dialysis treatment is delivered. It is well known that family and social support greatly affects the quality of life of patients by improving their approach to life and therefore also to dialysis. However technologically advanced, no procedure can succeed unless it is performed in the context of humanized health care directed toward the needs of the patient. In this context, the difficult decision about whether to prolong life become easier if it is shared between attending physicians and families or surrogates working together to understand the correct information and organize the delivery of appropriate end-of-life care.

REFERENCES

1. Excerpts from the United States Renal Data System 1998 Annual Data Report. Am J Kidney Dis 1998;32(Suppl 1):S38–41.
2. Collins AJ, Foley RN, Herzog C, et al. United States Renal Data System 2008 annual data report abstract. Am J Kidney Dis 2009;53(1 Suppl):S8–374, vi–vii.
3. Kurella M, Covinsky KE, Collins AJ, et al. Octogenarians and nonagenarians starting dialysis in the United States. Ann Intern Med 2007;146(3):177–83.
4. Jager KJ, van Dijk PC, Dekker FW, et al. ERA-EDTA Registry Committee. The epidemic of aging in renal replacement therapy: an update on elderly patients and their outcomes. Clin Nephrol 2003;60(5):352–60.
5. European Dialysis and Tranplant Association Registry. 2006 annual report. July 2008. Available at: http://www.era-edta-reg.org/index.jsp?p=annrep. Accessed June 5, 2009.
6. Locatelli F, Marcelli D, Conte F, et al. 1983 to 1992: report on regular dialysis and transplantation in Lombardy. Am J Kidney Dis 1995;25:196–205.
7. 1997 Annual Report of Registro Lombardo Dialisi Trapianto, Regione Lombardia. Milan (MI): Direzione Generale Sanità; 1998.
8. Jungers P, Chauveau P, Descamps-Latscha B, et al. Age and gender-related incidence of chronic renal failure in a French urban area: a prospective epidemiologic study. Nephrol Dial Transplant 1996;11:1542–6.
9. Centers for Disease Control and Prevention (CDC). Prevalence of chronic kidney disease and associated risk factors – United States, 1999–2004. MMWR Morb Mortal Wkly Rep 2007;56(8):161–5.
10. Muntner P, Coresh J, Powe NR, et al. The contribution of increased diabetes prevalence and improved myocardial infarction and stroke survival to the increase in treated end-stage renal disease. J Am Soc Nephrol 2003;14(6):1568–77.
11. Malberti F, Conte F, Limido A, et al. Ten years experience of renal replacement therapy in the elderly. Geriatr Nephrol Urol 1997;7:1–10.

12. US Renal Data System: 2002 annual data report. Bethesda (MD): The National Institutes of Health, National Institute of Diabetes and Digestive and Kidney Diseases; 2002.

13. Locatelli F, Marcelli D, Conte F, et al. Patient selection affects end-stage renal disease outcome comparisons. Kidney Int 2000;57(Suppl 74):S94–9.

14. Rajagopalan S, Dellegrottaglie S, Furniss AL, et al. Peripheral arterial disease in patients with end-stage renal disease: observations from the Dialysis Outcomes and Practice Patterns Study (DOPPS). Circulation 2006;114(18):1914–22.

15. Silberg JS, Barre PE, Prichard SS, et al. Impact of left ventricular hypertrophy on survival in end-stage renal disease. Kidney Int 1989;36:286–90.

16. Parfrey PS, Griffiths SM, Harnett JD, et al. Outcome of congestive heart failure, dilated cardiomyopathy, hypertrophic hyperkinetic disease, and ischemic heart disease in dialysis patients. Am J Nephrol 1990;10(3):213–21.

17. Nelson CB, Port FK, Wolfe RA, et al. The association of diabetic status, age and race to withdrawal from dialysis. J Am Soc Nephrol 1994;4(8):1608–14.

18. Foley RN, Parfrey PS. Cardiac disease in the diabetic dialysis patient. Nephrol Dial Transplant 1998;13:1112–3.

19. Nitsch D, Burden R, Steenkamp R, et al. Patients with diabetic nephropathy on renal replacement therapy in England and Wales. QJM 2007;100(9):551–60.

20. Mailloux LU, Bellucci AG, Napolitano B, et al. Survival estimates for 683 patients starting dialysis from 1970 through 1989: identification of risk factors for survival. Clin Nephrol 1994;42:127–35.

21. Stenvinkel P, Heimburger O, Paultre F, et al. Strong association between malnutrition, inflammation, and atherosclerosis in chronic renal failure. Kidney Int 1999;55:1899–911.

22. Murray AM, Tupper DE, Knopman DS, et al. Cognitive impairment in hemodialysis patients is common. Neurology 2006;67(2):216–23.

23. Kurella M, Mapes DL, Port FK, et al. Correlates and outcomes of dementia among dialysis patients: the Dialysis Outcomes and Practice Patterns Study. Nephrol Dial Transplant 2006;21(9):2543–8.

24. Sekkarie MA, Moss AH. Withholding and withdrawing dialysis: the role of physician specialty and education and patient functional status. Am J Kidney Dis 1998;31(3):464–72.

25. Spike JP. Responding to requests for dialysis for severely demented and brain injured patients. Semin Dial 2007;20(5):387–90.

26. Couchoud C, Labeeuw M, Moranne O, et al. for the French Renal Epidemiology and Information Network (REIN) Registry. A clinical score to predict 6-month prognosis in elderly patients starting dialysis for end-stage renal disease. Nephrol Dial Transplant 2009;24:1553–61.

27. Joly D, Anglicheau D, Alberti C, et al. Octogenarians reaching end-stage renal disease: cohort study of decision-making and clinical outcomes. J Am Soc Nephrol 2003;14(4):1012–21.

28. McKenzie JK, Moss AH, Feest TG, et al. Dialysis decision making in Canada, the United Kingdom, and the United States. Am J Kidney Dis 1998;31:12–8.

29. Lambie M, Rayner HC, Bragg-Gresham JL, et al. Starting and withdrawing haemodialysis – associations between nephrologists' opinions, patient characteristics and practice patterns (data from the Dialysis Outcomes and Practice Patterns Study). Nephrol Dial Transplant 2006;21(10):2814–20.

30. Renal Physicians Association and American Society of Nephrology. Clinical practice guideline. Shared decision-making in the withhold and withdrawal from dialysis. Washington, DC 2000, Report No 2.

31. O'Hare AM, Bertenthal D, Walter LC, et al. When to refer patients with chronic kidney disease for vascular access surgery: should age be a consideration? Kidney Int 2007;71(6):555–61.
32. Murtagh FE, Marsh JE, Donohoe P, et al. Dialysis or not? A comparative survival study of patients over 75 years with chronic kidney disease stage 5. Nephrol Dial Transplant 2007;22(7):1955–62.
33. Brunori G, Viola BF, Parrinello G, et al. Efficacy and safety of a very-low-protein diet when postponing dialysis in the elderly: a prospective randomized multi-center controlled study. Am J Kidney Dis 2007;49(5):569–80.
34. Locatelli F, Andrulli S, Pontoriero G, et al. Supplemented low-protein diet and once-weekly hemodialysis. Am J Kidney Dis 1994;24(2):192–204.
35. Excerpts from the United States Renal Data System 1996 Annual Data Report. Am J Kidney Dis 1996;28(3 Suppl 2):S1–S165.
36. The Patient Service Committee: initiation or withdrawal of dialysis in end stage renal disease: guidelines for the health care team. Public Education Treatment Series 03-134-CM. New York: National Kidney Foundation; 1996.
37. Holley JL, Carmody SS, Moss AH, et al. The need for end-of-life care training in nephrology: national survey results of nephrology fellows. Am J Kidney Dis 2003; 42(4):813–20.

Index

Note: Page numbers of article titles are in **boldface** type.

Clin Geriatr Med 25 (2009) 555–561
doi:10.1016/S0749-0690(09)00067-6
0749-0690/09/$ – see front matter © 2009 Elsevier Inc. All rights reserved.

geriatric.theclinics.com

Moving?

Make sure your subscription moves with you!

To notify us of your new address, find your **Clinics Account Number** (located on your mailing label above your name), and contact customer service at:

Email: journalscustomerservice-usa@elsevier.com

800-654-2452 (subscribers in the U.S. & Canada)
314-447-8871 (subscribers outside of the U.S. & Canada)

Fax number: 314-447-8029

Elsevier Health Sciences Division
Subscription Customer Service
3251 Riverport Lane
Maryland Heights, MO 63043

*To ensure uninterrupted delivery of your subscription, please notify us at least 4 weeks in advance of move.